Religion and COVID-19 Vaccination in Zimbabwe

W0234697

This book analyses the role of religion during the COVID-19 pandemic and vaccination rollout in Zimbabwe.

Zimbabwe was listed by the World Health Organization (WHO) as one of thirteen African countries to have fully vaccinated more than 10% of its population against COVID-19 by the end of September 2021, but the country fell far short of the government's own target for achieving 60% inoculation by December 2020. This book analyses whether religion played a role in explaining why the government's pro-vaccine stance did not translate into high vaccination rates. Drawing upon various religions, including African indigenous religions, Christianity and Islam, the book considers how faith actors demonstrated vaccine acceptance, resistance or hesitancy. Zimbabwe offers a particularly interesting and varied case for analysis, and the original research on display here will be an important contribution to wider debates on religion and COVID-19.

This book will be useful to academics, researchers and students studying religious studies, sociology, health and well-being, religion and development.

Tenson Muyambo (DPhil) lectures in the Department of Teacher Development at Great Zimbabwe University in Masvingo, Zimbabwe.

Fortune Sibanda (DPhil) is a professor of Religious Studies in the Department of Philosophy and Religious Studies, Great Zimbabwe University, Masvingo & Department of Theology and Religious Studies, University of Eswatini, Eswatini.

Ezra Chitando (DPhil) serves as a professor in History and Phenomenology of Religion at the University of Zimbabwe.

Routledge Studies on Religion in Africa and the Diaspora

For more information about this series, please visit: www.routledge.com/series/routledge-studies-religion-africa-diaspora/RSRAD

Religion and COVID-19 Vaccination in Zimbabwe

Edited by Tenson Muyambo,
Fortune Sibanda and Ezra Chitando

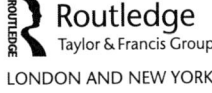

Routledge
Taylor & Francis Group
LONDON AND NEW YORK

First published 2024
by Routledge
4 Park Square, Milton Park, Abingdon, Oxon OX14 4RN

and by Routledge
605 Third Avenue, New York, NY 10158

Routledge is an imprint of the Taylor & Francis Group, an informa business

British Library Cataloguing-in-Publication Data
A catalogue record for this book is available from the British Library

ISBN: 978-1-032-48357-3 (hbk)
ISBN: 978-1-032-48360-3 (pbk)
ISBN: 978-1-003-38863-0 (ebk)

DOI: 10.4324/9781003388630

Typeset in Times New Roman
by Newgen Publishing UK

Contents

Editors

Tenson Muyambo earned a PhD from the University of KwaZulu Natal (UKZN), South Africa. He is a research fellow at the University of South Africa's (UNISA) Research Institute for Theology and Religion (RITR), College of Human Sciences. He lectures at the Great Zimbabwe University, and researches and publishes extensively on indigenous knowledge systems, religion (Ndau indigenous religion), gender, education, pandemics and African Spirituality. He has co-edited the books, *Religion and the COVID-19 Pandemic in Southern Africa* (2022) and *Re-imagining Indigenous Knowledge and Practices in 21st Century Africa: Debunking Myths and Misconceptions for Conviviality and Sustainability* (2022).

Fortune Sibanda (PhD) is a professor of Religious Studies in the Department of Philosophy and Religious Studies, Great Zimbabwe University, Masvingo and Department of Theology and Religious Studies, University of Eswatini, Eswatini. Professor Sibanda is also a research fellow in the Research Institute for Theology and Religion, UNISA, South Africa. He is a specialist in the History and Phenomenology of Religion; African Indigenous Religions and New Religious Movements (particularly Rastafari). His research interests include Indigenous Knowledge Systems, religion and health, religion and the environment, human rights issues, law and religion, religion and the culinary arts tackled from an African perspective. Sibanda has published edited books, book chapters and his work has also appeared in refereed journals. He is a member of a number of academic associations, including the American Academy of Religion (AAR), African Consortium for Law and Religion Studies (ACLARS), African Theological Institutions in Southern and Central Africa (ATISCA), Association for the Study of Religion in Southern Africa (ASRSA) and African Association for the Study of Religion (AASR). Professor Sibanda is a member of the ACLARS Publication Committee and ACLARS Board member.

Ezra Chitando (DPhil) is a professor of History and Phenomenology of Religion at the University of Zimbabwe. His broad research and publication interests include method and theory in the study of religion, as well as religion, health, gender, security, politics, development, climate change, and sexuality, among others.

Contributors

Makomborero Allen Bowa (PhD candidate) is a lecturer in the Department of Philosophy, Religion and Ethics at the University of Zimbabwe. His research interests include the appropriation of biblical text in the analysis of issues relating to poverty, disability, gender, social death, politics, human rights, health and wellbeing in African societies. His approach to the Biblical text is scientific in that he treats Old Testament themes as models for Africa, to either emulate or reject in addressing its religious, socio-economic and political challenges.

Excellent Chireshe is an associate professor of Religion and Gender in the Department of Philosophy and Religious Studies, at the Great Zimbabwe University. She is also a research fellow in the Department of Religion Studies, University of the Free State, South Africa. She holds a PhD in Religious Studies from the University of South Africa. She has published widely on religion and gender and has presented several papers at national and international conferences.

Mutsawashe Chitando is currently pursuing a PhD in Public Health with a specialisation in Health Economics at the University of Cape Town, South Africa. Her research interests revolve around the convergence of public health and various social categories such as economics, gender, climate change and religion. As a researcher, she strives to contribute to the achievement of the Sustainable Development Goals 3 and 5, which aim to promote good health and well-being, as well as gender equality, through policy and advocacy efforts.

Sophia Chirongoma (PhD) is a senior lecturer in the Religious Studies Department at Midlands State University, Zimbabwe. She is also an academic associate/research fellow at the Research Institute for Theology and Religion (RITR) in the College of Human Sciences, University of South Africa (UNISA).

Edmore Dube (PhD, University of Zimbabwe) is a senior lecturer in the Department of Philosophy and Religious Studies, Great Zimbabwe

University. His research interests are in the areas of religion, health and justice resonating with the common good.

Anniegrace Hlatywayo (PhD) is an Indigenous Knowledge scholar and a lecturer at the Midlands State University, Zimbabwe. Her research focuses on Indigenous Knowledge Systems-based Approaches to Sexual and Reproductive Healthcare. She researches in the areas of: African indigenous sexual and reproductive health practices; African indigenous approaches to adolescent sexual and reproductive health (ASRH); African indigenous conceptualisation of food behaviour for pregnancy and postpartum. Her research interests include Gender, Religion and Development; HIV and AIDS; Theology and Development; and Indigenous Knowledge and Biodiversity (Traditional medicines). Anniegrace has experience in research and publication; postgraduate training; community engagement initiatives and project management. She has co-edited *Reimaging Indigenous Knowledge and Practices in 21st Century Africa: Debunking Myths and Misconceptions for Conviviality and Sustainability (2022)*.

Bernard Pindukai Humbe is a PhD holder in Religion Studies from the University of Free State, South Africa. He is a lecturer in the Department of Philosophy and Religious Studies at Great Zimbabwe University, Masvingo. Currently he is a research fellow at the University of South Africa (UNISA). His areas of research interest include: Religion and COVID-19, African Indigenous Religious Knowledge Systems (AIRKS), Traditional Law and Social Development, Religion and Entrepreneurship, Religion and Social Transformation, and Religion and Power.

Mavis Thokozile Macheka (PhD) is a lecturer in the Department of Development Studies at the National University of Lesotho. She is also an avid researcher, consultant, development practitioner, political ecologist and qualitative research methodology expert. Her research straddles the fields of social research, political ecology, community development and human development. She has experience in research formulation, data collection, analysis and report writing. She is also a qualitative research expert who coordinates research, including designing online and offline qualitative data collection tools such as interview guides, focus group discussions guides and questionnaires guides.

Etwin Machibaya is a lecturer at the Great Zimbabwe University in the Teacher Development Department. She holds a doctoral degree in African Languages from the University of South Africa (UNISA). She has published a number of articles in refereed journals and has also presented conference papers locally and internationally. Her main research interests are in Literature, Onomastics, Language Teaching, Gender and Indigenous Knowledge Systems.

Tobias Marevesa is a senior lecturer in New Testament in the Department of Philosophy and Religious the Great Zimbabwe University, where he teaches New Testament Studies, and New Testament Greek. He holds a PhD from the University of Pretoria in South Africa. He is also a research fellow at the Research Institute for Theology and Religion (RITR) in the College of Human Sciences, University of South Africa (UNISA), a research associate with the University of Pretoria (UP) and a postdoctoral fellow with the University of KwaZulu Natal in South Africa (UKZN). His areas of interest are New Testament studies and politics, Pentecostal expressions in Zimbabwean Christianity, culture, human rights, gender-based violence, COVID-19 pandemic and pedagogical issues. He has also published in the area of New Testament studies and conflict resolution on the Zimbabwean political landscape. He has attended and presented a number of papers at both regional and international conferences and has published articles and book chapters in reputable international journals and book projects. He is a member of the New Testament Society of Southern Africa (NTSSA), Reading Association of Nigeria (RAN), Association for the Study of Religion in Southern Africa (ASRSA), African Consortium for Law and Religion Studies (ACLARS), and the International Consortium for Law and Religion Studies (ICLARS).

Rev Henerieta Mgovo is a lecturer in the Department of Philosophy and Religious Studies at the Great Zimbabwe University. Her areas of research interest are the New Testament, Gender, as well as the New Testament and socio-political transformation. She holds an MA in Religious Studies (UZ) and is a PhD student in the New Testament at the University of Zimbabwe.

Silas Nyadzo is a PhD Candidate at Roehampton University. He holds an MA Theology and Biblical Studies. He is affiliated to Apostolic Faith Mission International Ministries UK (AFMIM UK). His research interests include Pentecostal Missions.

Tarsisio M. Nyatsanza is an academic and researcher with a BA Hons (Religious Studies & Philosophy), MA (Philosophy), Graduate Certificate of Education (from the University of Zimbabwe), an ESRC-funded PhD in Education from the University of Glasgow and is also an associate fellow of the Higher Education Academy (AFHEA–UK). He is an experienced teacher in the Humanities areas, University lecturer and Graduate Teaching Assistant in Africa and the UK. He has also worked in various community-based NGOs that focus on community learning and participatory action research that promotes the social justice agenda. Tarsisio has been a facilitator and a presenter at a number of distinguished seminars, workshops and conferences both locally and internationally.

Cuthbert Pisirai is a lecturer at Great Zimbabwe University in the Robert Mugabe School of Heritage and Education. He specialises in Curriculum

Studies and teaches both undergraduate and postgraduate students in the Teacher Development and Curriculum Studies departments respectively. He earned a Masters Degree in Curriculum Studies at Great Zimbabwe University. His research interests are in emerging issues in curriculum and education.

Nomatter Sande holds a PhD in Religion and Social Transformation from the University of KwaZulu Natal (South Africa). Nomatter is a Practical Theologian. He is a research fellow at the Research Institute for Theology and Religion (RITR) in the College of Human Sciences, University of South Africa (UNISA). His research interests include disability studies, Pentecostal theology, religious violence, peace and gender.

Wisdom Sibanda is a PhD student in the Department of Geography at the University of the Free State and a humanitarian practitioner with a number of national and international organisations. His research interests include Political Theory, Development Studies, Environmental Politics, Human Geography and Migration, Environmental Policy and Planning, Environmental Governance, Water, Sanitation and Hygiene, Social Theory, Environmental Management, Climate Change, Disaster Risk Management, Public Policy and Management, Monitoring and Evaluation and Results Based Management. He has experience in community development that includes conducting participatory baseline surveys, participatory, monitoring and evaluation and participatory reporting through the use of participatory approaches.

Beatrice Taringa holds a PhD in Education, Master of Education Degree, Bachelor of Education Degree in Curriculum and Arts Education specialising in Indigenous Language Education, ChiShona, all from the University of Zimbabwe and Diploma in Education specialising in ChiShona and History from Gweru Teachers College. She is a lecturer in the Department of Languages and Arts Education at the University of Zimbabwe. She is a postdoctoral research fellow at UNISA Department of Language Education, Arts and Culture. She has research interests in Curriculum issues in Education, Gender, Culture and Human Rights in Education.

Josiah Taru (PhD) is an anthropologist whose work explores the intersection between Pentecostalism, political processes and development in postcolonial Zimbabwe. His work is expanding into health and medical humanities, exploring the role of religion in reproduction processes among migrants. Josiah is a postdoctoral fellow in a Wellcome Trust-funded Reimagining Reproduction in Africa (ReRe) project at the Centre for the Advancement of Scholarship at the University of Pretoria in South Africa. Josiah is a faculty member at the School of Social Sciences at Great Zimbabwe University, Zimbabwe.

Maradze Viriri holds a doctoral degree in Onomastics from the University of KwaZulu Natal, South Africa. He has published several articles in refereed journals and book chapters. He has also presented papers at international conferences. Currently, he is a lecturer at Great Zimbabwe University. His main research interests are in Onomastics, language policy, gender and indigenous knowledge systems.

1 Introduction

Religion and COVID-19 Vaccination in Zimbabwe

Tenson Muyambo, Fortune Sibanda and Ezra Chitando

Instigating exasperation among many public health officials and confounding some politicians, religion has emerged as a significant factor in the global response to COVID-19 (see among others, Sing, 2020; Kaunda, 2021; Osei-Tutu et al., 2021; Paweł et al., 2022; Marshall & Wilkinson, 2022; Sibanda et al., 2022). Religion, a ubiquitous phenomenon, has demonstrated remarkable tenacity. After its critics in the secularisation thesis wrote its epitaph and others questioned its authority (Chavez 1994), religion has refused to go away quietly. It continues to influence the beliefs and practices of millions of people across the world. In particular, the COVID-19 pandemic reminded critics and admirers of religion of its relevance. For better or for worse, religion featured prominently in discourses on COVID-19. This presence of religion in the global response to the pandemic has generated interest among scholars and activists, giving rise to some strategic questions and themes.

In this volume, contributors focus on one of the most striking aspects of the religion and COVID-19 interface, namely, religion's response to COVID-19 vaccines, alongside other themes. Embracing a contextualised approach, namely, concentrating on the Zimbabwean setting (but drawing out wider implications), contributors explore how religion engaged with COVID-19 in the wake of the rollout of vaccines. They also interrogate religion's role in responding to related COVID-19 themes. We are convinced that the Zimbabwean case study provides valuable insights into religion's interface with COVID-19, particularly in relation to diverse responses to vaccines. Although Zimbabwe's performance in promoting the uptake of COVID-19 vaccines was satisfactory (as at 11 May 2022, 40.2% of the population had had at least 1 dose; 26.8% had been fully vaccinated and 5.7% had received the booster[1]), more needed to be done to encourage vaccination.

We recognise that our engagement with the Zimbabwean context will be one among several publications on religion and the pandemic. It does appear certain that the existential crisis wrought by COVID-19 will continue to generate numerous publications relating to the role and impact of religion. This volume contributes to the ongoing reflections on religion and COVID-19 by focusing more consistently on the dynamics associated with vaccination (and related

DOI: 10.4324/9781003388630-1

themes). Religion was one of the most significant variables in the vaccination drive that the global health institution, namely, the World Health Organization (WHO), governments and other health promoters embarked on in the wake of COVID-19. The volume reviews the responses by faith actors to the vaccination drive, alongside other related themes. It confirms the ongoing relevance of religion on the global stage (see for example, McDonagh et al., 2021). Before delving into relevance of religion and the emerging themes in light of COVID-19, we first interrogate the definitional issues relating to the notions of religion and vaccines.

Religion and Vaccines: Navigating the Definitional Considerations

In this section, we conceptualise how 'religion' and 'vaccines'/'vaccination' were understood in this volume. By and large, this volume centres around 'religion' and 'vaccines' as the two leading concepts. Despite the fact that the different chapters in this volume explored these concepts in their own way, we consider it as critical to some of the key elements related to them. First, in humanistic studies in general and in religious studies in particular, the need for and the nature of definitions is an enormous and audacious act characterised by confusion (Smith 1987: 32). Indeed, critical terms for religious studies (Taylor 1998; Chitando, 2013: 5) are fluid, possess misleading connotations and cannot be universalised regarding their meaning and application. Therefore, the term 'religion' is open to debate since an attempt to hazard a universal, exhaustive and binding definition results in a sterile academic exercise (Cox, 1996). In his book, *The Meaning and End of Religion*, the term 'religion' is "notoriously difficult to define" (Smith 1964:17) because it is culture-specific, whilst Jonathan Z. Smith (1998: 281) asserts that religion was a product of scholars' creation for their intellectual purpose, but we are also certain that it is a public observable phenomenon practised by human beings. Platvoet (1999) also usefully observes that scholars are unable to say what religion has been in the past, is currently and shall be in the future, for all the people elsewhere. Nevertheless, it is useful to realise that what is problematic is not necessarily defining, but, rather, "*explicitly* defining" (Smith 1987: 33, italics in original). On this basis, open or working definitions of religion can be conceived, whereby to define is not meant to finish, but an anchor upon which to make useful reflections (Smith, 1987). In this volume, the term religion is used in a flexible and non-normative way in order to facilitate the understanding of discussions sustained in the various essays.

Second, the concept of 'vaccines' just as that of 'religion' is equally slippery and like an elusive butterfly (Smith, 1987), despite having a long history of use and application. Today, vaccines have become an integral part of human existence as a proven defence against viruses through immunisation of children, adults, domesticated and wild animals (https://health.ec.europa.eu/sys tem/files/2018-05/glossary_en_0.pdf). Therefore, a vaccine is a biological preparation that improves immunity to a particular disease. Etymologically, the word 'vaccine' can be traced to the Latin *Variolae vaccinae* (cowpox), which Edward Jenner demonstrated in 1798 could prevent smallpox in humans. The term 'vaccine' applies to all biological preparations, produced from living organisms, and from weakened or killed forms of the microbe, its toxins or one of its surface proteins, that enhance immunity against disease. Administered in liquid form, either by injection, by oral, or by intranasal routes, vaccines are used to prevent (prophylactic vaccines) or, in some cases, to treat disease (therapeutic vaccines) (www.phrma-jp.org/wordpress/wp-content/uploads/old/library/vaccine-factbook_e/1_Basic_Concept_of_Vaccination.pdf). In the pre-COVID-19 era, a number of vaccines were in use against viruses such as yellow fever, influenza and child-killer diseases like Measles, Rubella and Hepatitis. The COVID-19 vaccines were introduced as an intervention against coronavirus disease. People responded variedly with some showing acceptance whilst others were hesitant.

The two concepts, that of religion and vaccines, occur in space and time in Zimbabwe. Whilst earlier studies on religion and vaccination (see, for example, Machekanyanga et al., 2017) remain relevant and informative, there is need to analyse the changing context brought by new challenges and responses to the COVID-19 vaccination. Chapters in this volume seek to address this changing context by focusing on religion and the COVID-19 vaccination in Zimbabwe. It can be asserted that both religion and vaccines are essential in promoting human flourishing as they are systems of survival. Whereas religion thrives on non-human support from the divine realm, the vaccines are a scientific remedy. For the interface of religion and science also see Muyambo et al. (2022) and Muyambo and Tendere (2023). Both religion and vaccines endeavoured to empower individuals, families, communities and nations. Just as religion has often been utilised as "a coping and survival strategy in many social settings" (Mapuranga 2014: 236), the acceptance or hesitancy towards COVID-19 vaccination was also preoccupied with the need to survive. Thus, this volume operates with open or working definitions of religion and a particular focus on COVID-19 vaccines. We now turn to an overview of the emerging themes in relation to religion and the COVID-19 pandemic.

Religion and COVID-19: An Overview of Emerging Themes

Although COVID-19 is a very young pandemic (according to the current, available scientific information, the virus was first discovered in Wuhan City, China, in 2019), it has attracted considerable scholarly interest. This is significant, given the fact that the pandemic is still unfolding, as well as the fact that the literature is being produced "in the heat of the struggle". We will not be able to review the extant literature within the context of this introductory chapter. However, we will draw attention to some of the emerging and key themes that are relevant to this volume.

In particular, scholars from within religious studies, biblical studies, theology, ethics and others have already invested considerably in clarifying its implications. For example, in *Christianity and COVID-19: Pathways for Faith* (Kaunda et al., 2021), contributors interrogate the meaning of suffering and faith in the context of COVID-19 in global Christianity. Some of the emerging themes and questions include the impact of religion and conspiracy theories on COVID-19 vaccination in different contexts. While public health officials were keen to promote COVID-19 vaccination, some religious actors were hesitating or actively resisting the vaccines (Nagar and Ashaye, 2022). On the other hand, some religious actors were promoting COVID-19 vaccination on the basis of religious teachings (see for example, Mardian et al., 2021). The implications of conspiracy theories in/and religion (Dyrendal et al., 2018) and their impact on the global COVID-19 vaccination drive the call for deeper analysis. Further, the need to counter vaccine hesitancy within faith communities and to mobilise religious actors to join others to promote COVID-19 vaccine confidence (Harisson and Wu, 2020) has emerged as a critical issue requiring ongoing engagement.

Another theme that has drawn the attention of some scholars relates to the relationship between the restrictions associated with COVID-19, for example, the ban on mass gathering, and religious freedom (see for example the special issue of the journal, *Fides Es Libertas: The Journal of the International Religious Liberty Association*, 2021 Special Edition on COVID-19 and Religious Liberty). With followers of various religions keen on expressing their independence from state control, COVID-19 presented fresh challenges to the theme of religious freedom. There is ongoing debate over the notion of freedom of religion, as well as the extent to which states can curtail this freedom in the wake of public health concerns (Martínez-Torrón, 2021). This has direct relevance to the church-state interface (Berkmann, 2020). We also add the interest in indigenous knowledge systems, gender-based violence, racism, as well as the implications of COVID-19 to the academic study of religion/boundaries of the disciplines (Sexton, 2021), and engaging in feminist pedagogies during the pandemic (Scharnick-Udemans, 2021). See also, Ramrathan et al. (2020) for reflections on rethinking the Humanities curriculum in the context of COVID-19. Other researchers have focused on the turn towards digital platforms (Kilonzo and Omwalo, 2021), highlighting how the ban on physical gatherings influenced the migration of religious performances to online platforms. Beyond the contribution of religion, other researchers have sought to examine the economic impact of COVID-19 globally (Faghih and Forouharfar, 2022).

Maseno (2021) has examined the extent to which one female Pentecostal-Charismatic preacher in Kenya, namely, Jane Ndegwa of Hope Evangelistic Ministries (HEM), used prophecy as a resource for self-legitimacy in the competitive religious sector. By uttering prophetic words regarding the impact of COVID-19 and forewarning citizens of the trouble ahead, she was asserting her credentials as a legitimate sacred practitioner, Maseno argues. Mahiya and Murisi (2022) reflect on the reconfiguration and adaptation of churches in Zimbabwe in the face of COVID-19, while Chukwuma (2021) examines the changes to doctrine and liturgy in the context of the pandemic in Nigeria.

In relation to COVID-19 vaccines, earlier research has identified low trust in vaccines in general, concerns about side effects of vaccines, distrust in government and healthcare professionals, the need for closure and conspiracy beliefs. Recognising the difference between vaccine hesitancy and being anti-vaccine, Pertwee et al. (2022) have underscored the importance of trust in promoting COVID-19 vaccines. While indicating that the WHO had already noted worrying levels of vaccine hesitancy before COVID-19, World Vision (2021: 7) identifies a number of factors contributing to COVID-19 vaccine hesitancy. These include misinformation through social media, fatalism (the idea that those who will die will do so, anyway), as well as concerns regarding the side effects of COVID-19 vaccines. However, trusted community leaders, such as faith leaders, could play a critical role in promoting the uptake of COVID-19 vaccines (World Vision 2021: 7). Matikiti (2021) reflects on the need to consider traditional medicine alongside COVID-19 vaccines in Zimbabwe. The following section looks at the interface of religion and COVID-19 vaccination with the intent to demonstrate how religion reacted when the COVID-19 vaccines were introduced.

Religion and COVID-19 Vaccination

Admittedly, COVID-19 came and has had an undeniable impact on the lives of people globally. Its advent has put the socio-economic, political, religious, as well as educational prospects of humanity in a precarious situation. Sibanda et al. (2022: 1) admitted that "within a short period of time, the pandemic became the world's most pressing emergency, exposing the limitations of biomedicine and highlighting the vulnerability of human beings in different parts of the world". The first COVID-19 case in Africa was reported in Egypt on 4 February 2020 (Anjorin, 2021). By 22 June 2021, Africa had recorded more than 5.1 million cases, with over 137,000 deaths (WHO, 2021). As of 14 April 2020, Zimbabwe had recorded eighteen cases and three deaths (Muyambo 2022). As the pandemic continued and still continues to alter "the way we live, interact and socialise" (Jaja et al., 2020), governments' initial efforts to combat the pandemic focused and continue to focus on controlling the spread of the pandemic through well-publicised public health measures (Anjorin et al., 2021).

As the pandemic mutates and takes different forms, scientists cannot watch humanity at the mercy of the COVID-19 pandemic. Efforts have been made in coming up with vaccines as another dimension to controlling the pandemic. Lessons learnt from the vaccination of diseases such as Polio, Smallpox, Yellow Fever and others that previously killed millions of people gave hope that the only way to effectively deal with the pandemic was through vaccines. Humanity's experiences from previous vaccination of pandemics has brought a lot of hope and trust in vaccination worldwide. Given the successes recorded in previous diseases' vaccination programmes, stakes are high that the COVID-19 vaccination is the only hope that remains at our disposal in the fight against the pandemic. Wiysonge et al. (2021) concur when they argue that vaccines could have a similar impact on COVID-19 if there is optimal and equitable uptake of the COVID-19 vaccines worldwide. Anjorin et al. (2021) opine that there has been an accelerated development and approval of COVID-19 vaccines. Cook et al. (2022) are of the view that the successful development and implementation of vaccines are currently our most effective defence against the COVID-19 pandemic.

Matikiti (2021: 127) admits that "in Africa health is grounded in and informed by religious and cultural practices that emerge from the values and beliefs held by particular communities or groups of people". It is for this reason that this volume seeks to unravel how people of different religious orientations relate to COVID-19 vaccination basing on their value and belief systems. Having accelerated the development and approval of the vaccines, low-income and middle-income countries (LMICs) have been at the receiving end due to vaccine nationalism. There is what is now commonly referred to as 'vaccine apartheid' where richer countries are either keeping large quantities of the vaccines for themselves when needy countries do not have enough and/or are over-pricing the vaccines beyond the reach of many LMICs. It has been noted that where the few vaccines have been available and accessible, vaccine acceptance by different religious groupings has been ambivalent. The nexus between religion and COVID-19 in general is complex to the extent that different religious orientations diametrically differ as to how they relate to the pandemic. While some religions have come to terms with the 'new normal', others are still battling to understand this novel pandemic. Most religions, globally, view COVID-19 vaccination as one way among many that can be used to curb the spread of the pandemic. However, it must be noted that within the same religion, for example, Christianity, not all Christians believe in and have faith in COVID-19 vaccines. While some Christian movements have come to terms with COVID-19 vaccination, others like some of the Apostolic movements shun vaccination, particularly COVID-19 vaccines. The belief by some of these Apostolic movements is that while all of us are in some way wounded by COVID-19, Jesus as a great healer, is the one who heals, *not vaccines*. They argue that it is through Jesus' healing abilities that he attracted people to him. The underlying understanding by these Apostolic believers is that they shall be healed by faith, which is the core of the Christian belief.

This religious ambivalence towards COVID-19 vaccination accounts for the need to understand deeply how different religious orientations receive, interpret and appropriate the vaccine information available to them. Literature has indicated that religion accounts for most COVID-19 cases in the world (Rashid, 2020; Roth et al., 2020; Winiger, 2020). Religious practices such as using a single spoon for distributing wine to congregants (Roth et al., 2020), kissing, touching and washing of dead bodies as practised in Judaism and African religions, presented and continue to present ready pathways for the spread of the virus. On the other hand, religious organisations were and are still found to be central in mitigating the pandemic. Winiger (2020) opines that religious organisations play a major role in saving lives and reducing illness related to COVID-19 by providing a primary source of support, comfort, guidance, and direct healthcare and social service for the communities they serve. It is against this background that religion, as an important cog in human life, has a stake in the 'vaccine willingness' and 'vaccine hesitancy'. Due to the infodemic, that is, 'mis–and disinformation' (Winiger, 2020) about COVID-19 vaccines, religious organisations have received, interpreted and appropriated vaccine information differently. While some religious organisations have embraced the need to have their members get the jab, others, owing to a lot of conspiracy theories, have not only backed off but have been very sceptical about the vaccines. The next sections are an examination of the positive and negative responses by religious faiths to the vaccines.

Religion and COVID-19 Vaccination in Zimbabwe: Positive Responses

As the foregoing section highlights, the discourse on religion and COVID-19 vaccination has been prominent in diverse settings, globally and in Africa. In this section, we seek to highlight the positive responses to COVID-19 vaccination by religious actors in Zimbabwe. We will draw attention to the complexity of trying to establish hard-and-fast categories in relation to trying to link particular responses to specific denominations, as the situation was fluid (and remained so at the time of writing). Thus, for example, while some might casually declare that Zimbabwean Pentecostals were more susceptible to accepting COVID-19 conspiracy theories, in reality many Pentecostals were getting vaccinated while some members of mainline churches refused to get vaccinated. Below, we outline some of the main reasons why some religious actors promoted COVID-19 vaccination in Zimbabwe.

First, there were positive responses to COVID-19 vaccination (and other related public health messages regarding the pandemic such as handwashing, observing physical/social distance, observing restrictions on public gatherings, etc.) by many religious actors due to theological convictions. These theological convictions could be regarded as both an interfaith and personal stance, namely, that many religious actors regarded the availability of COVID-19 vaccines as a decisive intervention from the spiritual realm to respond to the pandemic. In this regard, the vaccines were interpreted as a gift from God (for believers from theistic religions), God and the ancestors (for followers of African Traditional/ Indigenous Religions), or simply from the Sacred (see Eliade, 1959). Followers of diverse religions in Zimbabwe who supported or promoted COVID-19 vaccination used faith as the frame for interpreting the vaccines. For them, the Sacred realm was intervening strategically to release creation from the grip of an unrelenting pandemic.

In particular, Christians who supported COVID-19 vaccination had numerous biblical texts that they used to defend their positions. They cited passages where God promises security and prosperity to the faithful. In addition, they cited texts where God is a source of refuge and a deliverer in times of trouble to support the COVID-19 vaccine uptake. This confirmed the importance of the Bible to African and Zimbabwean Christianity. Here, the Bible was mined, not as an ancient text addressing events in the long past, but as a contemporary text speaking to current realities (see for example, West and Dube, 2000). Passages that maintain that God created the world and put humans in charge (Genesis 1: 26) and gave the earth to them (Psalm 115: 16); as well the use of medicine in the Bible (I Timothy 5: 23) were used to support COVID-19 vaccines. However, as we shall illustrate below, the same Bible was appealed to by those who opposed COVID-19 vaccines.

Second, religious supporters of COVID-19 vaccines understood and presented themselves as forces of good locked in mortal combat with forces of darkness that spewed and spawned conspiracy theories. In this scheme, conspiracy theories are regarded as not just some mischief by keyboard warriors, but as an evil scheme to lead the elect of God on the path to death and destruction. Although this theme is still related to the foregoing one on theological motivation, the notion of fighting in God's name (see for example, Adogame et al., 2020) is deployed in the quest to defeat vaccine hesitancy and promote the uptake of COVID-19 vaccines. Some champions of COVID-19 vaccines presented themselves as engaged in the sacred task of defeating conspiracy theories, while promoting truth and light.

Third, some religious actors, particularly from within mainline Christianity in Zimbabwe, were pro-vaccines due to the long history of their denominations in the provision of healthcare. Mission churches have been heavily involved in setting up health centres across many parts of the country (see Zvobgo, 1986; Chirongoma, 2020; and Muyambo et al., 2022). This close relationship between mainline churches and biomedicine has enabled many members of mainline churches to accept vaccines, including COVID-19 vaccines. Equally, many traditionalists and Muslims consider their religions to have been always open to and accepting of vaccines. It is this background that enabled many religious actors in Zimbabwe to come out in support of COVID-19 vaccines.

Fourth, many Zimbabweans recall the high death rate the country experienced due to HIV/AIDS, especially in the early 1990s when there was no medication for HIV (Chitando 2007). These were the days when getting infected with HIV was understood as a death sentence, as many infected people died due to the lack of treatment options. With the introduction of Antiretrovirals (ARVs) , there was greater hope for people living with HIV. As a result, there is a general appreciation of the efficacy of biomedicine, even if it is often supplemented by, or used alongside, indigenous medicine. This provided a sound basis or platform for accepting COVID-19 vaccines.

Fifth, the religion-state partnership, established over many years (Hallencreutz and Moyo, 1988; Chitando, 2013), enabled many religious leaders to join public health officials and government functionaries in promoting COVID-19 vaccines. Although sometimes there is tension between the state and religious leaders, for the most part cordial relations exist between the two. In many instances, political leaders are members of mainline churches (although they actively seek to cultivate favourable relations with other religious formations) and they expect the cooperation of church leaders in rolling out government policies and programmes. This also applies to religious leaders from other communities in Zimbabwe. They generally seek to partner with government and they regarded popularising COVID-19 vaccines as consistent with the partnership stance.

Sixth, and finally for this section, we can concede that some religious actors might have regarded the task of promoting COVID-19 vaccines as a strategic opportunity for self-promotion. We do not raise this possibility as a critique or to doubt the convictions of religious actors who promoted COVID-19 vaccines. However, we are aware of the intensity of competition within the religious sector in Zimbabwe (in the region, on the continent and globally). In this regard, it is strategic for religious actors to present themselves as progressive, reasonable and acting in sync with public health messaging. Consciously or otherwise, they need to present themselves as superior to their competitors on the market (who might be championing the anti-COVID-19 vaccines). This is due to the reality that:

> religious products … have become branded in much the same way that consumer products have been branded. Religious organisations have taken on names, logos or personalities, and slogans that allow them to be heard in a cluttered, increasingly competitive marketplace … Faith brands, like their secular counterparts, exist to aid consumers in making and maintaining a personal connection to a commodity product. Introducing, sustaining, and perpetuating the brand across product lines allow these faith brands to be "top of mind" in an overcrowded commercial environment.
>
> (Einstein 2008: xi)

We should reiterate, however, that although many religious actors supported the rollout of COVID-19 vaccines, this did not imply that they did not simultaneously utilise complementary and indigenous medicines. As shown by various studies, including, for example, Dahlin (2002) and Batisai (2016), Zimbabwe (and Sub-Saharan Africa more generally) is characterised by medical pluralism. Communities, families and individuals choose from a wide array of health options and often utilise a number of them simultaneously. In other instances, however, religious actors either openly or quietly contested the drive towards COVID-19 vaccines in Zimbabwe. We turn to this theme below.

Religion and COVID-19 Vaccination in Zimbabwe: Resistance

A survey conducted in July–August 2020 in South Africa shows that about 36% of South Africans were reluctant to be vaccinated against COVID-19. These statistics differ from country to country. Several factors have been cited as having been responsible for the low COVID-19 vaccination uptake. Vaccine hesitancy is said to be one of the greatest threats to global health (Wiysonge et al., 2022). For purposes of avoiding ambiguity and clumsiness, we attempt to define vaccine hesitancy/resistance/unwillingness. Cooper et al. (2018: 2355) conceptualise vaccine hesitancy as "the continuum between vaccine acceptance and refusal". The World Health Organization (WHO) defines vaccine hesitancy as "a delay in acceptance or refusal of vaccines despite the availability of vaccination services" (Aborode et al., 2021: 1). This is the unwillingness to receive vaccines when vaccine services are available and accessible (Wiysonge et al., 2022). Put simply, vaccine hesitancy is that doubt whether one should get vaccinated or not when vaccines are available and accessible. It is the dilemma that people find themselves in regarding taking or not taking the vaccine, resulting in COVID-19 vaccination resistance.

Vaccine hesitancy poses a substantial risk for both people who delay or refuse to be vaccinated and the larger community. It must be noted that vaccine resistance, that is equally understood as vaccine hesitancy, did not start with the COVID-19 pandemic in Zimbabwe, but has been there for a long time. For example, vaccine hesitancy has been largely expressed by people of different religious orientations, particularly the 'white garments' Apostolic congregants and from indigenous religion whose adherents are delaying vaccination owing to conspiracy theories that are awash on social media. To substantiate that vaccine hesitancy has been with the Zimbabwean populace for a long time, Machekanyanga et al. (2017) link the rise in measles in Zimbabwe to objections among Apostolic Church members. It is on record that the Johanne Marange's religious grouping flatly refuses to get vaccinations against various diseases. For example, the grouping is known for rebuffing government's immunisation programmes in schools. They hold on to their children from going to school on immunisation days.

When the Zimbabwean government introduced the vaccine against the COVID-19 programme in 2020, there were ambivalent reactions to it, as indicated earlier on. The government had a target of 10 million people to be vaccinated, which constitutes 60% of the population. The understanding then was that having 60% of the population vaccinated, the country would achieve herd immunity, a condition where the pandemic's spread would have been curtailed. Alas, the uptake of the vaccines was and still continues to be very slow and this slowness can be explained by a number of factors, chief among them being religious.

One major setback the Zimbabwe government confronted was that the pandemic hit when, generally, people had little faith and trust in the government owing to the highly polarised political arena. It is at this point in time this volume wishes to repeat asking two cardinal questions once asked in a study by Kugarakuripi and Ndoma (2022): First, how do Zimbabweans feel about COVID-19 vaccination? Second, among those who are vaccine hesitant, what is driving their reluctance? In an Afrobarometer survey in Zimbabwe, it was found out that about half of the citizens are reluctant to take the COVID-19 vaccines. More surprisingly in this survey was that among those who resisted or refused the vaccines were mostly the highly educated. One would expect the less educated to do this due to either lack of understanding or suspicion of getting orders from the elite. The more educated people's reluctance to take the vaccines, despite their vantage position in understanding the efficacy of vaccines, is generally explained by their religious positioning. Besides the distrust that comes from doubting government's ability to ensure vaccine safety (Kugarakuripi and Ndoma, 2022), religious people either listened to their religious leaders who were sceptical of the vaccines or followed the conspiracy theories that were awash on social media. To illustrate how vaccine hesitancy was caused by religious actors, one prominent religious figure dismissed the vaccines as the 'mark of the beast' (Gleeson and Gilbert 2021) and went viral on social media that he and his family would defy government policy on COVID-19 vaccination. When a religious leader with a high social standing openly denounces the vaccines, he or she has the potential to discourage members of his or her congregation and other members of society to resist COVID-19 vaccination.

Coupled with the haphazard manner in which the vaccine education programme was undertaken in Zimbabwe, religious actors shun vaccination due to COVID-19 vaccination conspiracy theories. For instance, in African indigenous religion, most of the followers turned to social media misinformation and disinformation such as (1) getting vaccinated makes one sterile, a calamitous condition in African perspective where procreation is not only a perpetuation of one's family lineage but an expression of the continuity of life itself, (2) vaccination subjects the vaccinated to a two-year life-span after vaccination, and (3) vaccination is a ploy by the West to wipe Africans from existence. For example, Edmore Dube in this volume alludes to Muslims' suspicion of vaccines that come from countries that are perceived as adversaries to Islam as a religion. Given all this social media misinformation, which unfortunately the Zimbabwean government did not or could not counter, African indigenous religion adherents and other religious actors tended to resist or reject the vaccine. These and other themes are the preoccupation of this volume which range from vaccine acceptance and resistance in a context where the government took it for granted that people would go *en masse* to vaccination centres. No clear and concerted efforts were made to ensure that the COVID-19 vaccination programme succeeded, save making the information available through a language and media not accessible to the majority. Thus, the slow uptake of the vaccine jabs was partly due to lack of information and partly due to distrust in the government by religious actors. Religious actors saw and still see a government that is not up to the task owing to a plethora of failures by the same government in the socio-economic and political lives of the people. This explains why even at this time of writing herd immunity has not been achieved despite the different COVID-19 vaccination blitz action plans employed by the government, including church, street and school vaccination programmes.

In desperation, owing to the high vaccine resistance by the population, the Zimbabwe government has said one thing and does quite the opposite. It has been on record that COVID-19 vaccination is not compulsory but what has been witnessed is the government engaging in vaccination coercion at the very least, thereby raising human rights issues. For example, when the ban on church gathering was lifted it was replaced by the directive that only the vaccinated could attend face-to-face church services, a situation that unfortunately divided the church. Because any people would want to access church services they had to get the jab against their wish. Although lack of knowledge on COVID-19 vaccines equally shares a substantial percentage towards vaccine hesitancy, religious beliefs, practices and norms are comparatively more responsible for the vaccine delay and/or refusal. In a study, well before the advent of COVID-19, by Machekanyanga et al. (2017), poor knowledge of vaccines, lack of understanding and appreciation of the effectiveness of vaccinations, religious teachings that emphasise prayers over the use of medicine, lack of privacy in a religiously controlled community and low levels of education were found to be the main contributing factors towards vaccine hesitancy among key community members and leaders. The next section is a summary of the chapters that constitute this volume.

Chapters in this Volume

The volume consists of sixteen chapters in all. It commences with this chapter, 'Introduction: Religion and COVID-19 Vaccination in Zimbabwe', by the editors, Tenson Muyambo, Fortune Sibanda and Ezra Chitando. The chapter serves to put the readers into perspective by first theorising on the phenomenon of vaccination from the global and local experiences. In this way, the chapter examines the various responses by different players such as religion, health sector and the government in light of the COVID-19 pandemic, vis-à-vis the problem of vaccine hesitancy, positive responses (by the 'pro-vax'), and the negative responses (by the 'anti-vax'. All in all, the chapter provides a window for peeping into the complex gamut of responses to vaccination by different stockholders and stakeholders, with particular focus on how religion and spirituality influence the obtaining standpoints and narratives.

Subsequent to Chapter 1, the volume is divided into three clusters, under which fall the different chapters reflecting on the diverse responses to COVID-19 vaccination in Zimbabwe, namely, the positive (COVID-19 vaccine acceptance), negative (COVID-19 vaccine resistance/hesitancy) and both (COVID-19 vaccine and hesitancy) clusters. Under the first cluster on vaccine acceptance, in Chapter 2, Mutsawashe Chitando and Ezra Chitando examine the interface between public health and religion, while Anniegrace Hlatywayo and Sophia Chirongoma analyse the Ndau Indigenous Knowledge Systems and COVID-19 in Chapter 3. In Chapter 4, Beatrice Taringa and Sophia Chirongoma explore how the Shona vaccine acceptance was characterised by repackaging the funeral and post-burial rites. Tenson Muyambo, Josiah Taru and Fortune Sibanda situate mainline Christian Churches' responses to

COVID-19 vaccination in Masvingo and Bikita Districts, in Chapter 5, while in Chapter 6 Tobias Marevesa and Fortune Sibanda ask the question whether anything good can come out of Nazareth (Apostolic churches) by exploring the relevance of apostolic women's empowerment trust in the context of COVID-19 vaccination in Zimbabwe.

Having explored the cluster of chapters on vaccine acceptance, the second cluster concentrates on vaccine hesitancy and resistance. In Chapter 7, Edmore Dube focuses on the Mberengwa Muslim Ummah's response to COVID-19 vaccination, while in Chapter 8 Wisdom Sibanda analyses the negative responses of migrant communities towards COVID-19 vaccination at Tongogara Refugee Camp. In Chapter 9, Tarsisio M. Nyatsanza regards COVID-19 vaccination as a site and scene of power contestation under the aegis of spirituality and uncertainty. Henerieta Mgovo examines Johanne Marange Apostolic Church's negative response to the COVID-19 vaccination rollout, in Chapter 10, while in Chapter 11, Nomatter Sande and Silas Nyadzo tackle the experiences of diasporic Zimbabweans in the United Kingdom as 'disconcerting vaccination voices'. The second cluster is capped by Chapter 12 where Excellent Chireshe and Mavis Thokozile Macheka explore the vaccine uptake in African Initiated Churches and traditional healers in Masvingo Province.

The third and last cluster focuses on both COVID-19 acceptance and hesitancy. Accordingly, in Chapter 13, Makomborero Allen Bowa analyses how the Bible influenced both vaccine acceptance and hesitancy, while in Chapter 14, Bernard Pindukai Humbe highlights how vaccination was a catalyst for church ideological bisection in some African Initiated Churches. Similarly, the trio, Maradze Viriri, Etwin Machibaya and Cuthbert Pisirai trace the appropriation of Shona Traditional Religion and gender to COVID-19 vaccination in Buhera South, Manicaland province, in Chapter 15. In the concluding chapter, Chapter 16, Ezra Chitando, Tenson Muyambo and Fortune Sibanda review the theme of vaccination acceptance and resistance through the matrix of religion and development.

Conclusion

The responses towards COVID-19 vaccination in Zimbabwe is far from being homogenous. Notwithstanding that there are some overlaps in the various responses of people to the vaccination rollout, this introductory chapter has placed the chapters as accounts to responses that fall under three clusters, namely, vaccine acceptance (by the 'pro-vaxxers'), vaccine hesitancy (by the 'anti-vaxxers') and those that towed the middle way. Essentially, while the chapters in this volume explore the various responses towards vaccination, they provide only a glimpse of the experiences in contemporary Zimbabwe. Arguably, further research encompassing more religious traditions in different parts of the country is necessary. However, the chapters in the volume have demonstrated that religion remains an indispensable cog-wheel in imagining Zimbabwe's future responses to health emergencies.

Note

1 https://ourworldindata.org/covid-vaccinations?country=ZWE, accessed 13 May 2022.

References

Aborode, A.T., Fajemisin, E.A., et al. 2021. Vaccine hesitancy in Africa: Causes and strategies to the rescue. *Therapeutic Advances in Vaccines and Immunotherapy*, 9, 1–5. https://journals.sagepub.com/doi/10.1177/25151355211047514 (Accessed 16 March 2022).

Adogame, A., Adeboye, O., and Williams.C. (Eds). 2020. *Fighting in God's Name: Religion and Conflict in Local-Global Perspectives*. London: Lexington Books.

Anjorin, A.A., Odetokun, I.A., Abioye, A.I., Elnadi, H., Umoren, M.V., Damaris B.F., et al. 2021. Will Africans take COVID-19 vaccination? *PLoS ONE* 16(12), e0260575. https://doi.org/10.1371/ journal.pone.0260575

Batisai, K. 2016. Towards an integrated approach to health and medicine in Africa. *SAHARA J*, 13(1), 113–122. DOI:10.1080/17290376.2016.1220323; PMID:27538792; PMCID: PMC5642441.

Berkmann, B.J. 2020. The COVID-19 crisis and religious freedom: The interaction between state and church norms in Germany, especially in Bavaria. *Journal of Law, Religion and State*, 8(2/3), 179–200.

Chavez, M. 1994. Secularization as declining religious authority. *Social Forces*, 72(3), 749–774.

Chirongoma, S. 2020. Church-related hospitals and health-care provision in Zimbabwe. In Ezra Chitando (Ed.), *The Zimbabwe Council of Churches and Development in Zimbabwe*. Cham: Palgrave Macmillan, 125–147.

Chitando, E. 2007. *Living with Hope: African Churches and HIV/AIDS*. Vol. 1. Geneva: World Council of Churches.

Chitando, E. (Ed.). 2013. *Prayers and Players: Religion and Politics in Zimbabwe*. Harare: SAPES Books.

Chukwuma, O.G. 2021. The impact of the COVID-19 outbreak on religious practices of churches in Nigeria. *HTS Teologiese Studies/Theological Studies*, 77(4), a6377. https://doi. org/10.4102/hts.v77i4.6377

Cook, E.J., et al. 2022. Vaccination against COVID-19: Factors that influence vaccine hesitancy among an ethnically diverse community in the UK. *Vaccines (Basel)*, 10(1), 106. DOI:10.3390/vaccines10010106. PMID:35062768; PMCID:PMC8780359.

Cooper, S., Betsch, C., Shambala, E.Z., Mchiza, N. and Wiysonge, C.S. 2018. Vaccine hesitancy: Apotential threat to the achievements of vaccination programmes in Africa. *Human Vaccines & Immunotherapeutics*, https://doi.org/10.1080/21645 515.2018.1460987

Cox, J.L. 1996. *Expressing the Sacred: An Introduction to Phenomenology of Religion*. Harare: University of Zimbabwe Press.

Dahlin, O. 2002. *Zvinorwadza: Being a Patient in the Religious and Medical Plurality of the Mberengwa District, Zimbabwe*. Frankfurt am Main: Peter Lang.

Dyrendal, A., Robertson, D.G. and Asprem, E. (Eds). 2018. *Handbook of Conspiracy Theory and Religion*. Leiden: Brill.

Einstein, M. 2008. *Brands of Faith: Marketing Religion in Commercial Age*. New York: Routledge.

Eliade, M. 1959. *The Sacred and the Profane: The Nature of Religion*. New York: Harper and Row.

Faghih, N. and Forouharfar, A. (Eds). 2022. *Socioeconomic Dynamics of the COVID-19 Crisis Global, Regional, and Local Perspectives*. Cham: Springer.

Gleeson, S. and Gilbert, A.C. 2021. Some say COVID-19 vaccine is the 'mark of the beast'. Is there a connection to the Bible. www.usatoday.com/story/news/nation/2021/09/26/covid-vaccine-mark-beast-what-book-revelation-says/8255268002/

Hallecreutz, C.H. and Moyo, A. (Eds). 1988. *Church and State in Zimbabwe*. Gweru: Mambo Press.

Harisson, E.A. and Wu, J.W. 2020. Vaccine Confidence in the time of COVID-19. *European Journal of Epidemiology*, 35, 325–330. https://health.ec.europa.eu/system/files/2018-05/glossary_en_0.pdf "Vaccination Glossary"

Jaja, I.F., Umunna, M., and Jaja, C.J.I. 2020. Social distancing: How religion, culture and burial ceremony undermine the effort to curb COVID-19 in South Africa. *Emerging Microbes and Infections*, 9(1), 1077–1079.

Kaunda, C.J. et al. (Eds). 2021. *Christianity and COVID-19: Pathways for Faith*. New York: Routledge.

Kilonzo, S.M. and Omwalo B.O. 2021. The politics of pulpit religiosity in the era of COVID-19 in Kenya. *Front. Commun*, 6, 616288. DOI: 10.3389/fcomm.2021.616288

Kugarakuripi, J. and Ndoma, S. 2022. Lack of trust in government, reliance on social media may drive hesitancy in Zimbabwe. *Afrobarometer*, 500, 1–8.

Machekanyanga, Z., Ndiaye, S., Gerede, R., Chindedza, K., Chigodo, C., Shibeshi, M.E. Goodson, J., Daniel, F., Zimmerman, L., and Kaiser, R. 2017. Qualitative assessment of vaccination hesitancy among members of the Apostolic Church of Zimbabwe: A case study. *Journal of Religion and Health*, 56, 1683–1691. https://doi.org/10.1007/s10943-017-0428-7

Mahiya, I.T. and Murisi, R. 2022. Reconfiguration and adaptation of a church in times of COVID-19 pandemic: A focus on selected churches in Harare and Marondera, Zimbabwe. *Cogent Arts & Humanities*, 9(1), 2024338, DOI: 10.1080/23311983.2021.2024338

Mapuranga, T.P. 2014. Surviving the urban jungle: AICs and women's socio-economic coping strategies in Harare (2000–2010). In E. Chitando, M.R. Gunda, and J. Kuegler (Eds), *Multiplying in the Spirit: African Initiated Churches in Zimbabwe*. Bamberg: University of Bamberg Press, pp. 227–239.

Mardian, Y. et al. 2021. Sharia (Islamic Law) perspectives of COVID-19 vaccines. *Front. Trop. Dis.*, 2, 788188. DOI: 10.3389/fitd.2021.788188

Marshall, K. and Wilkinson, O. 2022. Two years and counting: COVID-19 through a religious lens. Working Paper 22. Berkeley Centre for Religion, Peace, and World Affairs.

Martínez-Torrón, J. 2021. COVID-19 and religious freedom: Some comparative perspectives. *Laws*, 10, 39. https:// doi.org/10.3390/laws10020039

Maseno, L. 2021. Eschatological prophecies before and during COVID-19: Female Pentecostal-charismatic preachers self-legitimation through prophecy in Kenya. *Pharos Journal of Theology*, 102, Special Edition 2, 1–12.

Matikiti, R. 2021. Confessing Jesus Christ in cultural context: The one-sided politics of COVID-19 vaccination in Zimbabwe. *History Research*, 9(2), 127–135.

McDonagh, P. et al. 2021. *On the Significance of Religion for Global Diplomacy*. New York: Routledge.

Muyambo, T. 2022. Social distancing in the context of COVID-19 in Zimbabwe: Perspectives from Ndau religious indigenous knowledge systems. In F. Sibanda, T. Muyambo, and E. Chitando (Eds), *Religion and the COVID-19 Pandemic in Southern Africa.* London/New York: Routledge, 37–51.

Muyambo, T., Sande, N., and Tendere, J. 2022. 'Wash and Pray': The nexus of African Christianity and science in the context of COVID-19 in Zimbabwe. *Journal of Religion in Africa*, 52, 348–378. https://doi:10.1163/15700666-12340234

Muyambo, T. and Tendere, J. 2023. Beyond the COVID-19 pandemic: Is rethinking the interface of religion and science possible in the Zimbabwean context? In M. Manyonganise (Ed.), *Religion and Health in a COVID-19 Context: Experiences in Zimbabwe*, 285–304.

Nagar, S. and Tomi, A. 2022. A shot of faith: Analyzing vaccine hesitancy in certain religious communities in the United States. *American Journal of Health Promotion* (IF2.87), Pub Date: 2022-01-02, DOI: 10.1177/08901171211069547

Osei-Tutu, A. et al. 2021. The impact of COVID-19 and religious restrictions on the well-being of Ghanaian Christians: The perspectives of religious leaders. *Journal of Religion and Health*, 60, 2232–2249.

Paweł, Ł. et al. 2022. Does religion predict coronavirus conspiracy beliefs? Centrality of religiosity, religious fundamentalism, and COVID-19 conspiracy beliefs. *Personality and Individual Differences*, 187, https://doi.org/10.1016/j.paid.2021.111413

Pertwee, E., Simas, C., and Larson, H.J. 2022. An epidemic of uncertainty: Rumors, conspiracy theories and vaccine hesitancy. *Nat Med*, 28, 456–459. https://doi.org/10.1038/s41591-022-01728-z

Platvoet, J.G. 1999. To define or not to define: The problem of the definition of religion. In J.G. Platvoet and A.L. Molendijk (Eds), *The Pragmatics of Defining Religion: Contexts, Concepts & Contests.* Leiden: Brill, pp. 245–266.

Ramrathan, L. et al. (Eds). 2020. *Re-thinking the Humanities Curriculum in the Time of COVID-19.* Durban: CSSALL.

Rashid, R. 2020. Being called a cult is one thing, being blamed for an epidemic is quite another (online). The New York Times (Date of citation: 07.05.2020), available at www.nytimes.com/2020/03/09/opinion/coronavirus-south-korea-church.html. [Google Scholar]

Roth, A.W.S. and Philips, D. 2020. Churchgoers all over world come to terms with physical distancing advice (online). The Guardian (Date of citation: 07.05.2020), available at www.theguardian.com/world/2020/mar/29/church-goers-around-the-world-ignore-social-distance-advice. [Google Scholar]

Scharnick-Udemans, L-S.S. 2021. Feminist pandemic pedagogies: Podcasting and the study of religion. *Journal for the Study of Religion*, 34(1), 1–22.

Sexton, J.S. 2021. The critical study of religion and division in the age of COVID-19. *International Journal of Public Theology*, 15, 157–176.

Sibanda, F., Muyambo, T., and Chitando, E. (Eds). 2022. *Religion and the COVID-19 Pandemic in Southern Africa.* London: Routledge.

Sibanda, F., Muyambo, T., and Chitando, E. 2022. Introduction: Religion and public health in the shadow of the COVID-19 pandemic in Southern Africa. In F. Sibanda, T. Muyambo, and E. Chitando (Eds), *Religion and the COVID-19 Pandemic in Southern Africa.* London/New York: Routledge, pp. 1–24.

Singh, D.E. 2020. Role of religions in the spread of COVID-19. *Journal of Ecumenical Studies*, 50(2), 289–310.

Smith, B.K. 1987. Exorcising the transcendent strategies for defining Hinduism and religion. *History of Religion*, 27(1), 32–55.

Smith, J.Z. 1998. Religion, religions, religious. In M.C. Taylor (Ed), *Critical Terms for Religious Studies*. Chicago, IL: University of Chicago Press, pp. 269–284.

Smith, W.C. 1964. *The Meaning and End of Religion*. New York: Mentor.

Taylor, M.C. (Ed.). 1998. *Critical Terms for Religious Studies*. Chicago, IL: University of Chicago Press.

West, G. and Dube, M.W. (Eds). 2000. *The Bible in Africa: Trajectories, Transactions, Trends*. Leiden: Brill.

Winiger, F. 2020. More than an intensive care phenomenon: Religious communities and the WHO Guidelines for Ebola and Covid-19. https://doi.org/10.1515/spirc are-2020-0066

Wiysonge, C.S., Ndwandwe, D., Ryan, J., Jaca, A., Batouré, O., Anya, B.P.M, and Cooper, S. 2021 . Vaccine hesitancy in the era of COVID-19: Could lessons from the past help in divining the future? *Human Vaccines & Immunotherapeutics*, 18(1), e1893062 https://doi.org/10.1080/21645515.2021.1893062

World Health Organization (WHO). 2021. Ten health issues WHO will tackle this year. www.who.int/news-room/spotlight/ten-threats-to–global-health-in-2019 (Accessed 16 March 2022).

World Vision. 2021. *Faith in Action: The Power of Faith Leaders to Fight a Pandemic*. London: World Vision.

Zvobgo, C.J. 1986. Medical missions: A neglected theme in Zimbabwe's history, 1893–1957. *Zambezia*, 13(2), 109–118.

2 Bridging the 'Social Distance' between Public Health and Religion

Insights from Responses to COVID-19 Vaccines in Zimbabwe

Mutsawashe Chitando and Ezra Chitando

Introduction

In the face of the challenges posed by some ultra-conservative religious actors who challenged the rollout of the COVID-19 vaccines in Zimbabwe (as was the case in other parts of the world), there is an urgent need to reflect on the relationship between public health and religion. The potent combination of conspiracy theories and religion (see e.g. Dyrendal et al., 2019) led to some religious leaders and their followers resisting the COVID-19 vaccination efforts in Zimbabwe (and other parts of the world). On the other hand, it emerged that religious sources were deemed reliable for COVID-19 vaccine information and information authentication (Adetayo et al., 2022). Such developments necessitate reflecting on how public health and religion could be brought closer together in order to respond more effectively to current health challenges, as well as to prepare more effectively for future health emergencies. In this chapter, we contend that it is strategic to review the teaching of Medicine and Religion[1] to enable practitioners from these fields to communicate more effectively when they will be serving in the field. We utilise the case of responses to COVID-19 vaccines in Zimbabwe to illustrate the need for the two fields to reach a rapprochement and facilitate greater understanding between them. We propose that public health specialists must strive to acquire religious literacy (see e.g. Parker, 2020), while religious leaders need to acquire health literacy (see e.g. Okan et al., 2019). This is for both those who are still studying, as well as for those who are now in the field.

We recognise that in most African settings, the teaching of Medicine and Religion takes place in two distinctive, mutually exclusive and 'socially distancing/distanced' Faculties. Typically, Medicine is taught in Colleges of Health Science, while the teaching of Religion takes place in Faculties of Arts and Humanities or Social Science. In most instances, students in the College of Health Science do not interact with religion, while students of Religion do not interface with those in the Health Sciences. Although the era of HIV and AIDS challenged this separation in a profound way (see for example, Azetsop, 2016) and there is growing interest in the interface between religion and health (Chatters, 2000), the disjuncture continues to be observed in Zimbabwean and

DOI: 10.4324/9781003388630-2

many other African institutions of higher learning. The International Religious Health Assets Programme (IRHAP) at the University of Cape Town in South Africa represents a creative and promising effort to bridge this divide (see for example, Cochrane et al., 2011). The struggle to bridge the divide has meant that when there are public health emergencies, such as COVID-19 and the attendant issue of vaccination, the two fields have struggled to communicate effectively.

We are persuaded that the COVID-19 pandemic, particularly as expressed through vaccine hesitancy and vaccine rejection (as well as through the world religion's interpretation of the pandemic (see e.g. Chryssides and Cohn-Sherbok, 2023) reignited the urgency of approaching public health and religion in a more creative and dynamic way. The COVID-19 pandemic made it crystal clear that public health and religion are constantly conjoined. To teach or discuss one without the other is deeply unsatisfactory. This is because public health has serious implications for religion. In turn, religion has serious implications for public health. Religion frames health norms (Mpofu, 2018), and the behaviour of religious people has a bearing on public health. This generates the debate on religious exemptions, whereby some religious people or groups argue that they should be allowed to proceed with their beliefs and practices, even when such have implications for public health (Ogolla, 2015). This tension became very clear during the COVID-19 pandemic where some ultra-conservative religious groups sought to continue with their religious observances in defiance of public health directives. Further, some religious groups and individuals resisted COVID-19 vaccines on religious grounds (Musoni and Chitando, 2022).

However, it would be unfair to reduce the interface between religion and public health during the COVID-19 pandemic in Zimbabwe to resistance by a few religious groups (see e.g. Matikiti, 2021). If anything, the dominant story must be one of the positive interaction between public health practitioners and religious leaders. The progress that has been achieved between the sectors in the response to HIV and AIDS (see e.g., Kurian, 2016) has been solidified during the COVID-19 response. Although there were pockets of resistance, the major, and striking, dimension has been the mutual respect and coordination between public health officials and religious leaders. In many countries, there has been a seamless transition from public health messaging to religious proclamations. Many religious leaders promoted the uptake of COVID-19 vaccines, regarding them as a sign of God's intervention to address the public health challenge. In this chapter we are arguing that this bodes well for the relationship between Public Health and Religion as closely related fields. Religious leaders and public health officials can influence a person's belief in a health threat together with a person's belief in the effectiveness of the recommended health interventions (Janz and Becker, 1984). According to the Health Belief Model (HBM) theory, these perceptions influence the likelihood of a person's adoption or non-adoption of the recommended behaviour (Janz and Becker, 1984). We maintain that this has definite implications for the teaching and practice of the two fields in Africa.

In order to bring the chapter into its proper perspective, the first section provides an overview of reflections on public health and religion in general. This is to facilitate an appreciation of how scholars have approached the two fields. The authors conducted an in-depth review of literature in Google and Semantic Scholar, guided by the key words (vaccines, public health, religion, religious leaders, COVID-19, and Zimbabwe). We contend that in order to appreciate the dynamics surrounding the religious response to COVID-19 vaccines, there is a need to understand the general context where religion and public health interact. The second section is divided into two. The first part discusses the tension between public health practitioners and religious leaders in response to COVID-19 with special reference to vaccines, while the second part focuses on the positive interactions in relation to the same. In conclusion, we reflect on the main issues emerging from the reflections and make some recommendations regarding public health and religion in Zimbabwe, with implications for Africa. One point worth noting is that in this chapter we shall be moving freely between 'public health and religion,' and 'religion and public health' due to our complementing specialisations.

Religion and Public Health: An Overview

In this section, we review some of the extant literature relating to religion and public health (although we summarise the emerging trends). This will lay the foundation for understanding how these fields interface in the Zimbabwean context in the sections that follow. It is critical to acknowledge that our review is not intended to be exhaustive. Rather, it is indicative. It seeks to draw attention to some of the key and abiding issues between religion and public health, globally. This will help in putting the Zimbabwean religious responses to COVID-19 vaccines into their proper context.

Religion as a Determinant of Health

Public health professionals and religious leaders over the years have realised the need to engage at different levels to enable the success of public health interventions. Amongst this group of actors are the religious leaders who assume a role of authority and have earned a level of respect and trust in their various communities (Oluduro, 2010). Religion is not only about religious practices or identities, but also about norms, values and beliefs (Idler, 2014). From this angle, religion is, therefore, a social determinant of health as it falls under "the non-medical factors that affect both the quality and distribution of health within populations" (Shi et al., 2009, n.p.). In addition to religion, political, economic, education and social factors also contribute to the distribution of health in the society. According to Gross (2015), an individual's belief about their health is often inseparable from their religious beliefs, and as such, it is imperative to understand the interface that exists between religion and public health in order to improve population health. For Makoka (2020), churches, for example, are well-placed to inculcate awareness of health issues through commemorating strategic days on the calendar through religious eyes. In relation to COVID-19, this places us on high alert to seek to respond to the question: "How did religious leaders interpret the pandemic, and were these interpretations consistent with, or at variance with public health guidelines?" In the specific case of COVID-19 vaccines in Zimbabwe, we ask, "How did religious leaders respond to COVID-19 vaccines and how can relations between religious leaders and public health practitioners be improved to respond to current and future health challenges?"

The responses of faith communities in Zimbabwe to COVID-19 vaccines would be largely influenced by, for example, how some African Indigenous/Initiated/Instituted Churches (AICs) have resisted biomedical approaches (see e.g. Maguranyanga, 2011). However, there are notable shifts within the sector, as some beliefs are being dropped or modified in response to overtures by various activists, including faith-based organisations (see e.g. Musevenzi, 2017). Some members of Pentecostal churches have also placed emphasis on miracles, with emerging movements using healing as the arena for securing a comparative advantage (see e.g. Chitando, 2021). On the other hand, although there was a close connection between the setting up of the mainline churches and medical missions in Zimbabwe (see e.g. Zvobgo, 1986), many members of the mainline churches continue to be influenced by indigenous beliefs. As a consequence, medical pluralism is a reality in Zimbabwe, as it is in other African contexts (see e.g. Hampshire and Owusu, 2013). Thus, there is biomedicine, indigenous medicine, prophetic healing from AICs and Pentecostal churches, as well as creative blending of the various therapeutic systems. All these had an impact on the reception of COVID-19 vaccines from religious perspectives.

The Role of Religious Entities in Response to Health Emergencies

For decades, religious institutions have played a pivotal role in the provision of health services in low-middle income countries. These institutions have played a role in challenging social inequalities through their provision of public health infrastructure in hard-to-reach communities (Kagawa et al., 2012). Their efforts also include health education and promotion as evidenced by their response to the HIV pandemic where the faith-based organisations took up the role of creating community awareness and promoting behaviour change (Kidia, 2018). Religious institutions also play a key role in caring for the people living with HIV, as well as offering psychosocial support for the affected individuals and their families. These efforts have proven to be key in confronting the stigma and demystifying the myths associated with the disease (Blevins et al., 2019).

In times of catastrophe, many people rely on the religious narrative to explain the seemingly uncontrollable and life-threatening events (Idler, 2014). For example, in the 2009 H1N1 pandemic, religious leaders played a pivotal role communicating the risks that were associated with the pandemic to their various communities. Similarly, the world's religions have sought to respond to COVID-19 (Chryssides and Cohn-Sherbok, 2023). Risk communication has been cited as being critical in minimizing the adverse social, political and economic impacts that are typical of a pandemic (WHO, 2018). During the Ebola outbreak (2014), religious leaders assumed a similar role as they took up the responsibility of behavioural change and communication (BCC) in their various communities (Manguvo and Mafuvadze, 2015). Initially, their efforts were limited to burying the dead and consoling the living, but, as the deaths sky-rocketed, religious leaders began leading the initiatives to stop the practices that led to the transmission of the virus (Blevins et al., 2019). Amongst these practices were the burial rituals and the laying of hands on the sick which fuelled the spread of the Ebola virus. In addition, the religious leaders also took up the vital task of case finding followed by case monitoring.

From these different health emergencies, what has been observed is the mutual concern over the health of the affected population that is shared by both the public health practitioners and the religious leaders. The contributions made by the religious leaders and faith-based organisations towards community health are not only limited to the times when disaster strikes, but they are also evident in the provision of essential day-to-day health services, particularly in the low-middle income countries.

Religion and Health Systems Strengthening

In countries where government structures are weak and fail to provide basic services, such as social justice, protection, health and education, faith-based health providers (FBHPs) play a pivotal role filling the gap between what is and what should be (UNDP, 2014). Globally, the focus is on achieving universal health coverage in the form of quality health services that are available and acceptable without the individuals facing the risk of financial hardship or impoverishment (Ghaffar, 2018). In a bid to achieve this, many low-middle income governments have sought to optimise the contributions of non-state actors (e.g. FBHPs) in improving health coverage. Estimates from the WHO suggest that FBHPs provide 30%–70% of health care in low-middle income countries (Magezi, 2018). In this light, FBHPs are critical in ensuring availability (they operate even in the most remote communities), affordability (cost of services to individuals is not profit-driven) and acceptability (messages from FBHPs often resonate with the community) of health services.

In Zimbabwe, in 2008, a period which was characterised by severe social, economic, and political hardships, the government turned to FBHPs for the provision of primary health care services. Primary healthcare forms an integral part in addressing the main community health needs which include promotive, preventive, curative and rehabilitative services. This is not unique to Zimbabwe, but in many sub-Saharan countries, more than 50% of primary health service delivery is through FBHPs (Marshall and Aylward 2013). For governments with weaker health systems, there is a need to meaningfully engage with non-state actors to address some of the challenges faced within the health system. In countries where the governments have partnered with FBHPs, the service delivery and health workforce building blocks of the health system have largely benefited (Maulit, 2017).

There are some concerns that governments have when it comes to involving FBHPs in the health service delivery for a country. These are often to do with measuring the quality of care provided by these non-state actors. When it comes to public health practice, while the trust and influence that religious leaders have over their communities is a resource to tap into, it is at times considered an obstacle when the religious and public health messages are contradictory (Manguvo and Mafuvadze, 2015). The religious and public health communities are not innately at odds, but over the years there are topics that have stirred a lot of debate. Topics around sexual and reproductive health (contraception and abortion), vaccination, and other essential medicines are some of the topics that the two groups have had to and are still trying to find common ground. Gender bias is also a phenomenon that is present in some of the religious doctrines and this often leads to the predisposition of women to some preventable diseases (Oluduro 2010). Having different agendas and finding a common language between the public health professionals and religious leaders are some of the barriers that the two groups need to overcome for the successful implementation of public health interventions. This can be illustrated from the responses to COVID-19 vaccines by the religious community in Zimbabwe. We turn to a discussion of this theme below.

Public Health, COVID-19 Vaccines and Religion in Zimbabwe

In this section we seek to highlight some key issues relating to the responses of Zimbabwean religious leaders to the pandemic, with special reference to the COVID-19 vaccines. Did the religious leaders uphold the protocols relating to COVID-19 as articulated by public health practitioners, as well as promoting the uptake of COVID-19 vaccines? If they did not do so, what were some of the key factors that led to this clash of approaches? If there was harmony between the two categories of professionals, what facilitated this? The first section addresses the first question, while the second section focuses on the second question. These questions and sections are guided by constructs of the HBM, and will explore the perceived barriers and benefits of the COVID-19 vaccines in the purview of religious leaders and public health officials. However, we provide a brief introduction to the centrality of religion in Africa/Zimbabwe first so as to assist the reader to appreciate our focus on religious leaders and COVID-19.

The late doyen of African theology, John S. Mbiti (1969), bequeathed the very strong idea that Africans are notoriously religious and that religion permeates every aspect of African life. This underscores the important role that religion occupies in the lives of most Africans. Indeed, although there is rapid social change, religion remains central to the lives of most Africans in the contemporary period (Grillo et al., 2019). African Traditional Religions, Christianity, Islam and various other religions of the world shape the beliefs and actions of millions of Africans, including Zimbabweans. Therefore, it would be expected that when a crisis of the magnitude of COVID-19 appeared, religion would feature prominently in terms of interpreting the pandemic and guiding responses to the protocols relating to the pandemic.

As Ninian Smart (1996) explained, religion has many dimensions that are relevant to various aspects of the lives of believers. Religion provides an explanatory framework regarding why events happen, and offers hope in the context of fear and desperation. Therefore, with COVID-19, religion accentuated its relevance globally. In this section, we analyse the interface between public health and religion, paying particular attention to the theme of COVID-19 vaccines.

Tensions and Contradictions between Public Health Practitioners and Religious Leaders in Zimbabwe over COVID-19 Vaccines

There were some religious leaders (admittedly, a minority, but a significant one) who adopted a non-compatibilist stance regarding COVID-19 public health messages (including the uptake of vaccines) and faith. In this section, we reflect on a number of reasons why they gained some followership. First, public health and religion interfaced in a strained way when the pandemic began to be reported in different African contexts, particularly in the week 13–20 March 2020. As we note below, this strand of resistance continued, admittedly at a lower level. Although most politicians, acting on advice from public health experts, had given directives to regulate the number of people attending religious activities (some countries began with a maximum of 100 people and moved down to 50), a notable number of religious leaders did not adhere to the protocols. This was not limited to Zimbabwe, as some Christian churches, for example in parts of Kenya, Ghana, Nigeria, Malawi, Zambia, South Africa and other countries, continued to have their weekly services as usual. Although some churches observed some of the protocols, such as using hand sanitisers and maintaining social distance, the majority had proceeded with a 'business as usual approach'. Similarly, attendance at many mosques for Muslims, temples for Hindus and at the sacred sites of other religions had remained normal during the first week. This earlier reaction by religious actors was to colour the response to COVID-19 vaccines, hence it is necessary to reflect on it. There are a number of reasons for this.

Historically, religion has been about faith and, for some, insisting on a public and defiant performance of religion in the public sphere is the ultimate expression (and confirmation) of faith. In some religions of the world, persecution, defiance and martyrdom are deemed signifiers of true religiosity. In Christianity, the declaration, 'the blood of the martyrs is the seed of the Church' has been popular as it associates martyrdom with the growth of the Church. This dimension of celebrating defiance is found in other religions of the world (Okeke, 2012). In this scheme, a believer's level of commitment is measured against his or her willingness to defy the authorities for the sake of his or her religion. As the pandemic progressed, resisting public messages that sought to promote COVID-19 vaccines could be interpreted as demonstrating unshaken faith on the part of those who questioned the origin, intention and efficacy of vaccines (Musoni and Chitando, 2022).

This dimension (of resistance as an expression/mark of faith) of religion is very difficult to deal with from a public health perspective. The more the authorities seek to force compliance, the more they run the risk of igniting the fanatical flame which always lurks within every religion. It is important for us to underscore the point that no single religion is without the capacity to gravitate towards sacralising or baptising violence, including indigenous religions. There have been examples of different religions adopting a militant outlook (Juergensmeyer, 2000). Thus, in the face of the directive to begin worshipping from home and being encouraged to be vaccinated, some ultra-conservatives in the different religions in Zimbabwe (and other parts of Africa) cried out that they were being persecuted and that their faith was under attack. They fell on the pre-existing template that in the last of days, those who did not recognise the legitimacy of religion would appear and persecute the faithful.

The initial resistance or lack of co-operation during the earliest phase of the COVID-19 pandemic, as well as resistance to vaccines in the latter phase of the pandemic in many parts of Zimbabwe and other parts of Africa/the world where there is religious pluralism was also due to inter-religious, as well as intra-religious competition. The former refers to competition between two (or more) different religions, particularly Christianity and Islam, in many African contexts (including Zimbabwe). These two religions are often locked in mortal combat. Co-operating too quickly with public health authorities and retreating from the public space would be seen as suggesting lack of robust and high-level faith by followers of one religion. Similarly, hurrying to accept COVID-19 vaccines could be interpreted as accepting the failure of one's Supreme Being to facilitate miraculous healing. This could lead to taunting by one's religious competitors. In Zimbabwe, Christianity and Islam are engaged in low-level conflict, although the public posturing goes a long way in minimising the competition.

Intra-religious competition among churches was another factor that could account for the refusal or failure to collaborate with public health authorities regarding observing lockdowns and accepting vaccines at both the onset and height of COVID-19 in Zimbabwe and other African contexts. African Christianity is very broad, consisting of the historic mainline churches (Catholics and Protestant), AICs and the newer/younger African Pentecostal Churches. All these forms of Christianity are engaged in an intense struggle for members, influence and power. Anthropologist Francis Nyamnjoh and historian Joel Carpenter have articulated this competition well and we cite their observation below:

The fact that religion does not occur in a social, political and cultural vacuum should necessarily alert the attention of scholars – who provide for and are sensitive to the suggested approach – to the categorical imperative of the role of power, money, poverty and the cultures they engender and perpetuate in what form religion and religiosity assume in the lives of individuals and in the institutions and everyday relations of a given society.

(Nyamnjoh and Carpenter, 2018: 290)

Another challenge that persisted in terms of resistance by some religious actors to public health guidelines during the COVID-19 pandemic in Zimbabwe were the declarations by some religious leaders that cast suspicion on the vaccines. In particular, one highly influential Pentecostal church leader had an initially extremist stance towards vaccines. He charged that the politicians have never had the welfare of the citizens at heart: why would they now be so keen to protect them by rolling out the COVID-19 vaccines? He was joined by some leaders of AICs who adopted a deeply Africanist position and averred that the COVID-19 vaccines were part of an elaborate ploy to eliminate black Africans from the face of the earth. After all, they continued, the slave trade, colonialism and the skewed global financial systems confirmed that the world was essentially anti-black Africans.

Finally, tension between public health practitioners and religious leaders also emerged over the interpretation of the pandemic. As was the case with HIV and AIDS when some religious leaders abandoned the biological/scientific explanations, in COVID-19 some religious leaders promoted spiritual or mystical explanations, as well as conspiracy theories. They generated fear, alarm and despondency by describing COVID-19 in apocalyptic terms. In this scheme, the end of the world had begun and the vaccines represent the last stage in God's decisive plan to annihilate the earth and usher a new era. However, there were other religious leaders, who were the majority, who belonged to the compatibilist camp where the vaccines were consistent with faith.

Positive Engagement between Religious Leaders and Public Health Practitioners in Response to COVID-19 Vaccines in Zimbabwe

Despite the tensions outlined above, on the whole religious leaders in Zimbabwe and other parts of Africa struck a very good rapport with public health officials in the wake of COVID-19, including in promoting vaccines. In this section, we highlight some of the key areas of positive engagement. Once again, space considerations imply that we are unable to offer detailed analyses of these points. First, most religious leaders were quick to suspend physical religious services as soon as the public health restrictions were spelt out and to encourage their members to be vaccinated. Although we have drawn attention to the initial resistance, once most governments indicated seriousness in restricting interactions, most religious leaders moved immediately to implement these measures and to promote the uptake of vaccines. This cut across the different religious traditions in Zimbabwe. For example, the leadership across the denominations moved to suspend public religious events and moved to online services. Similarly, Muslim leaders also encouraged the faithful to pray at home, and not at the mosque. Globally, even one of the most important Muslim rites, namely, the pilgrimage to Mecca (*hajj*) was suspended for 2020. Thus, by shifting most religious activities online, many religious leaders in Zimbabwe were acting in sync with public health messages.

Second, many religious leaders in Zimbabwe became key sources of knowledge and information relating to COVID-19, including the benefits of getting vaccinated. Religious leaders were integral to information dissemination regarding COVID-19. As we noted above, the HIV pandemic prepared the religious leaders to be visible on the frontlines and provide accurate information to counter denial and stigmatisation. They transferred the knowledge and skills gained in the HIV response to the COVID-19 response. Further, this was leveraging on the perception of religious leaders as trusted health messengers (see Wiginton et al., 2019).

Third, and related to the foregoing, many religious leaders in Zimbabwe were promoting biomedicine. Although, as discussed above, there were some religious leaders in the country who were insisting on faith healing, the majority were recommending that individuals had to utilise the established health facilities, many of which were owned by the faith communities themselves. This was a very important step, as claims of faith healing have endangered the lives of many people in Africa during the time of HIV and AIDS (Chitando and Klagba, 2013). In this regard, therefore, religious leaders were promoting positive health-seeking behaviour in the context of COVID-19. This was highly strategic, as their voice is listened to by many people and this went a long way in promoting harmony with public health practitioners.

Fourth, FBHPs played a complementary role to public and private health facilities. As we noted in the literature review, FBHPs are integral to health delivery in Africa, including Zimbabwe. Due to the emergency precipitated by COVID-19, it was critical that religious leaders ensured that their health facilities were up to the required standard in the face of COVID-19. Church-owned health facilities, for example, were used as vaccination centres, alongside other public health facilities. In this regard, Church Health Associations (CHAs) in Africa were actively involved in preparing to respond to the pandemic. This confirmed the strategic role that FBHPs play in health delivery in Africa, including Zimbabwe.

Conclusion

We began this chapter by drawing attention to the 'social distancing' between Public Health and Religion in Africa. We are persuaded that the foregoing description and analysis of African religious leaders' response to COVID-19 with special reference to vaccines lays bare the urgency of conceptualising the two fields together. We also applied the HBM theory to explore the relationship between these fields. The two fields must transcend the perceived distance between them and interact in ways that promote mutual enrichment. We contend that public health officials in Africa and everywhere else, therefore, need religious literacy. This implies that they must have a deep understanding of how religion functions. On the other hand, religious leaders in Africa need to have a deep understanding of health through the acquisition of health literacy. This can be achieved by teaching students of Medicine and Religion together, as well as promoting healthy interactions between them when they would have entered the field. This is a very strategic way of preparing for future pandemics, since effective collaboration between the two sets of professionals is critical to the attainment of positive outcomes.

The dominant idea of religion as irrational, emotional and antithetical to progress has been challenged by Zimbabwean (and other African) religious leaders with high levels of public health awareness in their response to COVID-19, including vaccine promotion. For example, in Tanzania and Zambia, when the presidents were adopting a populist stance and encouraging religious activities during the pandemic, some religious leaders stood firm. They maintained that there would be no public worship services till the danger posed by the pandemic had passed. This is highly commendable and confirms the strategic role of informed and competent religious leaders. Religious leaders who have acquired health literacy are assets to their communities and countries. In turn, public health officials who have religious literacy are valuable resources to their profession and beyond.

Given the extent to which religion permeates all aspects of life in Zimbabwe and Africa, it would be conceivable to argue that most public health practitioners on the continent are themselves religious. Some of the public health practitioners even hold high positions within their faith communities. In this regard, they are religious leaders! Future studies could explore the extent to which this shared religious outlook between public health practitioners and religious leaders facilitates (or frustrates) effective communication between these two categories of strategic actors on Zimbabwe's/Africa's health scene. In closing, we strongly recommend serious investment in the joint training of students of Public Health and Religion in Zimbabwe and Africa. As we have highlighted through the case study of Zimbabwean/African religious leaders and COVID-19 with special reference to vaccines and through the prism of the HBM theory, these two categories of professionals must have ongoing and mutually enriching conversations to ensure a healthy and robust Zimbabwe and Africa.

Note

1 We use the capital letters to designate the respective (but intersecting) fields of study and practice.

References

Adetayo, A.J., Williams-Ilemobola, O.B., and Asiru, M.A. 2022. Religious sources of COVID-19 vaccine information, authentication and vaccination acceptance among students in selected universities in Nigeria. *Journal of Consumer Health on the Internet*, 26(2), 157–170.

Azetsop, J. (Ed.) 2016. *HIV & AIDS in Africa: Christian Reflection, Public Health, Social Transformation*. Maryknoll, NY: Orbis Books.

Blevins, J.B., Jalloh, M.F., and Robinson, D.A. 2019. Faith and global health practice in Ebola and HIV emergencies. *American Journal of Public Health*, 109(3), 379–384.

Chatters, L.M. 2000. Religion and health: Public health research and practice. *Annual Review of Public Health*, 21, 335–367.

Chitando, E. (Ed.). 2021. *Innovation and Competition in Zimbabwean Pentecostalism: Megachurches and the Marketization of Religion*. London: Bloomsbury.

Chitando, E. and Klagba, C. (Eds). 2013. *In the Name of Jesus! Healing in the Age of HIV*. Geneva: World Council of Churches.

Chryssides, G.D. and Cohn-Sherbok, D. (Eds). 2023. *The Covid Pandemic and the World's Religions*. London: Bloomsbury.

Cochrane, J.R., Schmid, B., and Cutts, T. (Eds). 2011. *When Religion and Health Align: Mobilising Religious Assets for Transformation*. Pietermaritzburg: Cluster.

Dyrenda, A., Robertson, D.G., and Asprem, E. (Eds). 2019. *Handbook of Conspiracy Theory and Contemporary Religion*. Leiden: Brill.

Ghaffar, A. 2018. *The Role of Non-State Actors in Strengthening Health Systems*. Geneva: World Health Organization.

Grillo, L.S., van Klinken A., and Ndzovu, H.J. 2019. *Religions in Contemporary Africa: An Introduction*. London: Routledge.

Gross, C.L. 2015. *Spirituality and Religion as a Social Determinant and Social Mediator of Health*. Master of Arts Dissertation. Nashville, TN: Graduate School of Vanderbilt University.

Hampshire, K.R. and Owusu, S.A. 2013. Grandfathers, Google, and dreams: Medical pluralism, globalization, and new healing encounters in Ghana. *Medical Anthropology*, 32(3), 247–265.

Idler, E.L. 2014. *Religion as a Social Determinant of Public Health*. New York: Oxford University Press.

Janz, N.K. and Becker, M.H. 1984. The health belief model: A decade later. *Health Education Quarterly*, 11, 1–47.

Juergensmeyer, M. 2000. *Terror in the Mind of God: The Global Rise of Religious Violence*. Berkeley, CA: University of California Press.

Kagawa, C.R., Anglemyer, A., and Montagu, D. 2012. The scale of faith based organization participation in health service delivery in developing countries: Systemic review and meta-analysis. *PLOS ONE* 7(11), https://doi.org/10.1371/annotation/1e80554b-4f8a-4381-97f1-46bf72cd07c9

Kidia, K.K. 2018. The future of health in Zimbabwe. *Global Health Action*, 11, 1496888.

Kurian, M. 2016. *Passion and Compassion: The Ecumenical Journey with HIV*. Geneva: World Council of Churches.

Magezi, V. 2018. Church-driven primary health care: Models for an intergrated church and community primary health care in Africa (a case study of the Salvation Army in East Africa). *SciFlo*, 74(2), 1–11.

Maguranyanga, B. 2011. *Apostolic Religion, Health and the Utilization of Maternal and Child Health Services*. Harare: UNICEF.

Makoka, M. 2020. *Health-Promoting Churches: Reflections on Health and Healing for Churches on Commemorative World Health Days*. Geneva: World Council of Churches.

Manguvo, A. and Mafuvadze, B. 2015. The impact of traditional and religious practices on the spread of Ebola in West Africa: Time for a startegic shift. *The Pan African Medical Journal*, 22(9).

Marshall, K., and Aylward, L. 2013. *Health in Africa and Faith Communities: What Do We Need to Know?* Washington DC: Berkley Center for Religion, Peace & World Affairs.

Matikiti, R. 2021. Confessing Jesus Christ in cultural context: The one-sided politics of COVID-19 vaccination in Zimbabwe. *History Research*, 9(2), 127–135.

Mbiti, J.S. 1969. *African Religions and Philosophy*. Nairobi: Heinemann.

Mpofu, E. 2018. How religion frames health norms: A structural theory approach. *Religions*, 9(4), 119: https://doi.org/10.3390/rel9040119

Mualit, J.A. 2017. *Partnerships that support health systems resilience over time: A study of non-state, faith-based health providers in Africa*. Cape Town: University of Cape Town.

Musevenzi, J. 2017. The African Independent Apostolic Church's doctrine under threat: The emerging power of faith-based organisations' interventions and the Johanne Marange Apostolic Church in Zimbabwe. *Journal for the Study of Religion*, 30(2), 178–206.

Musoni, P. and Chitando, E. 2022. Spiritualization of the causes of illness: An analysis of the Zimbabwean-born White Garment Churches' theological position on the origin and treatment of COVID-19. *Exchange*, 51(4), 361–376.

Nyamnjoh, F. and Carpenter, J. 2018. Religious innovation and competition in contemporary African Christianity. *Journal of Contemporary African Studies*, 36(3), 289–302.

Ogolla, C. 2015. The public health implications of religious exemptions: A balance between public safety and personal choice, or religion gone too far? *Health Matrix*, 25(1), 257–308.

Okan, O. et al. (Eds). 2019. *International Handbook of Health Literacy: Research, Practice and Policy Issues across the Life Span*. Bristol: Policy Press.

Okeke, E.C. 2012. Persecution and martyrdom of Christians in the Roman Empire from AD 54 to 100: A Lesson for the 21st century church. *European Journal of Scientific Research*, 8(16), 175–190.

Oluduro, O. 2010. The role of religious leaders in curbing the spread of HIV/AIDS in Nigeria. *SciFlo*, 13(3), 208–236.

Parker, S. 2020. Religious literacy: Spaces of teaching and learning about religion and belief. *Journal of Belief & Values*, 41(2), 129–131.

Shi, L., Tsai, J., and Kao, S. 2009. Public health, social determinants of health, and public policy. *Journal of Medical Science*, 29(2), 43–59.

Smart, N., 1996. *Dimensions of the Sacred: An Anatomy of the World's Beliefs*. Berkeley, CA: University of California Press.

UNDP. 2014. *UNDP Guidelines on Engaging with Faith-Based Organizations and Religious Leaders*. Vienna: United Nations.

WHO. 2018. *Managing Epidemics: Key Facts about Major Deadly Diseases*. Geneva: World Health Organization.

Wiginton, J.M., King, E.J., and Fuller, A.O. 2019. 'We can act different from what we used to': Findings from experiences of religious leader participants in an HIV-prevention intervention in Zambia. *Global Public Health*, 14(5), 636–648.

Zvobgo, C.J. 1986. Medical missions: A neglected theme in Zimbabwe's history, 1893–1957. *Zambezia*, 13(2), 109–118.

3 Indigenous Knowledge Systems and COVID-19

A Case Study of the Ndau in Eastern Zimbabwe

Anniegrace Hlatywayo and Sophia Chirongoma

Introduction

In December 2019, a highly contagious pneumonia associated with the coronavirus disease (COVID-19) broke out in Wuhan, Hubei Province in China (Lone and Ahmad, 2020; Zhou et al., 2020). On 7 January 2020, the etiological cause of the unexplained pneumonia cases was identified as a novel severe acute respiratory syndrome coronavirus-2 (SARS-CoV-2) (Lone and Ahmad, 2020). The clinical manifestation of the disease was termed coronavirus disease 2019, also known as COVID-19 (Paintsil, 2020). Within the period of one month, COVID-19 had globally spread to the rest of the world. On 30 January 2020, the World Health Organization declared a public health emergency of international concern for the novel COVID-19 outbreak (Hui et al., 2020; Chen et al., 2020; CDC, 2020). This novel COVID-19 virus has been considered to be one of the biggest pandemics in human history (Du Toit, 2020). The number of infections continued to rise and the pandemic posed a major threat to public health across the globe.

COVID-19 is a highly communicable respiratory disease that is caused by a new strain of coronavirus. It may be transmitted from symptomatic persons to others particularly through respiratory droplets, direct contact with infected persons or through contact with contaminated surfaces and/or objects (Liu et al., 2020; Huang et al., 2020). An infected person is more contagious at the onset of the symptomatic stage as compared to later developmental stages of the disease (WHO, 2020). The virus has an incubation period of between 1 and 14 days and this represents the time between exposure to becoming contagious as well as the onset of symptomatic presentation. During this particular period, pre-symptomatic transmission can occur (WHO, 2020). This entails that COVID-19 infected persons can transmit the virus before developing significant symptoms (Chan, 2020).

In the absence of a cure, the management of the disease is mainly supportive. This entails best health practices through prevention and control measures. The World Health organization (WHO) issued guidelines aimed at reducing the risk of transmission of the novel coronavirus. These are listed as (i) frequent and careful washing of hands with soap and running water; (ii)

DOI: 10.4324/9781003388630-3

avoid touching the face including the mouth, nose and eyes; (iii) covering the mouth and nose when coughing or sneezing; (iv) maintain social distance by keeping a distance of two (2) metres from other people and (v) self-quarantine if sick and (vi) wearing a face mask (WHO, 2020). Infection can be prevented by observing and maintaining personal hygiene practices. Traditional public health outbreak response through isolation, quarantine, social and/or physical distancing, community containment, national lockdowns and travel bans, and restrictions were globally adopted as containment and mitigation measures against the novel COVID-19 infection. Other strategic measures enforced for reducing and controlling the spread of COVID-19 included the closing of schools, companies and offices. A ban on large gatherings in the form of religious, sports and social events was also globally enforced. Since funeral gatherings have been identified as one of the COVID-19 super spreaders, measures were put in place to revisit some death and burial rituals in order to reduce the chances of spreading the virus.

While the global village was frantically searching for a cure against the novel virus, it was imperative for countries to adopt a multifaceted approach as containment measures aimed at mitigating the spread of COVID-19. This entailed the promotion of indigenous knowledge and home-grown creative solutions as preventive, curative and protective measures aimed at mitigating disease transmission. In the context of China and the origin of the COVID-19 outbreak, Chinese medicinal approaches to mitigate against the novel pandemic were adopted as prevention and treatment measures. These included the oral administration of herbal concoctions, wearing of Chinese Medicine (CM) sachets and indoor herbal medicinal fumigation (Wang, 2011). Hence, China adopted historical and indigenous methods of responding to disease outbreaks. It is against this background that this chapter focuses on how people in Southern African, with particular reference to the Ndau in eastern Zimbabwe, were resorting to indigenous methods for preserving health and well-being (Durie, 2004; Levers, 2006) in the wake of the COVID–19 epidemic and the implications of the same to the uptake of COVID-19 vaccines.

COVID-19 in Southern Africa: The Ndau People's Interface with the Epidemic in Zimbabwe

Despite Africa being the last continent to be affected by the novel COVID-19 pandemic, it was highly susceptible to becoming the most vulnerable continent with high mortality rates wrought by the epidemic. The postulations made by the WHO in April 2020 warning that Africa could be the next epicentre for COVID-19 (BBC News, 2020) fortunately did not materialise. It was feared that due to the continent's poor quality of biomedical healthcare systems (Gbadamosi, 2020) the continent would be devastated. Additionally, some parts of the African continent are also characterised by a huge immuno-compromised population due to high prevalence rates of HIV and AIDS infection, Tuberculosis, Malaria and other chronic diseases (World Economic Forum, 2020). Africa's susceptibility to high levels of COVID-19 infection was also feared due to resource constraints in the form of limited testing capacity; inadequate ventilators and ICU facilities for severe cases; limited number of personal protective equipment (PPE) for healthcare workers and low levels of economic and socio-political stability. Overcrowding, high levels of poverty, poor nutrition as well as lack of sanitation facilities in most African urban and peri-urban areas were feared as worsening Africa's vulnerability to the pandemic.

The first case of COVID-19 infection in Africa was detected in Cairo, Egypt on 14 February 2020 through an asymptomatic individual who had travelled from China. The second case was reported in Nigeria on 27 February 2020 (Paintsil, 2020). Thereafter, the pandemic caused many deaths in various African countries, with South Africa the most affected. The impact of the severe lockdowns on Africa's economies was also very significant. However, the lack of specific antiviral drugs and vaccines for COVID-19 during the early phase, coupled with the African continent's vulnerability to the novel pandemic called for homegrown/local strategies as containment measures against the spread of the virus. The novel COVID-19 pandemic presented an opportune time for Africa to revitalise her indigenous knowledge systems and, where appropriate, interface them with other knowledge systems as well as blending them with modern technology in a bid to promote the fullness of life. It also called on the African continent to improve the already compromised, dilapidated and ill-equipped biomedical healthcare systems (Chirongoma, 2016).

Methodology

This chapter is based on secondary sources of data collected from the Internet, research articles as well as social media and news outlets related to COVID-19. Google Scholar and PubMed were searched for English articles on COVID-19. Search words included COVID-19, COVID-19 in Africa, Indigenous Knowledge Systems and COVID-19, Indigenous Conceptualisation of Health and Sickness, Traditional Medicine and COVID-19 and Responses to COVID-19 Vaccines in Zimbabwe. The authors also tapped into their knowledge reserves acquired through their ongoing research on the role of indigenous knowledge systems in preserving health and well-being in Africa, including attitudes towards biomedicine and vaccines.

African Indigenous Conceptualisation of Health and Illness

Within the African perspective, religion and healing are intertwined. Hence, in order to address the health and well-being of African people, one has to understand their religious worldview (Shoko, 2007). Indigenous beliefs and practices are an integral part of the religious life of the African people. African indigenous healing procedures are interlinked with the socio-cultural, epistemological, ontological and cosmological considerations (Hlatywayo, 2017). This ultimately gives rise to holistic healthcare practices. As such, indigenous healing practices do not only focus on the physical, rather, it also pays attention to the psychological, spiritual as well as the social dimension of individuals, families and communities in an all-inclusive way (Chirongoma, 2014). The holistic nature of indigenous healthcare is evidenced through its services that incorporate treatment and management of disease as well as prevention and health promotion strategies and for further promotion of good health (Harfield et al., 2018).

Additionally, indigenous healthcare services also pay attention to the social determinants of health. Based on this understanding, religious beliefs and practices are major determinants in the recovery process of a sick individual (Aziato et al., 2016). Hence, "a person's well-being depends on his/her harmonious relationship with the community and supernatural forces as well as the maintenance of necessary equilibrium between relationships" (Oguamanam, 2006: 112). As such, health practitioners should take into account the health-seeking behaviours of their patients (Chirongoma, 2020). Kahissay et al. (2017) rightly point out that it is vital to understand the perceptions of illness and health that is common in indigenous communities. This is equally important for health workers as well as policy makers as this understanding will help them to strategise and design holistic healthcare models that are culturally acceptable within indigenous communities (Murove, 2009).

Within indigenous communities, therapeutic intervention is holistic and involves both diagnostic and curative rituals embedded in religio-cultural and psychosocial underpinnings (Oguamanam, 2006). Notwithstanding this, the effects of religion on illness and health are often overlooked (Gaydos et al., 2010), especially within the biomedical discourse (Hlatywayo, 2017). Within indigenous communities, treatment modalities are culturally specific. One's choice of treatment is not always determined by financial constraints and/or accessibility of biomedical health care but by one's perception of the aetiology of illness based on one's religious beliefs (Asare and Danquah, 2017). Hence, despite the modes of transmission and one's susceptibility to infection, spiritual/religious beliefs always come into play. Therefore, in some cases when a person falls sick, consultation with a traditional healer or a priest is made to determine causal factors for one's susceptibility to ill health (Chavunduka, 1994). All these factors had a bearing on whether and the extent to which indigenous communities responded to COVID-19 vaccines when they became available and were being promoted by public health experts and political actors.

African Indigenous Communities' Response to Transmittable Diseases, Isolation and Social Distancing

In the absence of a vaccine and/or treatment for a highly infectious disease such as the COVID-19 pandemic, social distancing was considered as one of the most vital strategies to contain transmission. From a universal perspective, social distancing, also referred to as physical distancing, is a strategy employed to minimise physical contact between individuals in a bid to curb the spread of highly infectious or contagious diseases (ECDC, 2020; Jaja et al., 2020; Musinguzi and Asamoah, 2020). Social distancing measures included but were not limited to, the suspension or closure of social activities that promote social contact i.e. social and/or mass gatherings, business activities and public transport facilities.

Whilst social/physical distancing has also been globally adopted as one of the containment measures against the spread of COVID-19 infection, this practice clashed with indigenous beliefs and practices that are based on the social connectedness of family and community during sickness and/or health. The need for social connection is explained by Van Bavel et al who point out that social connection "helps people to regulate emotions, cope with stress and remain resilient during difficult times" (2020: 466).

Social distancing is interpreted differently within indigenous settlements and/or rural settings where homesteads are dispersed thereby allowing families to stay at a distance from the other but close enough to be able to engage in daily care, support and cooperation (Chirikure, 2020). Therefore, during a disease outbreak or pandemic, the infected were isolated and housed in temporary structures on the outskirts of the homestead or demarcated community. A traditional healer or health practitioner was assigned to offer treatment and monitor the progress of the patient whilst taking precautionary measures against infection. After the patient's recovery or demise, the temporary structure is burnt as a way of destroying any particle that can lead to contamination. This was especially the case during the era when leprosy was still widespread in Africa. In the era of the COVID-19 pandemic, the rate of transmission was lower in rural settings as compared to urban settings due to the physical set-up of dwelling places. Good hygiene, sanitation and environmental control are part of daily practices within most indigenous communities. Adherence to these is guided by social/community taboos. For instance, among the Ndau of south-eastern Zimbabwe, common utility places like water springs have guidelines for maintenance. Certain objects are allowed for drawing water, it is believed that there are territorial spirits that protect the wells or springs (Muyambo and Maposa, 2014). Misfortune is believed to befall those who fail to uphold community maintenance guidelines. Water for consumption and domestic use is usually drawn from different wells as a measure to prevent pollution. Additionally, there are set periods of time for cleaning the community public spaces. Hence, indigenous communities have long-term community set procedures for maintaining the health and well-being of its members. This is also augmented by a diversified indigenous diet that includes fruits, roots and vegetables that strengthen the immune system. While social coherence was the glue that held society together, social distancing was inbuilt, in a supportive way (Chirikure, 2020).

COVID-19 and African Traditional Medicine

Traditional medicine refers to the sum total of knowledge, skills and practices based on the theories, beliefs and experiences indigenous to different cultures that are used to maintain health, as well as to prevent, diagnose, improve or treat physical and mental illnesses. Shoko (2018: 1) points out that African traditional medicine (ATM) is "at the heart of African people" and there has been a global resurgence of the use of natural and herbal medicines for primary healthcare. It is duly acknowledged that 80% of the global populace use traditional medicine. Whilst traditional medicine (TM) is taken as alternative and complementary to biomedical healthcare in the European context, within the African context, TM is the first choice of healthcare. This is equally argued by White (2015) who posits that ATM is not the same as alternative or complementary medicine but it is an African indigenous system of healthcare, hence, it cannot be referred to as alternative. In many African indigenous communities, biomedical health services are sought either as an alternative solution or after referral by a traditional healer. Coupled with the exorbitant costs associated with biomedical healthcare, ATM is increasingly gaining popularity because it is readily available, easily accessible, affordable and culturally acceptable (Chepkwony, 2006).

The lack of specific antiviral drugs and vaccines coupled with poor quality of healthcare and resource restraints in Africa calls for homegrown/indigenous strategies to safeguard against the novel virus infection. Gbadamosi (2020) argued that since COVID-19 is a viral infection, indigenous antiviral medicinal plants can be used for safeguarding against infection. Furthermore, the common use of botanical detoxifiers, immune boosters and natural antioxidants as constituents of traditional medicine that are used for managing infectious diseases can be adopted as preventive medicine against COVID-19 infection. Additionally, since the novel virus was a viral infection, Gbadamosi (2020) proposed the use of antiviral medicinal plants against COVID-19 infection.

Within the context of Zimbabwe, common indigenous medicinal plants for the treatment of colds and flu were recommended as prevention and control measures against COVID-19 infection. Commonly cited indigenous herbal medicines include *mugwavha (Psidium guajava L.)*; *muvhinji (euclea crispa)*; *musekesa (piliostigma thonningil)*; *muonde (ficus sycomorus L.)*; *mukute (Syzygium cordatum)*; *Zimbani (Lippia javanica [Burm.f. Spreng]) and Citrus limon* (Maroyi, 2013). The roots, leaves and/or bark of these plants are used as cough and fever medicine and for the treatment of chest pains, pneumonia, tuberculosis and throat inflammation. Concoctions from any of these plants are recommended as a daily dose for preventive measures against COVID-19 infection. In South Africa, the indigenous African potato (*Hypoxis*) is traditionally utilised as an immune booster that strengthens the body's natural immune system (Kaya, 2007). The African potato is also used for treating chronic viral and bacterial diseases. Therefore, this is an indigenous plant that can also be used as preventive medicine against COVID-19 infection due to its pharmacological activity as an immune booster. The University of Stellenbosch in South Africa has, through extensive research on the African potato, innovatively developed the plant into easy to take tablets and these are available in local pharmacies in the country.

Similarly, in the South African context, a study by Mehrbod et al. (2018) indicated the presence of antiviral activity in two indigenous medicinal plants, the *Rapanea melanophoeos* and *Pittosporum viridiflorum*. These plants may be used for the treatment of influenza. The authors further argue that the large repertoire of medicinal plants that are used for the treatment of various disorders contain useful biological activities that can be used to manage infectious diseases (Mehrbod et al., 2018). Another study carried out by Semenya and Maroyi (2018) presents a number of medicinal plants and the most notable include the botanical families of *Astaraceae*, *Fabaceaea*, *Lamiaceae* and *Amaryllidaceae*. These plants comprise a number of species that are used as remedies for respiratory infections and their related symptoms, i.e. tuberculosis, cough, fever, chest pains and cold (Semenya and Maroyi, 2018).

In the same light, Gbadamosi (2020) notes that the use of herbal medicines for both treatment and management of infections and diseases is part of Nigerian culture and customs. The indigenous knowledge associated with this practice is passed from one generation to another. He further proposes that since the presenting symptoms of COVID-19 infection include fever, cough, body pain, flu, and shortness of breath, plants exhibiting anti-malarial properties, cough remedies and medicinal plants with pharmacological properties for treating respiratory tract infections can be used as preventive medicines against infection (Gbadamosi, 2020). In the same context of Nigeria, *Cassia fistula* (purging cassia), *Phyllanthus amarus* (stonebreaker), *Lagenaria breviflorus* (wild colocynth), *Citrullus colocynthis* (bitter apple) and *Syzygium aromatic* (clove) are used for treating and managing viral infections (Gbadamosi, 2015). *Garcinia kola* (bitter kola) and *Bryophyllum pinnatum* (miracle leaf) are used as traditional cough remedies. *Spondias mombin* (yellow mombin), *Garcinia kola*, *Calotropis procera* (apple of Sodom), *Nymphaea lotus* (water lily) and *Abrus precatorius* (water lily) are used for managing respiratory tract infections (Gbadamosi, 2020). Since these indigenous medicinal remedies are used for managing similar presenting symptoms of COVID-19, they were pertinently adopted for preventing and managing the novel viral infection. Additionally, the use of indigenous medicinal plants as immune boosters offers better resistance against infection as well as curtailing the progression of the disease for the infected (Wabo, 2020). It was in this context of the widespread acceptance and use of indigenous medicinal plants that COVID-19 vaccines were later introduced.

Africa boasts of a rich biodiversity, hence, the epidemic provided an opportunity for Mother Africa to turn to her natural ecosystems and to take into account her indigenous pharmacopoeia for primary healthcare. It has been documented that a greater portion of the inhabitants on the African continent have a vested interest in indigenous medical solutions (Wabo, 2020). Many inhabitants in indigenous communities, both young and old, are conversant with the knowledge of a number of medicinal plant-based formulations for primary healthcare. Indigenous medicinal plant knowledge is generated through long periods of experimentation, observation and trial and error methods. Based on inherited knowledge and long-term usage, traditional healers, community healers and community sages have their own indigenous scientific strategies of testing for medicinal plant toxicity, safety and efficacy. Gbadamosi (2020) highlighted the pertinent need for turning to nature and to explore the beneficial properties of Africa's medicinal plants that serve as immune boosters and anti-infectives to fight against COVID-19 infection. "There is no human culture or worldview that does not subscribe to the medicinal values of plants" (Oguamanam, 2006: 119). Apart from using indigenous medicinal plants to mitigate COVID-19 infection, other traditional practices inclusive of steam bathing, gurgling warm water mixed with either herbs or salt were also suggested as preventive measures against infection.

With the introduction of COVID-19 vaccines, although originally there was vaccine hesitancy among most indigenous communities not only in Zimbabwe but worldwide, gradually, the Ndau people in eastern Zimbabwe were also embracing the vaccination programmes. Although initially, the vaccination programme in Zimbabwe was more concentrated on the urban communities, once the programme started spreading into the rural settings, the traditional leadership and the local healthcare workers were diligently encouraging all those who are eligible to be vaccinated to take up the vaccine. As has been noted above, the Ndau people's acceptance of the COVID-19 vaccination was informed by the fact that they generally operate on a three-tier healthcare system, i.e., interfacing western biomedicine, indigenous healing systems and faith–healing (Chirongoma, 2014, 2016). Hence, for the Ndau people, COVID-19 vaccination is perceived as part and parcel of their integrated and holistic healthcare system.

Conclusion

COVID-19 is a highly transmittable virus that has spread across the globe in a very short period of time. Communities in Africa were drawing on indigenous knowledge as coping mechanisms and containment mechanisms against COVID-19 infection. Clearly, most indigenous African communities have always relied on indigenous medical therapies for maintaining their health and well-being since time immemorial, hence, tapping into this rich and diverse resource base will go a long way in addressing the COVID–19 epidemic in Africa. This is especially important in light of the fact that in most African communities, the biomedical healthcare sector was already battling to cope even before the outbreak of the COVID-19 epidemic. Also, making resolute efforts to come up with authentically African solutions to challenges confronting the African continent such as health and well-being will make an immense contribution towards liberating Africans from an over-reliance on foreign medical interventions such as Western or Chinese medicine which is often unaffordable or inaccessible for most of the ordinary Africans. Hence, the COVID-19 epidemic could have presented an opportune moment for the bulk of the African populace to return to the basics, where as Africans we come up with home-grown solutions to contemporary existential challenges. The embracing of COVID-19 vaccination by the Ndau people in eastern Zimbabwe is also a pointer in the right direction; it emphasises the ongoing indigenous people's integration of the threefold healthcare system which entails tapping into Western biomedicine, African indigenous healing systems and faith healing. This openness and dynamism demonstrated the flexibility of indigenous health delivery systems. Traditional healers, cultural leaders, family heads and others countered the myths and misinformation surrounding COVID-19 vaccines and actively encouraged people in their areas to be vaccinated. It confirmed the vitality and contextual sensitivity of indigenous healing systems.

References

Asare, M. and Danquah, S.A. 2017. The African belief system and the patient's choice of treatment from existing health models: The case of Ghana. *Acta Psychopathol*, 3(4), 49.

Aziato, L., Odai. P.N.A, and Omenyo, C.O. 2016. Religious beliefs and practices in pregnancy and labour: An inductive qualitative study among post-partum women in Ghana. *BMC Preg and Childbirth*, 16, 138. DOI: 10.1186/512884-016-0920-1

BBC News. 2020. Coronavirus: Africa could be next epicentre, WHO warns, www.bbc.com/news/world-africa-52323375 (17 April 2020) (Accessed 25 April 2020).

CDC. 2020. *Africa CDC establishes continent-wide task force to respond to global coronavirus epidemic*. Africa Centres for Disease Control and Prevention. https://africacdc.org/news/africa-cdc-establishes-continent-wide-taskforce-to-respond-to-global-coronavirus-epidemic

Chan, J.F., et al. 2020. A familial cluster of pneumonia associated with the 2019 novel coronavirus indicating person-to-person transmission: A study of a family cluster. *Lancet*, 395(10223), 514–523.

Chavunduka, G.L. 1994. *Traditional Medicine in Modern Zimbabwe*. Harare: University of Zimbabwe Publishers.

Chen, N., Zhou, M., Dong, X., Qu, J., Gong, F., Han, Y., et al. 2020. Epidemiological and clinical characteristics of 99 cases of 2019 novel coronavirus pneumonia in Wuhan, China: A descriptive study. *Lancet*, https://doi.org/10.1016/S0140-6736(20)30211-7

Chepkwony A.K. (Ed.).2006. *Religion and Health in Africa: Reflections for Theology the 21st Century*. Nairobi: Paulines Publications Africa.

Chirikure, S. 2020. *How Ancient African Societies Used Social Distancing to Manage Pandemic*. The conversation.com.

Chirongoma, S. 2014. *Navigating Indigenous Resources That Can Be Utilized in Constructing a Karanga Theology of Health and Well-Being (Utano): An Exploration of Health Agency in Contemporary Zimbabwe*. Unpublished PhD Thesis, University of KwaZulu-Natal, Pietermaritzburg Campus, South Africa.

Chirongoma, S. 2016. Exploring the impact of economic and socio-political development on people's health and well-being: A case study of the Karanga people in Masvingo, Zimbabwe in *HTS Theological Studies Special Issue on Engaging development: Contributions to a critical theological and religious debate*, 72(3), 1–9.

Chirongoma, S. 2020. Church-related hospitals and healthcare provision in Zimbabwe. In Ezra Chitando (Ed.), *The Zimbabwe Council of Churches and Development in Zimbabwe*. Palgrave: Macmillan, pp. 125–147.

Du, Toit A. 2020. Outbreak of a novel coronavirus. *Nat Rev Microbiol*, 18, 123. DOI:10.1038/s41579-020-0332-0

Durie, M. 2004. Understanding health and illness: Research at the interface between science and indigenous knowledge. *International Journal of Epidemiology*, 33, 1138–1143. https://doi:10.1093/ije/dyh250

European Centre for Disease Prevention and Control (ECDC). 2020. *Considerations relating to social distancing measures in response to COVID-19–second update.* Stockholm: ECDC.

Gaydos, L.M., Smith, A., Hogue, C.J.R., and Blevins, J. 2010. An emerging field in religion and reproductive health. *J. Religion Health*, 49, 473–484.

Gbadamosi, I.T. 2015. Antibacterial attributes of extracts of *Phyllantus amarus* and *Phyllantus niruri* on *Escherichia coli* the causal organism of urinary tract infection. *Journal of Pharmacognosy and Phytotherapy*, 7(5), 80–86.

Gbadamosi, I.T. 2020. Stay safe: Helpful herbal remedies in COVID-19 infection. *Afr. J. Biomed Res*, 23(2), 131–133.Harfield, S.G., Davy, C., McArthur, A. et al. 2018. Characteristics of indigenous primary health care service delivery models: A systemic scoping review. *Globalization and Health*, 14, 12.

Hlatywayo, A.M. 2017. *Indigenous Knowledge, Beliefs and Practices on Pregnancy and Childbirth of the Ndau People of Zimbabwe.* Unpublished PhD Thesis. University of KwaZulu-Natal, South Africa.

Huang, C., Wang, Y., Li, X. 2020. Clinical features of patients infected with 2019 novel coronavirus in Wuhan, China. *Lancet*, 395, 497–506.

Hui, L., Qiao-ling, T., Ya-xi, S. et al. 2020. Can Chinese medicine be used for prevention of coronavirus disease 2019 (COVID-19)? A review of historical classics, research evidence and current prevention programs. *Chin J Integr Med*, 26(4), 243–250.

Jaja, I.F., Madubuike, U., and Jaja, C.I. 2020. Social distancing: How religion, culture and burial ceremony undermine the effort to curb COVID-19 in South Africa. *Emerging Microbes & Infections*, 9(1), 1077–1079. DOI:10.1080/22221751.2020.1769501

Kahissay, M.H., Fenta, T.G., and Boon, H. 2017. Beliefs and perception of ill-health causation: A socio-cultural qualitative study in rural North-Eastern Ethiopia. *BMC Public Health*, 17, 124. https://doi.10.1186/s12889-017-4052-y

Kaya, H.O. 2007. *Promotion of Public Health Care Using African Indigenous Knowledge Systems and Implications for IPRs: Experiences from Southern and Eastern Africa.* Nairobi: African Technology Policy Studies Network.

Levers, L.L. 2006. Samples of indigenous healing: The path of good medicine. *International Journal of Disability, Development and Education*, 53(4), 479–488.

Liu, J., Liao, X., Qian, S. et al. 2020. Community transmission of severe acute respiratory syndrome coronavirus 2, Shenzhen, China, 2020, *Emerg Infect Dis*. https://doi.org/10.3201/eid2606.200239

Lone, S.A. and Ahmad, A. 2020. COVID-19 pandemic – An African perspective. *Emerging Microbes and Infections*, 9(1), 1300–1308. DOI:10.1080/22221751.2020.1775132

Maroyi, A. 2013. Traditional use of medicinal plants in south-central Zimbabwe: Review and perspectives. *Journal of Ethnobiology and Ethnomedicine*, 9(31), https://ethnobiomed.biomedcentral.com/articles/10.1186/1746-4269-9-31 (Accessed 15 July 2020).

Mehrbod, P. et al. 2018. South African medicinal plant extracts active against influenza A virus. *BMC Complement Altern Med.*, 18(1), 112. DOI: 10.1186/s12906-018-2184-y. PMID: 29587734; PMCID: PMC5872571.

Murove, M.F. 2009. "African bioethics: An exploratory discourse. In M.F. Murove (Ed.), *African Ethics: An Anthology of Comparative and Applied Ethics* Pietermaritzburg: University of KwaZulu-Natal Press, pp. 157–177.

Musinguzi, G. and Asamoah, B.O. 2020. The science of social distancing and total lock down: Does it work? Whom does it benefit? *Electron J Gen Med*, 17(6), em230. https://doi.org/10.29333/ejgm/7895

Muyambo, T. and Maposa, R.S. 2014. Linking culture and water technology in Zimbabwe: Reflections on Ndau experiences and implications for climate change. *Journal of African Studies and Development*, 6(2), 22–28.

Oguamanam, C. 2006. *International Law and Indigenous Knowledge: Intellectual Property, Plant Biodiversity, and Traditional Medicine*. London: University of Toronto Press.

Paintsil, E. 2020. COVID-19 threatens health systems in sub-Saharan Africa: The eye of the crocodile. *J Clin Invest.*, 130(6), 2741–2744.

Semenya, S.S. and Maroyi, A. 2018. Data on medicinal plants used to treat respiratory infections and related symptoms in South Africa. *Data in Brief*, 21, 419–423.

Shoko, T. 2007. *Karanga Indigenous Religion in Zimbabwe: Health and Well-Being*. Ashgate: Ashgate Publishing Limited.

Shoko, T. 2018. Traditional herbal medicine and healing in Zimbabwe. *J Tradit Med Clin Natur*, 7, 254. DOI: 10.4172/2573-4555.1000254

Van Bavel, J.J. and Baicker, K. et al. 2020. Using social behavioral science to support COVID-19 pandemic response. *Nature Human Behaviour*, 4, 460–471.

Wabo, G.K. 2020. *Health Crisis Linked to the COVID-19 Pandemic in Africa: Essay on Pragmatic Approach of Solutions*. African Union for Youth Development, 47120.

Wang, W.Y. and Yang, J. 2011. An overview of the thoughts and methods of epidemic prevention in ancient Chinese Medicine. *Jilin J Tradit Chin Med* (Chin) 31, 197–199.

White, P. 2015. The concept of diseases and healthcare in African traditional religion in Ghana. *HTS Teologiese Studies/Theological Studies*, 71(3), Art.#2762.

WHO. 2020. COVID–19 situation update for the WHO African Region, 01 July, 2020 www.afro.who.int/publications/situation-reports-covid-19-outbreak-sitrep-18-01-july-2020 (Accessed 15 July 2020).

Zhou, P. et al. 2020. A pneumonia outbreak associated with a new coronavirus of probable bat origin. *Nature*, 579(7798), 270–273.

4 Unpacking and Repackaging the Shona Funeral and Post-Burial Rites in the Context of the Novel Coronavirus (COVID-19) in Zimbabwe

Beatrice Taringa and Sophia Chirongoma

Introduction

COVID-19 has become a global catastrophe, wreaking havoc in diverse contexts across most parts of the world. It has taken the world by storm. Nations and communities have been left utterly shaken to the core. They have suddenly found themselves with no time to reflect upon their religious, cultural and traditional assets' contribution toward managing, controlling and containment of this global pandemic. In December 2019, COVID-19 initially broke out in the city of Wuhan, Hubei Province in China, on the Asian continent (Lone and Ahmad, 2020; Zhou et al., 2020). For several months, the city of Wuhan was its epicenter, then it eventually spread to Europe and then to Africa. Its death toll has been higher in Asia and Europe despite the fact that they have world-class health delivery systems and abundant resources. So the fact that the death toll skewed toward the First and Second World economies raises questions on how it is spread and controlled. Within a period of approximately seven months (December 2019–July 2020), the pandemic had paralyzed the world economies and more economic causalities continue to unfold. The whole world was in a panic mode. The world leaders were numbed by confusion and dilemmas as they intermittently imposed, lifted and re-imposed the national lockdowns. They also found themselves fumbling between closing, opening and re-closing institutions. The COVID-19 pandemic has unique traits, making it different from its predecessors HIV/AIDS, cholera, typhoid and others. The behavior and traits of the pandemic demand a multi-disciplinary approach in dealing with it.

In April 2020, the World Health Organization (WHO) made predictions that Africa would become the next epicentre of the pandemic as it was being predicted that Africa's COVID-19 death toll would reach alarming rates during the winter season (BBC News, 2020). Once the epidemic found its way into Southern Africa, particularly as numbers of those infected with the coronavirus began surging in South Africa which shares the border with Zimbabwe, facilitating constant movement between the two countries, inevitably, Zimbabwe had to adopt stringent restrictions in the movement of human communities. From 31 March 2020, Zimbabwe had been observing various

DOI: 10.4324/9781003388630-4

lockdown phases/levels. With the inception of these lockdown measures, the funeral, burial and post-burial processes and procedures that lie at the heart of the Shona, vaDuma of Chief Ziki in Bikita were heavily affected. Under normal circumstances, whenever death strikes, the first consideration for most Shona people is to make all the necessary effort to attend the funeral. Physical attendance will accord them an opportunity to express their condolences to the immediate family members and, more importantly, to bid farewell to the departed loved one. Hence, the policy that during the first phase of the lockdown, all deaths were treated as COVID-19 related, hence, busing, feeding and hosting mourners was restricted to only 50 people impacted heavily on the indigenous Shona people's understanding of death and mourning. What was even more heart-wrenching is the stipulation that the handling of the corpse had become a preserve for specialized personnel as well as the fact that the funeral processes and procedures had to be conducted within 24 hours. Such a policy restricted the capacity of several close family members and friends from attending the funeral as well as hindering them from actively performing the funeral rituals as they would have done under normal circumstances. Many saw the arrival of COVID-19 vaccines as an opportunity to enable them to revert to these normal circumstances.

The restriction in funeral attendees brought another dimension of virtual funeral attendance to the fore in the Shona and vaDuma funeral ritual. Prior to COVID-19, virtual funeral attendance and mourning used to be viewed as an anti-social practice done by people who lack *Unhu/Ubuntu*. Furthermore, for some funeral service companies, body viewing was now restricted either to immediate family members, or in some cases, it was completely skipped. It is against this background that this chapter seeks to discuss how the COVID-19 pandemic necessitated the reconfiguring of the funeral, burial and post-burial rituals among the Shona people, as well as their responses to COVID-19 vaccination, using the vaDuma under Chief Ziki in Bikita district, Zimbabwe as a case study.

Background

Since the attainment of Independence in 1980, the Zimbabwean government's thrust has been on the resuscitation of cultural and traditional beliefs and practices. The cultural and traditional practices and procedures to do with the facets of the Shona spiritual worldview have been revisited and revived. Hence, funerals, burial and post-burial practices and procedures were not spared. The traditional leaders are increasingly gaining recognition and prominence to the extent of having the president of the chief's council having representation in parliament. Just as it has always been during the outbreak of past epidemics, COVID-19 once again put the Shona funeral, burial and post-burial religious, cultural and traditional practices under scrutiny. This was necessitated by the need to assess their possible contribution toward either hampering the management, control or prevention of the epidemic. Now that the world communities had gained some experience on how to deal with some more or less similar pandemics like HIV/AIDS, cholera, typhoid, Ebola, influenza and SARS which occurred in the past, they did not need to take chances or waste time by risking lives through questioning standards of control measures against the spreading of the epidemic. The major lesson that was learnt in the past is that cultural isoloation is diminishing as we drift away from precolonial societies into globalization. While cultures are slowly merging into a globalized one, individuals are dispersing. If we are cultured, then we need to be re-cultured in line with COVID-19 management, control and prevention. The contents of the social reconstruction theory are once again under scrutiny in the interests of a sustainable and healthy future. The ethos should be guided by a maxim such as "towards a COVID-19 sensitive cultural frame of reference tailored to meet the needs of the vaDuma under Chief Ziki in Bikita district." This frame of reference had to face the challenge of COVID-19 vaccines.

Culture is a social construct (Haralambos and Holborn, 1995). In this case, it is a human discourse that the community input to its construction. Ngigi and Busolo (2018) also defined culture in terms of its characteristics, that it is an integrated pattern of human behavior, language, thoughts, communication actions, customs, beliefs, values, attitudes and institutions of racial, ethnic, religious and social groups. Culture defines human operations. It is a product of socialization that shapes personality from birth to death. It is a social and religious campus and as such, it had to be accurate to give correct directions to the vaDuma participants on safe routes in the COVID-19 era. Furthermore, culture as a lens was not expected to falsify or should misinform the participants about the reality of COVID-19 treatment, management, containment and prevention strategies. It had to serve as a frame of reference that would guide behavior and mental operations. Culture becomes rubbed in the person's mind such that it appears natural and biological (Taringa, 2014). In most circumstances, culture aids or even impedes mental operations and subsequently rationalization. This may lead people to think culturally and justify even unethical conduct that threatens survival under the guise of culture. In the same vein, there was a need for cultural rethinking, especially on issues surrounding funeral procedures. Ignoring rethinking about such issues would have been tantamount to leaving desirable beliefs and behavioral practice to chance, which would have been likely to disempower instead of empowering the participants in the COVID-19 era. There was a need for an all-stakeholder approach in debates to do with polishing cultural behavior, norms and attitudes in a bid to transform toward being COVID-19 sensitive, just like what was done in the past during the outbreaks of HIV/AIDS, cholera and typhoid.

Similarly, Kanu (2007) proffers that, as human beings, we are embedded in our cultural tradition. Furthermore, tradition cannot be treated as something which is 'Wholly Other', as if one would continue to be a person even if tradition is entirely rejected. Thus, to the vaDuma, going contrary to their funeral ritual framework had far-reaching repercussions on their identity and personhood. Based on such a view of tradition, it means that it was not going to be easy to have the vaDuma easily reject their funeral ritual framework that has served them for so long despite the COVID-19 scare. This is so since these funeral rituals are part of the vaDuma cultural tradition that defines the Duma identity. Kanu (2007: 70) further adds that becoming a person entails appropriating certain material of one's cultural tradition and continuing to be a person means working through, developing and extending this material and this always involves operating in terms of tradition.

Funeral, burial and post-burial processes and procedures are human creations and as such, they can be constructed, deconstructed and reconstructed in response to the social, economic and political environment of the day. In fact, it was pertinent for the Shona people to choose which of their funeral, burial and post-burial processes and practices had to be preserved and which ones needed to be modified in light of the COVID-19 epidemic in their midst. As noted by Lawton (1980), the curriculum, that is, a way of learning and being, is a selection from culture. The term 'selection' implies that humanity is continually revisiting culture's intangible heritage and in the process, they will be deconstructing existing frames and reconstructing the new cultural frames of reference. This means that cultural building is a continuous process where participants select the cream of their assets that should be transformed and reshaped in a bid to survive in the face of the COVID-19 pandemic and other challenges, including COVID-19 vaccines.

There is a need for cultural sensitivity and a recognition of the fact that culture is porous and adjustable. Globalization has opened up the borders which makes it impossible to localize pandemics. This inevitably calls for cultural dynamism, mutation, evolution and reconfiguration. Clearly, even the most valued funeral, burial and post-burial processes and procedures could not remain untouched in the COVID-19 era. There would have been no need for the African communities, particularly, the Shona people, to remain with the old cultural traits. Such rigidity would have ended up keeping them entrapped in a cultural frame of reference to do with funeral, burial and post-burial processes and procedures that threatened their survival. This kind of inflexibility would have inadvertently put their future at stake, particularly in the face of pandemics. The cultural norms, values, attitudes and behavior systems to do with funeral, burial and post-burial processes and procedures had to be fashioned in a way that enabled the participants to remain afloat in the face of turbulent waters. This implies that it needed to be life-saving.

The Shona people have their own way of managing funerals, burial and post-burial processes and procedures. As explained by Shoko (2007) for ritual and practical purposes such as feeding the guests, usually a domestic animal is slaughtered at a funeral. Various rituals follow the funeral itself; the deceased's belongings will be distributed among those who are eligible to inherit. Some kill an ox at the burial to accompany the deceased. Others kill another animal sometime after the funeral (three months or two years later or even a longer period is observed) for the *kurova guva* (bringing back/domesticating the spirit of the dead) ceremony. According to Shoko (2007), if the correct funeral rites are not observed, the deceased's spirit may come back and trouble the living relatives.

It is against this background that the chapter seeks to examine the cultural resilience or the capacity of the religious, cultural and traditional system to continually change and adapt in line with COVID-19, including the response to COVID-19 vaccines, and yet remain within critical threshold that the dead will not come back and trouble the living among the vaDuma, a sub-group of the Shona under Chief Ziki in Bikita district. The main thrust of this chapter is that the Shona religious, cultural and traditional system had to be adjustable and demonstrate a long-term capacity to deal with change. Such flexibility would provide a platform for them to continue developing in the fast-mutating social, religious, cultural and political globalized terrain. This is informed by the reality of the matter that on the one hand, there are cases when change is gradual, where circumstances will be changing in a predictable way such that it allows systems ample time to adjust smoothly. On the other hand, change becomes so sudden, disorganizing and turbulent that it does not accord the system time to acclimatize; resultantly, it shocks the system. This is so since the COVID-19 situation was a matter of survival, a global dictate and an emergency.

The chapter now proceeds to examine the aspects surrounding funeral practices among the vaDuma under Chief Ziki in Bikita district so as to assess whether they threatened, exposed or shielded the participants from the adverse effects of COVID-19. Drawing insights from the case study of the vaDuma people under Chief Ziki in Bikita district, the chapter also seeks to examine whether the intervention programmes may have underestimated the impact of culture in the management, control and prevention of the spread of COVID-19 among the Shona people in Zimbabwe. COVID-19, just like its predecessors, called for the attention not only of the medical sector but multifaceted responses that required multi-sectorial, multi-dimensional and an all-stakeholder approach to holistically manage, control and prevent it from sweeping the world.

Theoretical Framework

The theoretical framework is an important component of the research study. It grounds the study and guides the methodological design (Mpofu, Otulaja and Mushayikwa, 2013).The main focus of this chapter was to examine how the Shona, in particular the vaDuma under Chief Ziki in Bikita district, become agents of cultural change in relation to COVID-19 management, control and prevention. It seeks to accommodate the Shona religious and cultural aspects to do with funeral, burial and post-burial in the context of management, control and prevention of the spread of COVID-19 using the VaDuma of Chief Ziki in Bikita district as a case study. The main argument raised in the discussion is that funeral, burial and post-burial processes and procedures among the vaDuma could not remain constant if the vaDuma community practices are and were meant to protect members from perishing during the COVID-19 era and beyond. We, therefore, argue that some of the indigenous practices surrounding death and burial had to be transformed in line with the COVID-19 safety protocols. The processes and procedures had to be unpacked and repackaged in a COVID-19 sensitive style that was life-saving. Hence, our study seeks to examine how the adoption of COVID-19 control measures could be done in line with the traditional African (Shona) culture.

The social reconstruction theory illuminates this chapter. According to Letsiou (2014), the process of social reconstruction seeks to make culture relevant to the day-to-day problems. It has a close connection with social matters and is progressive in outlook. In line with the social reconstruction theory, creativity and self-expression which enhance participant flexibility take centre stage in enabling the participants to conquer their environment. The social construction theory is characteristic of post-modernism as it is a cultural and ethnic framework that emerges to compete with existing norms and powers of the world that sacrificed Africans and their social rights on the altar of monopolizing power and authority in Western modes of knowing. Thus, based on Letsiou's (2014) view, social reconstruction is relevant for this study. It is liberating as it is a critique to the Eurocentric view of intervention programmes that are entirely biomedical while understating the religio-cultural factors in epidemic containment. In tandem with the social reconstruction theory, our chapter calls for the reconstruction of the Shona and vaDuma religio-cultural value framework for survival in the COVID-19 era.

Kanu (2007) defines tradition as a set of beliefs, practices, values and modes of thinking that are inherited from the past and that may organize and regulate ways of living and making sense of the world. Furthermore, Kanu (2007) argues that tradition exists only in constant alteration and as such it can be rethought, transmuted and recreated in novel ways in response to the meanings and demands of emergent situations. In the same vein, there was a need for vaDuma to undergo reframing and rethinking of their inherited funeral rituals and traditions in light of the emergent COVID-19 epidemic containment framework. This chapter argues that the vaDuma religio-cultural framework had to be an empowering tool that could contribute to the health and well-being of the society in the COVID-19 era. Through the social reconstruction theory, the vaDuma religio-cultural value framework could fashion and prepare the participants to cleverly manage not only epidemics but various situations in their lives. This could be possible through making the vaDuma flexible and adaptive for continuous change of social, economic and political situations in their lives when the need arises. Thus, the ideology of social reconstruction can be linked to collective production of meaning and knowledge through interaction. We concur with Kanu (2007) who, in concurrence with the social reconstruction theory, upholds the view that tradition is neither monolithic nor is it merely preserved and handed down to subsequent generations. Similarly, we contend that as cultural values are handed down consecutively over time, they undergo change as the realities that a receiving generation faces are never exactly the same as those of the transmitting one. Our standpoint is informed by the fact that the vaDuma ancestors who handed down the funeral rituals had been COVID-19 free, hence, in line with the social reconstruction theory, the contemporary vaDuma needed to unpack and repackage the funeral ritual framework cognizant of the COVID-19 constraints. Thus, any shift in the religio-cultural terrain, no matter how small, can lead to a recasting, reconfiguring and reconstituting of the traditional frameworks. Thus, these changes were bound to influence the vaDuma response to COVID-19 issues, including vaccinations.

Research Methodology

The chapter sets to explore the resilience of the vaDuma under Chief Ziki in Bikita in their funeral, burial and post-burial processes and procedures in light of the COVID-19 pandemic, including their responses to COVID-19 vaccination. The inductive theory has been adopted in the chapter. According to Bryman (2012: 6), the inductive theory "implies that a set of theoretical ideas drive the collection and analysis of data." "It also adopts interpretivist epistemology. Thus, reality is a social construction phenomenon and there are multiple realities" (Morgan and Sklar, 2012: 73). In this case, the study participants' experiences of adjusting to COVID-19 funeral, burial and post-burial processes and procedures is understood from the viewpoint of the vaDuma themselves.

Ontologically, the chapter is informed by constructivism which further adds that, "there are varied and multiple truths, leading the researcher to look for complexity of views rather than narrowing the few categories or ideas" (Creswell, 2009: 8). In this case, there is no set standard of COVID-19 sensitive funeral and burial processes and procedures that were adopted worldwide. In tandem with the constructivist ontology, the chapter uses the revelatory case study. This entails a selection of five headmen, one advisor for each of the headmen, one male and one female adult from each headman's area of jurisdiction in Chief Ziki's chiefdom. These twenty study participants were chosen as a representative sample to offer their insights on the resilience of the Shona vaDuma under Chief Ziki's jurisdiction in terms of how they renegotiated funeral, burial and post-burial processes and procedures, as well as responding to vaccination, in light of COVID-19. The selection is made in line with Punch's (2009:162) assertion that "we cannot research on everyone, everywhere, doing everything" as the scope may be too wide. Our vantage point for adopting this approach was influenced by the understanding that religious and cultural beliefs serve as a frame of reference in people's behavior and mental operations. This was also informed by the fact that in previous researches reviewed in this study, religious and cultural beliefs have been noted as major culprits that fueled the spread of epidemics in the past.

The study focused on how the vaDuma aligned their funeral and burial rituals to make them life-saving in the COVID-19 environment. The data were collected through electronic interviews, observation[1] and textual analysis of the Shona people's indigenous beliefs and practices surrounding death and funeral rites. The messages emerging from the selected excerpts of the purposively sampled key informants are analyzed on the basis of their resultant impact in curbing or fueling the spread of the deadly pandemic. For the collection and presentation of data, the chapter triangulated textual analysis of COVID-19 sensitization communications and interview excerpts. As noted by Punch (2009: 133), "data collection and analysis are done in cycles and stops after two repetitions and even continue until theoretical saturation is achieved." In analyzing the data collected for this chapter, the authors made use of the conventional content analysis of the excerpts on how the participants have come up with COVID-19 sensitive funeral, burial and post-burial processes and procedures. Besides the critical analysis, the data were also triangulated with discourse analysis to help in describing, interpreting and explaining such relationships as well as trying to account for the resilience of vaDuma funeral, burial, post-burial practices and responses to COVID-19 vaccination.

In organizing data, the chapter employed the thematic web-like data analysis and interpretation. Thematic networks allow the deriving of funeral, burial, post-burial and COVID-19 vaccination themes from the selected textual data and interview excerpts allow the unearthing of resilient themes salient in the texts at different levels. This also assisted the authors to extract themes that formed categories of basic themes on death, burial, post-burial rituals and COVID-19 vaccination among the Shona (Attride-Stirling, 2001). The dynamic translation theory was used as it allows relativity of equivalence of interview excerpts from the purposively sampled key informants.

Significance of the Chapter

Ngigi and Busolo (2018) emphasized that culture gives communities uniqueness. It should therefore not come as a surprise that in emergency situations or times of disaster, individual communities may require special attention, too, including the preparation of risk reduction and warning messages. This chapter seeks to understand how the Shona, with particular reference to the vaDuma community under Chief Ziki in Bikita district, become an agent of cultural transformation, with a special focus on the Shona funeral, burial, post-burial processes and procedures and responses to vaccinations in the face of COVID-19. This is motivated by the fact that these aspects could not remain constant as the context in which they were meant to serve had transformed. If definitions and contexts of funerals, burial, post-burial practices and responses to vaccines vary within, between and across cultures, it means that they are not monolithic. Similarly, cultures are not neutral and unchanging, as such; they should be revisited and realigned from time to time when the need arises. They can be unpacked and repackaged to be user-friendly and life-saving in the face of the prevailing social, religious, economic and political developments.

Brief Review of Related Literature

Reviewing of related literature is key in putting the chapter into the context of a related body of knowledge. Several scholars have examined how culture influences the management, control and prevention of the spread of pandemics. It is also important to bear in mind that each epidemic that hits the world communities has its unique characteristic traits that make it thrive and sometimes outclass previous learnt management, control and prevention styles. The world communities are anchored upon varied religious, cultural and social characteristics that make them respond differently even to the same epidemic. As such, the communities' uniqueness may hamper or foster life-saving behavior, attitudes, norms and values. Considering this uniqueness in communities, there is now a need to have differential treatment responses to these communities rather than a one-size-fits-all management, control and preventive strategy. This will help in guarding against imposing measures that may be alien to a specific community, which will make them resent or, worse still, to ignore life-saving information and services.

Tabane (2004) conducted an investigation that was aimed at establishing the influence of cultural practices of the Batswana on the transmission of HIV/AIDS in Botswana. The main question guiding the study was "To what extent do the cultural practices contribute to the spread of HIV/AIDS?" The study combined both qualitative and quantitative research approaches. It used the focus group discussions of 22 women and 26 male participants. The empirical findings confirmed that it is acceptable within the Batswana culture in Botswana that men can have multiple relationships even after marriage, making polygamy a common practice. Also, children are highly valued so that the use of condoms was generally unacceptable. Thus, the Tswana indigenous culture in Botswana was contributing to the spread of HIV/AIDS. Similarly, Arrey, Bilsen, Lacor and Deschepper (2017) concur with Tabane as they noted the vulnerability of women to HIV/AIDS in male-dominated Sub-Saharan communities where men have a culture of multiple and extra-marital relationships.

Ngigi and Busolo (2018) brought another dimension which reiterates the need for cultural competence training in addressing emergency situations and pandemics in communities. The approach brings a set of contingent behavior, attitudes and policies regarded as effective in cross-cultural situations as it is tailored to be culture-specific to communities. The approach is meant to ensure that services are respectful of and responsive to health beliefs and practices. The programmes informed by the cultural competency approach meet cultural and linguistic needs of diverse populations. It can also possibly improve individual and communities' management, control and prevention of spread of epidemics. Thus, health and related personnel should not be misled by global-ization into universalizing pandemic response programmes. This chapter there-fore propounds the need to promote culturally and linguistically appropriate management, control and preventive strategies for COVID-19 to ensure that the communities will benefit equally.

On another note, Oluga et al. (2010) draw the attention of intervention mechanisms to note deceptive cultural practices like wife inheritance which caused harm, in many cases leading to death. These scholars recommend basic teaching modes on Piaget's cognitive development theory. They note that the theory's three-staged cycle of assimilation, accommodation and adaptation may possibly help communities to discard negative cultural practices. In the same vein, this chapter proffers that the three-staged cycle may possibly make religious and cultural practices COVID-19 sensitive. There is a need to allow assimilation and adaptation where harmful funeral, burial and post-burial processes and procedures are noted and negotiate safer ones resulting in safe management as opposed to altercation. Apart from biological intervention, there is a need for a holistic approach which will ensure that specialists in cul-ture will constitute the intervention teams. Oluga et al. (2010) suggest that education is believed to be a "social vaccine." Based on that view, it becomes important for intervention programmes to regularly educate communities and to streamline the cultural practices that are now dangerous and have life–threatening consequences. The cultural approach should also be employed to carefully navigate the funeral, burial and post-burial processes and procedures. This will help to curtail cultural gatekeepers from banging the door against COVID-19 intervention programmes.

Ngigi and Busolo (2018) highlighted the need for a cultural approach to HIV/ AIDS prevention and care. They came to this conclusion after noticing that despite massive action to inform the public about the risk of HIV infec-tion, behaviour change was not occurring. The infection was said to be con-tinuing to rise. Through experience, researchers have learnt that HIV/AIDS is complex and multifaceted. They therefore came to the conclusion that it requires multidimensional strategies. So, it was only after abandoning a solely cognitive approach whilst taking a cultural approach which considers the population's characteristics, lifestyles and beliefs as essential references to the creation of an action plan that behavior change was noted and consequently, the HIV/AIDS prevalence rate began to diminish.

Similarly, Parker (2001) examined the development of an anthropological research in response to HIV/AIDS. He discovered that most of his predecessors focused on the behavioral correlates of HIV/AIDS infection among individ-uals but failed to examine the broader religious, social and cultural factors. Hence, Parker set out to answer the question on the importance of cultural systems in shaping sexual practices relevant to HIV/AIDS transmission, and prevention in relation to structural factors such as vulnerability. He therefore came to the conclusion that the intervention programmes were heavily biomed-ical in emphasis and a largely individualistic bias in relation to the ways social sciences may contribute meaningfully to the development and implementation of an HIV/AIDS research agenda. Since COVID-19 is a relatively new epidemic, our literature search failed to come up with any literature focusing on reconfiguring indigenous practices surrounding death and burial, as well as rural responses to vaccines in the face of the COVID-19 epidemic in Africa. This is the gap that our study intends to fill.

Having summarized the relevant literature, the next segment of the chapter focuses on presenting the key issues emerging from the content and discourse analysis as well as the field research to do with aligning funeral, burial, post-burial rituals and vaccines in light of COVID-19 among the indigenous vaDuma people in Bikita, Zimbabwe. These are presented in thematic form below.

Findings

This section aims to present the study's findings. The study describes the Shona, particularly the vaDuma community's funeral, burial, post-burial religio-cultural rituals and attitudes toward vaccines in the context of COVID-19. This is in response to Bohret's (2018) view that there is a lack of necessary qualitative research within public health and that the measures often rely on assumptions of culture and cultural practices. This is said to lead to public health responses being ineffective or even harmful. The participants were divided into two focus groups. The first group was that of community leaders; headsmen, headsmen's assistants and the community health workers. The second focus group was constituted by regular men and women from the selected headsmen's areas of jurisdiction. Like some of its predecessors, COVID-19 affected the funeral, burial and post-burial processes and procedures in a bid to curb the spread of the pandemic. These and other effects of COVID-19 have been explored under the following five sub-headings.

Knowledge about COVID-19

The participants were asked to talk about what they know about COVID-19 in terms of what it is, and what its symptoms are. The following insights came from the focus group discussions:

Chirwere chakatangira kuChina kuvarungu. Chirwere ichi chinopararira nokuchimbidza mukusangana vanhu vachisangana kubudikidza nokubatana. Munhu ane utachiona anotapurira vamwe nekukosorerwa nemunhu anacho. Vanhu vanogona kubata hutachiona pamadziro, chimbuzi, nhumbi kana midziyo yabatwa nemunhu ane utachiwana hwechirwere ichi. (The epicentre of COVID-19 is China, the land of white people. The disease spreads fast as people meet especially with physical contact with the infected person. If an infected person coughs, the virus can contaminate others. People may contract the infection through getting into contact with contaminated surfaces, toilet facilities, clothes and utensils.)

Chirwere ichi chine zviratidzo zvinoti; chinopinza kachando mumuviri, kukosora, kunetseka kufema, kuhotsira, kurwadziwa muchifuva, kupisa muviri nekupera simba. (The disease has these signs and symptoms, fever, coughing, difficulty breathing, sneezing, chest pains, rise in body temperature and fatigue.)

Chirwere ichi chine zvimwe zviratidzo zvakafanana nekuita manyoka, mabayo, kushaya chido nokudya nekupera simba uchinzwa kuneta. (The disease has other signs and symptoms that include diarrhea, pneumonia, loss of appetite and fatigue.)

Chirwere ichi chinotyisa. Hachitani kurwarisa kana kuuraya chaiko. Chinoparadzirwa nokushaya utsanana. Saka kuzvichengetedza vanhu vanokurudzirwa kugeza maoko nesipo nguva nenguva, kugara makataramukirana kuitira kuti anacho arege kutapurira mumwe. (This disease is frightening. It can quickly make a person sick and it even makes a person die within a short space of time. It spreads easily in unhygienic conditions. To be safe, people are encouraged to wash hands regularly with soapy water up to almost the elbows. People are also encouraged to maintain social and physical distancing in order to avoid the virus passed on from one person to another.)

The above insights by the participants are evidence that they knew what COVID-19 is. They even had details about the background to the outbreak of COVID-19, for instance, the fact that it originated from China which is its epicentre and how it spreads. They also showed that both community leaders, advisors to the community leaders and ordinary people were not only aware of the COVID-19 pandemic but they were equally afraid of the epidemic. On top of fearing it, they also stigmatized the victims which made the infected want to be secretive about their COVID-19 positive status. Having established that the participants, Shona vaDuma of Chief Ziki, were aware of COVID-19, the major question was whether their knowledge translated to casting a COVID-19 sensitive funeral, burial and post-burial ritual process and positive response to COVID-19 vaccines framework. In essence, our study was interested in finding out if the leaders, their assistants and the elderly were guiding their communities toward a resilient framework in safe handling and burial of their dead within the threshold of their religious and cultural norms and values.

When the participants were asked about how they could reduce the transmission of COVID-19 from the infected person to the community members, they responded as follows:

Aonekwa aine zviratidzo zveCOVID-19 anodanigwa vezveutano kuti abatsirwe kuti anofamba sei kunosvika kwaanonobatsirwa. (Whenever showing signs and symptoms of COVID-19, a person has to inform the village health workers so that he/she can be assisted on how to proceed to the quarantine centre for treatment.)

Anofungidzira kuti abatwa neCOVID-19 anofanira kuenda pake ega. Izvi kudzivirira kuti asatapurira vamwe. Vaange agere navo vakafanira kumbogara pavo voga kwenguva yakatarwa kuti vaonekwe kana vasina kutapurirwa. (Upon suspecting that one has contracted the COVID-19 infection, he/she should self-isolate to avoid passing on the virus to others. The rest of the members that have been staying with the infected person are also supposed to be isolated from the community for a given time until it is proven that they have not contracted the infection.)

Chirwere ichi chinonyanya kubva nevanenge vamboshanya kune dzimwe nzvimbo dzakanyanya kutekeshera chirwere cheCOVID-19. Saka vagari vemunharaunda tinovakurudzira kumhan'ara kwashabhuku kana vaona chiso chavasingasioni munharaunda mavo. (The disease mostly infects those that may have recently travelled to other areas or countries where the COVID-19 epidemic is prevalent. So the residents of each community are encouraged to report any new faces that they are not used to seeing in their communities.)

Kudzivirira COVID-19, vanhu vanokurudzirwa kubika kudya kwakafanana nenyama nemazai kuchiibva. Pane dambudziko pakukosorera pagokora nekumhoresana negokora. Isu kwedu takatobvumirana kuti zvokugunzvana chero nenhengo ipi zviregerwe. (To help reduce the spread of the disease, people are encouraged to effectively cook meat and eggs so that they can eat well-cooked food. There is a problem that we noted on coughing on an elbow while at the same time elbow greeting has replaced the handshake and hugs. In our community we agreed that there should be no physical contact of any kind.)

Chirwere ichi chinoti netsei kunzwisisa nokuti chinogona kubatira chero kubva pachitunha. Kana panhumbi dzomunhu anenge aine hutachiona hwacho. Chinogona kubatira nokuva pedyo nepedyo nomunhu anacho. Saka kudzivirira pane mitemo yakaiswa nehurumende nebazi reutano muZimbabwe kuderekedza kupararira kwechirwere ichi. Vanhu vanosungirwa kupfeka masiki yakavhara mhuno nomuromo nguva dzose vari paruzhinji vasingaderedze masiki pachirebvu. Vanhu vanokurudzirwa kutaramukirana zvinoita mamita maviri. Kuudza sabhuku kana paine hama yashanya ichibva kune imwe nzvimbo kana kunze kwenyika kuti iinde kwekunoongororwa. Kugara mudzimba uye kusafamba famba panguva dziri pakati penguva yetanhatu dzamanheru kusvika nguva dzenhanhatu dzemangwanani. (This disease is difficult to understand as it can even spread from the deceased's body. It can also spread through making contact with the clothes of the infected person. Failing to respect physical and social distancing with the infected person can also become a pathway for spreading the disease. As such, to prevent the spread of COVID-19, there are regulations that were put in place by government and the Ministry of Health and Child Welfare in Zimbabwe to reduce its spread. People are required to properly wear masks covering noses and mouths. They are also encouraged to maintain the social and physical distancing of about two meters all the time in public places. People have also been advised to inform the headmen about the arrival of a visitor from another area or country so that they [the visitor] can go to the quarantine centre for examination. People are also encouraged to stay indoors and to avoid movements during curfew times between 6:00 pm and 6:00am.)

Chirwere ichi chakaoma, chikaera chapinda munharaunda tinopera tose. Ibasa romunhu wose kuona kuti tadzivirira nharaunda yedu pamwechete. Munharaunda medu tine dambudziko revana vedu maJoni-Joni, vari kunzvenga vachidzoka kumusha. (This disease is complicated. Once it gets into our community, it will wipe out all of us. Therefore, it is everyone's responsibility to protect our community. In our community, we have a problem of our children working in South Africa who are evading quarantine measures, they come back home through skipping the border. There is therefore a high likelihood that without having undergone proper screening, if one is infected, they would spread the virus.)

The information that emerged from the focus group discussions revealed that the participants were not only aware of the dynamics of COVID-19 but they were also well aware of how to minimize or prevent its spread among communities. The participants must have had vivid imaginations after having heard, seen and read about the experiences of others, both in Zimbabwe and abroad. Some of the pronouncements were evidence of fear and forcible transformation since it was now a do-or-die situation. To the vaDuma, COVID-19 was a desperate situation that called for desperate measures where citizens had to comply or they were forced to comply without which they would die due to COVID-19. So with this in mind, it was possible for the community leadership and senior citizens to lead the effort to transform their funeral, burial and post-burial ritual processes and procedures, as well as taking up the COVID-19 vaccines in an effort to respond effectively to the pandemic.

This was in sync with Mogobe (2016) who notes that health literacy should give an individual the ability to access, process and comprehend health-related information with the goal of making an appropriate decision or set individual capacities in their four domains of cultural and conceptual knowledge, speaking and listening skills, writing, reading and numeracy skills. Thus, given that the vaDuma were aware of COVID-19 and its dynamics, this valuable knowledge had the potential of becoming a tool toward coming up with a lifesaving frame for care-giving and containment measures during funeral rituals.

Below, the chapter proceeds to discuss how the Shona vaDuma under Chief Ziki were reforming their funeral rituals and embracing safer burial practices in the face of COVID-19. The Shona vaDuma already had the culture of *kusengudza kuendesa kudumba* (quarantining the sick), especially those that had leprosy within their religio-cultural frame. Thus, the quarantining of COVID-19 infected people was not a problem as it was related to their religio-cultural conception. The only challenge is that the *kusengudza kuendesa kudumba* (quarantining the sick) used to be applied to the terminally ill who would have their relatives visit them. This is contrary to the COVID-19 quarantine system that was indiscriminate and involved the infected, those suspected to be infected and the sick.

Upon being asked about how COVID-19 could be cured, this is what the focus groups raised:

Uuuu! Ndinongonzwa vamiriri vebazi rehutano nekurerwa zvakanaka kwevana vachiti pari zvino, hapana mushonga. (Uuuu! I heard the Ministry of Health and Child Welfare representatives saying that at the moment, there is no cure.)

Vamwe vanoti vanoshandisa garlic, ginger, maremoni, mashizha emugwavha nemoringa. Vamwe tadohwa nokuzvishandisa kuti tifane tazvisimbisa kuitira kana COVID-19 ikavuya. (Some are saying they successfully used garlic, ginger, leaves of *moringa* and guava trees. Some of us we are already using them to strengthen our immunity in case the COVID-19 virus infects us.)

Ndizvozvo vamwe vanoti kufukira, kukarara nemvura ine munyu nemvura ine vinegar. Kana kungomwa mvura inopisa ina maremoni chero dzimwe nhambo isina neshuga zvayo. (True, some are saying steaming, gargling with warm salty water or apple cider vinegar. Or just drinking hot lemon water even without sugar are effective measures to cure COVID-19.)

Vamwewo ndivo vanoti utachiwana uhu hahurarami mumunyu. Saka unogona kuti uchibuda kuzhe kuruzhinji wongozvizorera munyu. Kana wadzoka wokarara nomunyu nokudira mvura ino munyu nomumhuno uchikwiza namaoko zvose usati wambobata zvinhu wapedza kugeza. Uye kuwacha zvipfeko nesipo usati wagara pasi nokubata zvinhu mumba mako. (Some are saying the virus does not survive in salt. So you can just rub your body with salt when going out in public. Upon coming back from public places, you then gargle with warm salty water, put some drops in the nose, rub the body and the hands with salt after taking a bath. Also wash the clothes with soap before sitting down or touching anything in your house.)

Vamwe vanoti paracetamol nemalaria drugs zvinoshanda. (Some are saying paracetamol and malaria drugs are effective in treating COVID-19.)

Vamwe vanoti urwere hwakurisa kuchipatara vane michina inobatsira kufema nokuisa kudya kubudikidza nemadhiripi. (Some are saying if the condition worsens, there are some ventilators and drip feeding in the hospitals which help to revive the patient.)

Ndizvozvo zvemushonga wokurapa COVID-19 takanzi tisanyeperana. Naizvozvi zviri nane kudzivirira nharaunda pane kuda kuzoedza kundorapwa pasina mushonga wokurapa. (As for the COVID-19 cure, we cannot lie as there is none. So it is better to prevent our communities rather than trying to cure when there is no cure.)

Chokwadi izvozvi ndaramo iri mumaoko edu isu savagari vomunharaunda kuti tivandudze mararamiro edu kuti tideredze kana kudzivirira kupararira kwechirwere ichi. Takadzidziswa kuzvidzivirira uye tikapiwa basa

rokushambadzira ruzivo rwezvekudzivirira chirwere ichi kunharaunda dzedu.
(At the moment, our survival is in our hands as the residents of communities to reduce or curb the spread of this disease. We attended workshops where we were taught about the prevention measures and we were given the responsibility to sensitize our communities about the prevention measures.)

The information emerging from the participants in the focus group discussions presented above reveals that the respondents had adequate knowledge about COVID-19 treatment and prevention measures. The major bone of contention is whether the knowledge was accurate or faulty and misleading and whether it could possibly curb or control the spread of COVID-19 among the Shona and vaDuma of Chief Ziki in particular. As noted by Taringa et al. (2019), in the early years of the HIV/AIDS epidemic, the Shona, just like any other communities, had to grapple with gaps in knowledge. The fact that there was no known HIV/AIDS cure led to gullibility as fake traditional healers and prophets capitalized on that gap. Similarly, the fact that there was no known COVID-19 is significant; it opened up the gap for rumors about homemade COVID-19 cure and concoctions to circulate as a survival strategy among communities. During the focus group discussions, some of the participants also revealed that there were knowledge gaps regarding the treatment regime for COVID-19 and others were also sharing information about the purported cures for COVID-19. The participants' facial expressions during discussions showed their near agreement to the circulating knowledge gap filler rumors. Some even confirmed that they were using some of the home-made therapies as part of prevention through strengthening their immunity in case they may be infected by the deadly COVID-19 virus. It is therefore important to find out if the COVID-19 knowledge gap filler rumors were likely to enhance or deter the smooth transition into COVID-19 sensitive funeral ritual practices and responses to vaccines that were life-saving in the face of the pandemic among the vaDuma of Chief Ziki of Bikita District. Below, we turn to discuss the funeral processes and procedures before and after COVID-19 among the vaDuma people.

Funeral Processes and Procedures: Before and During COVID-19

Upon being asked whether there were any differences in the pre-burial ritual processes and procedures, the respondents had this to say:

Vanhu vaingosvika vachibata maoko vachimhoresana nokudembedzana nokumbundirana vachichemedzana. (Mourners used to shake hands, consoling, hugging and crying together with the bereaved.)

Parufu paizara nehama neshamwari. Vanhu vaitakurwa kuuya nekubva parufu nemabhazi emainishuwarenzi. (Friends and relatives used to throng the funeral. People used to be ferried to and from the funeral by the funeral insurance buses.)

Chitunha chaibvumirwa kuvata mumba chisati chaenda kunovigwa nezuva raitevera. (The body of the deceased used to lie in state in the house before burial on the next day.)

Vanhu, kunyanya vakadzi, vaivata mumba mune chitunha vakagarira chitunha kusvika chabudiswa. (Mourners, especially women, would sleep in the room guarding the deceased's body until it is taken for burial.)

Vanhu vaipiwa zvokudya parufu. (The mourners used to be fed at the funeral.)

Hama nemadzisahwira vaigezesa mufi nokumuchinja hembe dzaanenge akafa nadzo. (Relatives and close friends used to bathe and dress the body of the deceased.)

Hama dzepedyo dzaivhura nokuona chitunha uye veruzhinji vaizotaridzwawo uso hwemufi. Mufi aivigwa zvine chiremerera. (Close relatives used to open the coffin and conduct body viewing before collecting it from the mortuary as well as upon arrival at the homestead. The mourners would also be given an opportunity for body viewing just before the deceased was taken for burial. The deceased used to be given a decent sendoff.)

The vaDuma had a religio-cultural framework that guided their funeral ritual processes and procedures. They had among their relationships people who perform certain rituals at a funeral depending on how they are related to the dead. Close relatives and friends had key roles to play in handling and burying the deceased. The vaDuma, just like all the other Shona ethnic groups, believe in life after death. Thus, they believe that if the handling and burial of the corpse is not properly conducted, the deceased will register his/her indignation by tormenting the living relatives from the grave.

As regards the belief systems, our chapter seeks to answer a question on the resilience of the vaDuma in transforming the funeral, burial and post-burial ritual processes and procedures and to ascertain their responses to COVID-19 vaccines. Another important dimension is the gendered aspect of bereavement and mourning of the dead. From the observations and focus group discussions, it is evident that it is women who spend the night(s) in the house where the deceased will be lying in state. Such a status was likely to induce women's vulnerability to COVID-19. This is regardless of whether the deceased is male or female. So, just like in the case of HIV/ AIDS, women have remained at the receiving end.

During the COVID-19 Pandemic

Upon being asked whether there were changes in the funeral, burial and post-burial procedures, this is what the participants in the focus groups said:

Vanhu vave kugeza maoko vachisvika panhamo uye vachibva kumakuva kunoviga mufi. (Mourners now wash hands upon arrival at the homestead where there is a funeral as well as when they are coming from the grave site after burial.)

Vekusvondo vaiisisimudza ndivo bhokisi romufi nokuviga vangove vaokeriwo sezvo zvose zvave mumaoko ana mazvikokota vezveutano. Chesvondo wangove munamato. (The church congregants who used to carry the coffin of their fellow believer have now become mere spectators as everything is now in the hands of the health personnel.)

Vanhu vave kungosvika pamakuva munhu odzikiswa mugomba votosiya vanopedzisa kuvakira nokufushira ivo votodzokera kumba vonogeza maoko nokuparara. (Mourners no longer stay long at the grave site, they will disperse soon after the coffin has been lowered into the grave. Only the builders will remain behind to finish up covering the grave. All the mourners will wash their hands before dispersing.)

Izvozvi vanhu vave kuenda parufu pamasaisai kubudikidza nekuona pavideo. Vanhu vaparufu havachafaniri kupfuura makumi mashanu. (For now, virtual mourning especially through video funeral attendance has become the new normal. Funeral gatherings have been curtailed to fifty members.)

Mabhazi haachatakuri vanhu kuenda nokudzoka kunhamo nokuda kweCOVID-19. (There is no more busing of mourners to and from the funeral venue because of COVID-19.)

Vanhu kana hama chaidzo hadzichafambi nemota ine chitunha kana kutungamirira chaiko. (Mourners or even relatives themselves no longer board the car carrying the body of the deceased or accompany the driver.)

Vanochema havachapiwi zvokudya parufu kana kugara kwenguva kunze vari hama dzepedyo. Zvakare zvekuuraya mombe zviya vanhu vachiita machikichori hapachina. (Mourners are no longer being fed at the funeral nor are they allowed to stay longer unless they are close relatives. The ritual of slaughtering a beast with people feasting at the funeral has automatically fallen off.)

Vanhu vave kuita zvokuti nematambudziko kwete kumhoresana mumaoko chaimo uye vakataramuka zvakatarwa nevehutano nehurumende. (Mourners now pass their condolences verbally and from a distance as stipulated by the health ministry and the government.)

Hapachina kumbundirana vanhu vachiwirana vachidembedzana. (No more hugging and embracing one another as mourners console each other.)

Chitunha chave kubatwa nevatorwa vezveutano. (The body of the deceased is now being handled by the strangers who are the health personnel.)

Vanhu vairara mumba vakagarira chitunha chave kungouya chichienda kumakuva. Hapachina zvokuti hama dzinogezesa nokupfekedza mufi. (The mourners are no longer holding a night vigil guarding the body of the deceased as it now comes and goes straight to the grave. The rituals of bathing and dressing the body of the deceased by the relatives is no longer being practiced.)

The information provided by the study participants presented above makes it apparent that all the relatives, friends and neighbors of the deceased observed the lockdown regulations. On arrival, they observe physical and social distancing, properly wearing masks, washing hands properly with soapy water and getting sanitized. However, it was also mentioned that in most instances, the close relatives quickly ignored the rules when they got into the house and saw the bereaved. They hugged and wept together. In the absence of the headsmen, advisors of headsmen and health personnel, they reverted to their old ways of mourning. If not closely monitored, there was a high likelihood of defeating all the efforts as such behavior opened loopholes for spreading COVID-19 in the community. The study participants also mentioned that there were some relatives who pretended as if upon getting into the funeral venue they were immune to COVID-19 and would override some safety precautions. This confirms what Bond and Brough (2007) and Fairhead (2016) noted in relation with HIV/AIDS, that sometimes biomedicalized measures regard culture as behavior, for example, hygienic practices and individual approaches led to victim blaming while the structural forces were neglected. This is the same with the COVID-19 situation where humanitarian responses unsettle practices regarding funeral rituals. Furthermore, there was a cultural knowledge gap to do with agreed homegrown substitutes of the behavioral practices in question.

However, it also needs to be acknowledged that the community leaders were playing a pivotal role in ensuring that the funeral gatherings remained curtailed. The funeral venues were no longer overcrowded. The headsmen, their advisors as well as health personnel closely monitored and dismissed the mourners who were not closely related to the bereaved in a bid to decongest the funeral venues. This position was in line with the ideology of social reconstruction which is based on the general belief that culture is a powerful resource which contributes to the improvement and wellbeing of communities. So this resonates well with Letsiou (2014) who argues that the social reconstruction of culture seeks to make culture relevant to the day-to-day problems.

Burial Processes and Procedures: Before and After COVID-19

During the burial processes and procedures, there were some notable changes that the participants raised in the focus group discussions. The following excerpts summarize some of the key issues that emerged:

> *izvozvi pangova nehama shoma dzinogona kuratidzwa kana kusatomboona mufi zvachose. izvi zvinoita kuti munhu anogona kutovigwa asiriye.* (Now there are few and, in some instances, not even one relative can view the deceased's body. Thus, it is possible that relatives may bury a stranger who is not their relative.)

> *vedzisvondo vaisibata rufu rwose vangovawo vaokeri kufanana nezvave kungoitwawo hama.* (The church congregants who used to run the funeral show for their members are just spectators, just like the relatives themselves.)

kuviga mufi hakuchina chiremerera. (Burying the deceased has lost its significance.)

kuti maringe nechibvumirano munharaunda medu, tave kutora mufi wose sokunonzi afa neCOVID-19 kuitira kuti tisimbise dziviriro yenharaunda dzedu. uye samasabhuku mudunhu takadodzidzisa vanhu vedu kuti vasasvora kana kutsamwira vakafafaidza misha yavo mushure mamagungano erufu nokuti hapana anoziva kana pakauya umwe aive neutachiwana hweCOVID-19 asi asati aratidza kurwara. takadovaudza kuti hai bodo hakusi kusema mufi kana vaimuchema asi kuti ndiyo nzira yekuchengetedza utano hwedu tose senharaunda. takadoti vanofafaidza varoverwe maoko uye vadzidzisewo vamwe maitiro akanaka anochengeta utano hwedu tose. (In line with our community agreement, we now consider all deaths as COVID-19 cases as a measure to prevent our communities from spreading the disease. As headsmen, we counsel our residents not to denounce the members that took the bold step of disinfecting their homes after funeral gatherings as it is not clear if some mourners may have been COVID-19 positive but not yet sick. We told our residents that those who disinfect their homesteads are not in any way showing disrespect for the dead and the mourners but rather they will be seeking to protect us as the community. We proposed that they should be given a round of applause and that they should teach others to practice safe funeral practices that enhance good health for all.)

vaya vachanzikwa kana kuonekwa vachivhura bhokisi kuti vaone chitunha, kuchipinza mumba kana kuchibata zvinorambidzana nezvakatarwa nevehutano vanotongwa voripiswa nokutyora chibvumirano choutano. (Those that are reported for or found conducting body viewing, keeping the corpse in the house or handling it contrary to the Ministry of Health and child welfare guidelines, they will be brought to the village court and charged for violating health standards.)

takabvumirana kuti mhiramudzimu dzose nezviera zvingada kuitwa zviitwe pasina chinotyora kutaramukirana nemamita maviri, kupfeka masiki nemazvo, kugeza maoko nemvura ine sipo nokushandisa sanitaiza, kusabata, kusapinza chitunha mumba, kusadya panhamo, kusagara mumba vanhu vanopfuura vatanhatu, kuona, kusabata kana kungovhura bhokisi munomufi kunze zvaitwa nevehutano. (We agreed that all the rituals and avoidances that might be performed should be done while observing two meters social and physical distancing, appropriately wearing the face mask, washing hands up to almost the elbow and sanitizing. There should be neither handling nor putting the corpse in the house. Mourners should not eat at the funeral, not more than six people should be in the house at once, there should be no body viewing, no touching of the corpse. Mourners should not open the coffin unless it is done by the health personnel.)

The issues raised by the participants are a testimony that the vaDuma are empowered. They took charge of their survival in the face of COVID-19.

Though there were still some challenges where some members who disinfected their homesteads after a funeral gathering were seen as abhorring the dead or members of their communities that came to console them; their peers intervened and the misconception was resolved easily. The vaDuma were suddenly forced to transform their funeral rituals and they were concertedly reforming it within the threshold they felt was reasonable. Granted, there is some evidence of agony whereby some study participants expressed that they felt as if death has lost significance. Nonetheless, the general picture is that the vaDuma were weaving the COVID-19 framework that was sensitive to religion and culture and that they were likely to comply and claim ownership. The ownership sense reduces the possibility of rejection that results when the intervention programmes are foreign and alien to religio-cultural contexts.

The adoption of the stance that all the deaths were perceived as COVID-19 by the vaDuma shows their flexibility. It fits well with globalization that calls for cultural dynamism, mutation and reconfiguration. The vaDuma adaptive traits helped them to survive as COVID-19 alignment of cultural intangible resources ensures survival. Thus, the rituals are products of human discourse, they are open to deconstruction and reconstruction in line with the social, cultural, political and economic developments of the time. Kargbo (2016) has shown how responses to Ebola included the transformation of rituals.

The agreed penalty measures by communities' leadership are evidence that there was some form of resistance whereby some members may violate the new stance. It is normal in communities that there is cultural lag where some isolated cases take time to change. The reality is that they will change over time. The resilience is usually as a result of the fear of the unknown. It is not easy to discard traditional and cultural resources as it has been rubbed into people to an extent that it erroneously appears natural and biological. This seemingly makes people think culturally rather than rationalizing, which risks people in light of COVID-19.

Post-Burial Processes and Procedures: Before and After COVID-19

In response to the question of how COVID-19 had affected their post-burial ritual processes and procedures, this is what the study participants said:

Hama dzaigara kwemazuva akati kuti dzichiita zvirango nokudzokera kuguva chifumi chamangwana vamwe vavo vave kungoparara pamwe neruzhinji. (Close relatives used to remain after the funeral for days to perform post-burial rituals. They would also go back to check if the grave site has not been tampered with. However, nowadays, most of the mourners are no longer staying, they usually disperse soon after burial.)

Vesvondo yaipinda mufi kana kuti afirwa vaipota vachiuya kuita munamato manheru oga oga kwamazuva akati kuti havachauyi. (The church congregants that used to visit the bereaved for several days after the funeral to conduct prayers and to comfort the bereaved are no longer coming.)

Nhaka yomufi yaizoparadzwa hama neshamwari vachiona izvozvi vave vashoma vanotora. Nedzimwe nguva nenhumbi dzacho dzomufi hadzina anotora zvichibva nokuti afa nei. (The belongings of the deceased used to be shared among relatives and friends. Unfortunately, with the advent of COVID-19, sometimes the belongings of the deceased have no takers.)

Vavakidzani vepedyo neshamwari dzomufi nedzanyakushaikirwa vaiita mazuva vachiuya kuzonyaradza nyakushaikirwa havachaiti nokuti vanotya COVID-19. (The neighbors and friends of the deceased and the bereaved who used to come to console the bereaved for days no longer do that for fear of COVID-19.)

Izvozvi vanhu munharaunda dzedu vanokurudzirwa kunyaradza vananyakufirwa panhare kubudikidza nekufona, pawatsiapu chati, pazumu, vhidhiyo koru, sikaipi kana imeiru. Izvaisionekwa sekusaremekedza vashakabvu avo vanenge vave vadzimu. (Now we encourage mourners in our communities to console the bereaved through Information Communication and Technology, like phone calls, WhatsApp chats, zoom meetings, video calls, Skype or even emails.)

For the first time in the history of the vaDuma, they were now consoling the bereaved virtually through zoom, glue, canvas, moodle, Edmodo, WhatsApp, Skype, emails and other electronic virtual platforms and means. For the first time in the history of the Shona vaDuma funeral rituals, electronic funeral attendance was being embraced. It ceased to be taken as a show off and a sign of lacking *Unhu/Ubuntu*. Physical attendance was no longer an issue. Information, Communication and Technology had since taken charge in almost all circles of the day-to-day running of the lives of the Shona. This resonates with Chirongoma and Mutsvedu (2021) who note that electronic mourning and funeral attendance has become more popular as the young generation of Zimbabweans are scattered across the globe for education and employment opportunities due to the Zimbabwean economic downturn. The vaDuma had revolutionalized their funeral rituals in line with global technological trends and sooner or later it is likely that they will normalize electronic attendance which was often regarded as deviance before the outbreak of COVID-19. The move is important in reducing overcrowdedness at funeral venues that may fuel the spread of COVID-19. This affirms Kanu's (2007) view that tradition only exists in constant alteration; it can be rethought, transmuted and recreated in novel ways in response to the meanings and demands of an emergent situation. In this case, the vaDuma funeral rituals were part of their intangible heritage that is not monolithic and needed refocusing in line with the COVID-19 environmental reality.

The Future of Shona vaDuma Funeral, Burial and Post-Burial Rituals

Upon being asked whether the vaDuma were going to revert to their old way of funeral rituals after COVID-19, the participants raised the following insights:

Kare haagari ari kare. Pakukutu hapaurayi. Hatichadzoki. Tatoona kuti hazviurayi. (Things change over time. Change never kills. We will not go back. We realized that these adjustments are not life threatening.)

Tatove nemabatiro matsva orufu. Handioni tichidzoka nokuti chirwere ichi chakati chee rukukwe. Chiri kuratidza kuti chiri pano zvachose. Chero chikaneta kunogona kuva nezvimwe zvinamaitiro acho. (We now have new ways of conducting funerals. I do not see us going back because the disease [COVID-19] has unrolled its mat [it's here to stay]. It appears as if it is going to be with us forever. Even if we conquer it, it is possible that another disease that has similar behavior traits will emerge.)

Kana chatisiya torarama tave vaDuma vatsva. Tinenge tave namaitiro matsva. (If it spares us, then we will live as the new vaDuma. We have already adopted new behavior, norms and values.)

Kana takasiya nhembe nezvireyi tinorega sei kusiya maitiro anotiisa panjodzi pamazino orufu neCOVID-19? (If we abandoned the traditional code of dressing whereby we were wearing animal skin and we were using sledges to transport goods, why can we not leave the religio-cultural rituals that endanger our lives through exposing us to the deadly COVID-19 virus?)

Ivo vezveutano vanoita basa rokuviga ngavatore mifanikiso yokupedzisira kuratidza hama dzomufi kuti dzigutsikane kuti ndiye ari mubhokisi. (The health personnel that are responsible for safe burial practices should take photographs of the deceased to be shown to the relatives of the deceased so that they can be assured that it is actually their relative who is lying in the coffin.)

Kuda zvimwewo zvakaita sokuona mufi tingangoti ngavaise girazi rinonjenjemera tione tisina kuvhura bhokisi romufi. Izvi ndinodaro nokuti kune vamwe vakaviga mutumbi usiri wavo vakazonofukunura ndokuzonovigwa nehama dzake chaidzo. (In order to guard against burying the wrong corpse, it might be better to adopt the use of glass-top coffins to allow the mourners to conduct body viewing without opening the coffin. This will guard against incidences whereby corpses get mixed up. For instance, there is a family that is reported to have buried a stranger who was later exhumed and was eventually buried by the real relatives.)

Kana zvaigoneka, zvaizonaka kana pakatsvagwa mushonga wokubaya mufi kuti chirwere chisatapukira, zvingatibatsira kuti tionekane nehama yedu zvitipe kutambira kuti akafa pachokwadi. (It would be helpful if the corpse can be administered an injection which pacifies the virus so that it will not be passed on to the other person. Such an intervention would help us to accord our loved ones a befitting send off. This will also assist us to come to terms with the reality that he/she has indeed passed on.)

From the insights raised by the study participants during the focus group discussions, it is clear that the COVID-19 induced religio-cultural transformation has affected most of the vaDuma people's deeply cherished death and burial rituals. It did not accord them ample time to acclimatize nor did it allow them time to calculate the transitional threshold that allows them to retain their identity as vaDuma in the funeral, burial and post-burial religio-cultural ritual framework reference. The top-down approach and the introduction of intervention strategies were overwhelming to the vaDuma people. Writing about the Shona people in general, Chirongoma and Mutsvedu (2021) also raise the same issues. Even though when conducting sensitization workshops, the community and health personnel adopted the bottom-up approach to enhance community ownership of the intervention processes, the general public in the vaDuma communities expressed that they felt that there is more that the community leadership could do to manage and prevent the spread of COVID-19. They also expressed willingness to embrace change within manageable threshold. Embracing change within the religio-cultural threshold minimizes religio-cultural shock as communities grapple with having to accept alien and foreign COVID-19 intervention measures. Cultural relevance reduces chances of tissue rejection when the communities show signs of behavioral change resistance. This confirms the view that if evolutions are not monitored and accepted, they may result in destabilizing the communities.

It is in this light that some of the study participants were suggesting interventions such as the need for funeral parlour personnel to give them a portrait of the deceased lying in the coffin, glass-top coffins to facilitate body viewing without having to open the coffin and injecting some chemical to ensure that the corpse does not spread the virus. The suggestions are evidence of religio-cultural lag which will vanish with time as the participants accept that change is here for good. Based on the insights from the focus groups and observations made, the vaDuma unpacked and repackaged their funeral rituals. In this case, when they hand it down, it will not be the same as it was when they inherited it. Thus, religio-cultural and traditional intangible heritage assets are accustomed accordingly so that they become life-saving. The vaDuma people fashion their inherited funeral rituals in light of COVID-19. The refashioning continues even in the future in light of unforeseen political, social and economic developments. The vaDuma, in suggesting a glass-top coffin, getting portraits of the deceased from the funeral parlor and the injection of safety drugs, are bidding to keep the body-viewing ritual alive even during the COVID-19 era. Thus, there are traditions that endure more or less intact, but primarily on the margins of the societies and with a greatly diminished sphere of influence (Kanu, 2007). Oluga et al. (2010), though writing in the context of HIV/AIDS, termed such risky cultural behaviors as deceptive cultural practices that harm and in many cases lead to death.

It was within the same paradigm of flexibility, change and realism that the vaDuma accepted COVID-19 vaccination. As they changed the rituals associated with death, burial and beyond, they also embraced COVID-19 vaccines when they were introduced. Study participants indicated that this shift happened because at its base, the indigenous culture seeks to promote life. The vaccines were interpreted in the context of a worldview that recognizes that cultures and their rituals are continually changing and shifting. Consequently, the vaDuma were in a position to accept COVID-19 vaccines when these became available. On a more pragmatic level, they regarded the vaccines as a strategic option that would enable them to honor their dearly departed in the amended rituals, but with greater freedom.

Concluding Analysis

Considering the above discussion, it is evident that the vaDuma funeral rituals have faced drastic transformative processes. Willingly or unwillingly, they found themselves engaging in a religio-cultural reconfiguration in line with COVID-19. The active participation of the vaDuma community from the grassroots in reshaping their intangible cultural heritage is central in ensuring compliance and it minimized the likelihood of fundamentalist rejection. Normally, when transition is too fast and abrupt and does not accord religio-cultural systems time to acclimatize, systems are subjected to cultural shock.

Learning Points

There are some learning points that the chapter raises. These are:

First, based on Piaget's cognitive development theory, assimilation, accommodation and adaptation are key ingredients in helping communities to discard negative cultural practices and adopt COVID-19 sensitive practices that are life-saving.

Second, religio-cultural intangible heritage assets are human discourses that guide communities' operations and they have to be correctly set in line with social, political and economic developments to avoid misinforming and misguiding the creators and benefactors.

Third, government and humanitarian epidemic responses and containment measures should not be single-handedly applied but they should be complemented by communities' contributions to help and accustom the efforts to communities' contexts which enhances ownership of new cultural frame.

Fourth, religio-cultural intangible heritage assets are not easy to discard, thus any efforts to ward out some deceptive practices should be carefully navigated and negotiated in order to avoid estranging community's gatekeepers who may close the doors against COVID-19's control, management and containment efforts.

Fifth, the positive response to COVID-19 vaccines confirms the dynamism and flexibility of indigenous cultures. Development practitioners must leverage on this dimension in order to register progress when working in communities that prioritize indigenous knowledge systems.

Note

1 The observations were conducted in line with COVID-19 safety protocols. One of the authors hails from Bikita, hence, the author attended two funerals for close family members and sought permission to collect data.

References

Arrey, A.E., et al. 2017. Perceptions of stigma and discrimination in healthcare settings towards Sub-Saharan African migrant women living with HIV/AIDS in Belgium: A qualitative study. *J Biosoc Sci.*, 49(5), 578–596. DOI:10.1017/s0021932016000468. EPUB:2017 oct 3. PMID:27692006.

Attride-Stirling, J. 2001. Thematic networks: An analytic tool for qualitative research. *Psychology*, 3(9), 385–405.

BBC News (2020) *Coronavirus: Africa could be next epicentre, WHO warns.* www.bbc.com/news/world-africa-52323375 (17 April 2020). Accessed April 25, 2020.

Bohret, I. 2018. *The Role of Culture in Response to Epidemics.* PGCert: Global Health Module. www.google.com/search?q=bohret%2C+i.+2018.+the+role+of+culture+in+response+to+epidemics&client=safari&channel=mac_bm&sxsrf=APwXEdc8YubCrD

Bond, C. and Brough, M.K. (2007). The meaning of culture within public health practice: Implications for the study of Aboriginal and Torres Strait Islander health. In Anderson, I. and Bentley, M. (Eds), *Proceedings Social Determinants of Aboriginal Health Workshop.* http://eprints.qut.edu.au. Adelaide: Cooperative Research Centre for Aboriginal Health, pp. 229–236.

Boushaba, S. 1988. *An analytic study of some problems of the literary translation: A study of 2 Arabic translations of K Gibran's the Prophet* (Unpublished PhD thesis). Manchester: University of Salford. Retrieved from Usir.Salford.ac.uk/14668/1/doi/136

Bryman, A. 2012. *Social Research Methods* (4th edition.). Oxford: Oxford University Press.

Bryman, A. and Bell, E. 2007. *Business Research Methods.* Oxford: Oxford University Press.

Charmaz, K. 2014. *Constructing Grounded Theory.* (2ndEd). London: Routledge, Taylor and Francis.

Chirongoma, S. and Mutsvedu, L. 2021. The ambivalent role of technology on human relationships: An Afrocentric exploration. In Beatrice Dedaa Okyere-Manu (Ed.), *African Values, Ethics and Technology: Questions, Issues and Approaches.* London: Springer International Publishing, pp. 155–172.

Creswell, J.W. 2009. *Research Design: Qualitative, Quantitative and Mixed Methods Approach* (3rd Education.). London: Sage Publications.

Elo, S. and Kyangas, H. 2008. The qualitative content analysis process. *Journal of Advanced Nursing*, 62(1), 107–115.

Fairhead, J. 2016. Understanding social resistance to the Ebola response in the forest region of the Republic of Guinea: An anthropological perspective. *Africa Studies Review*, 59(3), 7–31. DOI: 10.1017/asr.2016.87. Accessed 7/12/2019.

Haralambos, M. and Holborn, M. 1995. *Sociology: Themes and Perspectives.* London: Collins Educational.

Kanu, Y. 2007. Tradition and educational reconstruction in Africa post-colonial and global times: The case of Sierra Leone. *African Studies Quarterly*, 10(3), Spring 2007.

Kargbo, S. 2016. *How We Solved the Ebola Epidemic by First Understanding Culture.* Online TEDxMidAtlantic, YouTube. Available at www.youtube.com/watch?v. Accessed 7/12/2019.

Lawton, D. 1980. Curriculum planning and technological change. *Education + Training*, 22(4), 124. https://doi.org/10.1108/eb016710

Letsiou, M. 2014. *ART Intervention and Social Reconstruction in Education: Secondary Education.* ART Education Researched, Athens School of Fine Art, Greece.

Lone, S.A. and Ahmad, A. 2020. COVID-19 pandemic: An African perspective. *Emerging Microbes and Infections,* 9(1), 1300–1308. DOI:10.1080/22221751.2020.1775132

Mogobe, K.D. 2016. *Language and Culture in Health Literacy for People Living with HIV: Perspectives of Health Care Providers and Professional Care Team Members.* Research AIDS Treatment, June 2016.

Morgan, B. and Sklar, R. 2012. Sampling and research paradigms. In J.G. Maree (Ed.), *Complete your Thesis or Dissertation Successfully.* juta.co.za/pdf/23142/

Mpofu, V., Otulaja, F.S., and Mushayikwa, E. 2013. *Towards Culturally Relevant Classroom Science: A Theoretical Framework Focusing on Traditional Plant Healing.* Cultural Studies of Science Education. Springer. 10.1007_s11422-013-9508-5-1.pdf

Ngigi, S. and Busolo, D. 2018. Behaviour change communication in health promotion: Approaches, practices and promising application. *International Journal of Innovative Research and Development*, September 2018, 7(9), 84–95.

Oluga, M., Kiragu, S., Mussa, K., Muhamed, A., and Walil, S. (2010). Deceptive cultural practices that sabotage HIV/AIDS education in Tanzania and Kenya. *Journal of Moral Education*, 39(3), 365–380. DOI:10;1080/03057240:2010.497617

Parker, R. 2001. Sexuality, culture and power in HIV/AIDS. *Annual Review of Anthropology*, 30(2001), 163–179. Annual Reviews, www.jstor.org/stable/3069213. Accessed 07/05/2020.

Punch, K.F. 2009. *Introduction to Research Methods in Education.* London: Sage Publications.

Shoko, T. 2007. *Karanga Indigenous Religion in Zimbabwe: Health and Well-Being.* Aldershot: Ashgate Publishing Limited.

Tabane, E.M. 2004. *The Influence of Cultural Practices of Botswana People in Relation to the Transmission of HIV/AIDS in Botswana.* PhD Thesis. Pretoria: University of Pretoria. https://repository.up.ac.za/bitstream/handle/2263/28246/00front.pdf?sequence=1&isAllowed=y

Taringa, B. 2014. Implications of portrayal of women in Shona proverbs. *Zimbabwe Journal of Educational Research (ZJER)*, 26(3), 395–409.

Taringa, B., Nyawaranda, V., and Tatira, L. 2019. Rewriting the Feminine script: An exploration of women with wings in ChiShona literature prescribed for Ordinary Level Learners. *Zimbabwe Journal of Educational Research (ZJER)*, 31(1), 1–13.

Zhou, P., et al. 2020. A pneumonia outbreak associated with a new coronavirus of probable bat origin. *Nature*, 579(7798), 270–273.

5 Situating Mainline Christian Churches' Responses to COVID-19 Vaccination in Masvingo and Bikita Districts, Zimbabwe[1]

Tenson Muyambo, Josiah Taru and Fortune Sibanda

Introduction and Background

The advent of the COVID-19 pandemic in late 2019 and early 2020 – in Africa – brought with it uncertainties, shocks and anxieties. These ranged from people being unsure of the magnitude of the pandemic, its impact on the social, economic and religio-cultural milieu of communities and to the unpredictability of the future. These existential insecurities were exacerbated by both limited information and also misinformation about the properties and behaviour of the virus. For Bowa (2022: 186) "the COVID-19 pandemic … caused very serious social suffering across the globe and has exposed just how vulnerable our communities are". According to Okyere-Manu and Morgan (2022: 25), "the disease has had a global spread and led to many deaths". Given such tremendous impacts of the pandemic on humanity, governments were shaken to the core. While some governments speedily called into effect measures to curb the pandemic such as national lockdowns, the introduction of social distancing, wearing of face masks in public spaces and closure of non-essential sectors of the economy, some governments were clueless and adopted a wait-and-see attitude, just like what happened with the advent of the HIV and AIDS pandemic. The initial stages of the COVID-19 pandemic were characterised by denial, suspicion, myths, mistrust, inaction and conspiracy theories. Zimbabwe was no exception in this pandemonium caused by the pandemic.

In searching for solutions to deal with the pandemic decisively, countries relied on an uncomfortable deployment of science and religion (Muyambo et al., 2022; Muyambo and Tendere 2023). Most governments across the globe placed their trust in biomedical science as capable of delivering measures that could contain the spread of the virus. The Zimbabwean government adopted such a stance, tailor-making the World Health Organization measures to the local context. In Zimbabwe, church gatherings were banned as religious organisations were considered non-essential and as potential super spreaders of the virus. The role of the church was relegated to a spiritual and caring community in the face of many deaths. There were a few exceptions, for example, the government of

DOI: 10.4324/9781003388630-5

Madagascar introduced WHO measures while simultaneously promoting the use of an indigenous herbal tonic called COVID-Organics that had been developed by the Malagasy Institute of Applied Research (Desplat, 2022). In Tanzania, the then President John Magufuli oscillated between adopting the World Health Organization containment measures – informed by biomedical science – and relying on Pentecostal faith and prayer (Nakkazi, 2020). For the then President Magufuli, religious institutions –Christian and Islamic – were essential services in the intervention against COVID-19, thus had to remain open. In April 2020, the president declared three days of prayer, calling for divine intervention.

Zimbabwe presents an interesting case study for understanding the response of Christian organisations to COVID-19 and its containment measures. From the start, the government had side-lined churches in its response, before roping them in after the low vaccination rate among citizens. The government of Zimbabwe – informed by the Look East policy – procured COVID-19 vaccines from Chinese manufacturers. The two vaccines were Sinopharm and Sinovac. However, there was a scarcity of information about the trials, efficacy and safety of the two vaccines (Mundangowa et al., 2022). There was low vaccine uptake despite the availability of vaccines, with China donating more vaccines to Zimbabwe compared to other countries. Some citizens were suspicious of the vaccines. Some Pentecostal prophets worsened the citizens' suspicion through sermons that portrayed the vaccines as dangerous to human health and/or associated the vaccines with the devil's machinations (Kirby et al., 2020). Faced with such resistance, the government introduced measures to force people to receive vaccines. For example, unvaccinated people were not allowed on public transport. For civil servants, an ultimatum for vaccination was issued. Without vaccination, civil servants would be forced to take unpaid leave and would not access public transport. The government shifted its position by incorporating religious leaders in the fight against COVID-19. It is at the interstice of these shifts that we aim to discuss the role that religion played in Zimbabwe's response to COVID-19 vaccination following these government measures.

Studies have shown that most Zimbabweans trust and have more faith in religious leaders than in elected leaders (Afrobarometer, 2017). Lack of trust in government meant that the government had to involve leaders whom people trusted and had faith in. These were religious leaders. Kowalczyk et al. (2020) argue that spirituality is very important in the context of healthcare. They further argue that excluding spirituality in the healthcare of people, especially by leaders whom people have low trust in, is narrowing human desires to the physical sphere. It is against this background that this chapter explores the various responses to COVID-19 vaccination by different Christian mainline denominations in the Masvingo urban and Bikita rural districts of Zimbabwe. We aim to discuss how different Christian denominations responded, and also transformations in vaccination and concomitant containment measures. The focus on rural and urban settings is important in this discussion. There was militarised enforcement of COVID-19 regulation in urban centres while the same could not be said for rural areas.

COVID-19 and Methodological Issues

The data discussed in this chapter were collected between September 2020 and August 2022 as part of a larger research. This involved several visits to the field sites. The qualitative research methodology was selected as it is open and adapted to the field, especially during the COVID-19 pandemic. Furthermore, qualitative research captures experiences and lived reality within given contexts (Riessman, 2008; Clandinin and Connelly, 2000). To capture the responses to and approaches that some of the mainline Christian churches adopted in light of government-driven COVID-19 vaccination, qualitative research methodology informed the study. Two mainline Christian churches were purposively selected for the study, namely, the Roman Catholic Church (RCC) and Reformed Church in Zimbabwe (RCZ). The two religious movements have wider visibility and membership in Masvingo and Bikita districts. Through key informant interviews with members of the clergy at both churches, we obtained narratives of each church's response to calls by the government for people to be vaccinated against COVID-19. These narratives constitute official church positions on vaccinations and supporting mechanisms that the churches put in place as a response to the vaccination exercise. The key informant interviews were held over the phone or in person, depending on the COVID-19 situation and government regulations. To corroborate narratives from the clergy, fifty in-depth interviews were conducted with members from each church. Interviews with the laity provide narratives from below and chronicle what obtained on the ground with regard to vaccination, and mechanisms put in place to support or disregard the government's COVID-19 vaccination programme. Furthermore, congregants referred to statements made from the pulpit or sermons that discussed issues surrounding COVID-19 vaccines. Four focus group discussions (FGDs) were conducted with members of each church. Two focus group discussions were held via WhatsApp group. Focus group discussions aimed at capturing collective and general issues on COVID-19 knowledge, abidance to broader government COVID-19 containment measures such as observance of social distance during services, wearing of face masks, limiting the number of congregants to fifty or below were conducted.

Data analysis followed the steps outlined in Boeije (2010: 113–114). Data collected were categorised on the basis of broad themes that emerged from interviews, conversations, observations and focus group discussions. From the broad themes, axial coding was done with the aim of selecting conceptual abstractions from each theme. Axial coding helped in the selection of relevant categories for further analysis or require more data. Partly, axial coding informed conceptual abstractions upon which the chapter is structured. Lastly, selective coding determined connections between themes with the aim of understanding the bigger picture in the RCC and the RCZ's response to COVID-19 vaccination. Field data informed the narrative carried out in this chapter, with prominence given to data rather that theoretical underpinnings.

Fieldwork is inherently an ethical exercise (Delamont and Atkinson, 2018: 3). Permission to conduct research among the clergy and laity was sought and granted prior to the commencement of the study. Furthermore, individual consent was sought from all participants. The process of seeking individual consent in church spaces is complex in that while holding conversations with church members, ethnographically important issues can be raised or observed. In such instances, dynamic informed consent was sought verbally by researchers (American Anthropological Association, 2012). Some of the data collection was conducted during the COVID-19 lockdown. Government and the World Health Organization (WHO) regulations on COVID-19 were strictly adhered to. The research team strictly monitored participants and encouraged them to observe physical distance, and hand sensitisation before and after interviews and focus group discussions, restricting focus group discussions to sixteen people and the wearing of face masks. The Anthropology Southern Africa Ethical Guidelines (2005: 142) place the responsibility of protecting respondents from and anticipating harm that may emanate from partaking in the research on researchers. COVID-19 brought new dynamics and ethical dilemmas for researchers. As researchers, we were tested for COVID-19 before field visits as a way of protecting research participants. It was the researchers' responsibility to strictly adhere to government and WHO COVID-19 regulations for the safety of research participants.

Some of the key informant interviews and focus group discussions were conducted over the phone as either a way of limiting physical contact or continuing with data collection under the restrictive COVID-19 lockdown. The pandemic called for creative and innovative ways of collecting data (WHO, 2022). The use of social media such as WhatsApp groups to collect data among congregants was innovative and practical. This presented challenges and opportunities for the research team. Facilitating focus group discussion online came with a new dynamic to the researchers that was different from those conducted face to face. Facilitators had to keep steering the discussions towards research themes when participants digressed to other issues. As some group members tended to dominate during a discussion, as facilitators, we always found ways to invite other participants to give their views. Lastly, online focus group discussions took longer to conduct as participants were not online at the same time, and as facilitators, we kept the groups running for three days before closing them. Discussions that came a day later were rich and detailed, maybe because there were no limitations placed by questions that we posed to guide the discussions. Free conversations flowed and yielded information-rich narratives.

Conceptual Framework

Lived religion is the conceptual framework that informed data collection and analysis. Lived religion transcends the dichotomy between 'religion as prescribed' and the everyday experiences of members of a religious community.

The conceptual framework captures official positions on COVID-19 vaccination of the two mainline churches and goes beyond the institutional position by soliciting members' lived experiences and practices even within religious spaces. This allowed the study to capture discrepancies and congruences between the two. As Knibbe and Kupari (2020: 159) note, lived religion "enquires into how religion is encountered and experienced – how it comes into play – in different environments: public and private, official and informal, sacred, *and* secular". In this case, we aimed to understand how religion was experienced collectively and individually when it came to COVID-19 vaccination. The conceptual framework has the potential to bring to the fore how different mainline churches domesticated government regulation and vaccine programmes, and the differences that emerged from the domestication and operationalisation.

Mainline Christianity and Health Emergencies in Zimbabwe: A Historical Overview

Although the main focus of the chapter is on the experiences of the Roman Catholic Church and Reformed Church in Zimbabwe on COVID-19 vaccination, it is useful to provide a historical overview of mainline Christianity in the context of health from precolonial times to the present. Some of the mainline churches involved in the medical mission were from the London Missionary Society at Inyati and Hope Fountain; the Dominicans and Jesuits of the Roman Catholic Church established mission stations in Bulawayo, Harare and Masvingo; the Dutch Reformed Mission (now Reformed Church in Zimbabwe) at Morgenster; American Board Mission (now United Church of Christ in Zimbabwe) at Mt Selinda; United Methodist Church at Old Umtali (now Hartzell); the Wesleyan Methodist Mission at Waddilove and Kwenda; the Anglican Church at St Faith Mission, St Augustine and Bonda Missions, among others (Gelfand, 1973; Zvogbo, 1996). One of the earliest researchers on medicine and the Christian missions in the then Rhodesia/Southern Rhodesia (now Zimbabwe) was the medical anthropologist, Michael Gelfand, who in one of his writings, raised a question pertinent for this discussion, thus: "Did the Christian missionaries make any significant contributions to the health and welfare of the communities they served?" (Gelfand, 1973:109). We argue that this question is still relevant today as we grapple with existential realities in twenty-first-century Zimbabwe, including the debates on the health emergency of the COVID-19 pandemic. This suggests that the medical arm of Christian Mission services constituted a very important part of its contribution to society.

In some cases, the 'flag followed the cross', that is, the Christian missionaries preceded the establishment of the colonial state whilst in others, the cross (missionaries) followed the flag (colonial rule). In this way, there is a sense in which missionary Christianity is sometimes regarded as the "handmaid of colonialism" (Isichei, 1995). Therefore, the mission churches displayed the "ambivalence of the sacred" (Appleby, 2000) as they could be manipulated to oppress and could be used to liberate. In all this, the Christian missionaries risked their lives in the process of paving the way for the spiritual and social ministry of the church. Gelfand (1973: 109, 111) notes that the malaria fever was one of the tropical diseases that seriously threatened the progress and survival of missionaries in Central and Southern Africa, including Zimbabwe. Notably, whilst some missionaries were never trained in medicine, a handful of others were equipped with basic medical skills to administer simple medical treatments. In addition, the majority of Mission stations adopted a modified version of the broad "Livingstone concept of a missionary in Africa" (Gelfand, 1973: 112), which combined the teaching of Christianity with the dissemination of Western knowledge and skills, as well as the medical services. The Christian Missions pioneered the provision of medical services well before the colonial government started the construction of public hospitals and dispensaries. Christian medical services were popular among the African people in some places, but in other areas, the reverse was true out of scepticism in relation to Western medicine or because of their dependence on African traditional medicine. This is important in understanding the contribution of the mainline Christian churches in the health emergencies in Zimbabwe.

In the colonial and postcolonial eras, the mainline Christian churches have been handy in providing medical services at their health institutions and in promoting Christian values and principles relevant to human flourishing and development. Today, the mainline Christian churches, specifically, the Roman Catholic Church (RCC) and the Reformed Church in Zimbabwe (RCZ), are identified through religious bodies and platforms known as the Zimbabwe Catholic Bishops Conference (ZCBC) and the Zimbabwe Council of Churches (ZCC), respectively. Since colonial times, RCC and RCZ offered medical and other humanitarian services to the people. Whereas the RCC established a developmental arm known as the Catholic Development Commission (CADEC), churches under ZCC created Christian Care (CC) for emergency relief services and development to alleviate poverty, disease and hunger (Sibanda, 2017: 254). Therefore, the RCC and RCZ in collaboration with the government are committed to engaging all people in order to alleviate poverty and diseases and address misinformation and lack of understanding on health matters through the provision of medical services and information, education and communication. As the findings of the chapter show, the mainline Christian churches are resolute in upholding the value of human solidarity, care and accompaniment in times of health emergencies. This was the case at the height of HIV and AIDS where the church was found "listening with love" (Igo, 2005), thereby responding with care and support. Similarly, the response of the mainline Christian churches to the COVID-19 pandemic and the national vaccination programmes was arguably influenced by the lessons the churches gathered from the lived experiences of HIV and AIDS.

In line with the above, at this juncture, we add more flesh on the history of the RCC and the RCZ, which partly justifies why we chose to place them at the centre of the research. Pertaining to RCC, history says that in 1877 the first Roman Catholic Church Jesuits entered what is now called Zimbabwe. Initially, the Catholic Jesuits operated in the Southern region which was called the Zambezi Mission. In the 1980s, the RCC was the largest single denomination in postcolonial Zimbabwe (Chennells, 1980: 195). The Roman Catholic Church Diocese of Masvingo has several parishes in Masvingo province, where we find Masvingo and Bikita Districts. It is estimated that Catholics constitute 9% (1,145,000) of Zimbabwe's population. The church runs several schools and hospitals within the provinces.

The Reformed Church in Zimbabwe, historically, the Dutch Reformed Church (DRC), made its entry from South Africa into Zimbabwe in 1893. In 1952 it changed its name to Shona Reformed Church before changing again to Reformed Church in Zimbabwe (RCZ) in 1977. RCZ has huge presence in Southern Zimbabwe. Its headquarters is in Masvingo Province (Pretorius, 1999). It is one of the mainline churches that boasts of having done a lot in the development of Zimbabwe. They have a University, the Reformed Church University, a teachers' training college, Morgenster Teachers' College, Morgenster Hospital and several schools, among other facilities. It has a sizeable following, particularly in Masvingo province. What emerges from this history is that the RCC and RCZ are important cases/examples in understanding the contribution of mainline Christian churches to health emergencies such as the COVID-19 pandemic and the national vaccination programme.

Mainline Christian Responses to COVID-19 Vaccination

In the following sections, we discuss the ways in which RCZ and RCC leadership navigated measures that were put in place to contain the spread of the COVID-19 virus. The discussion focuses on how the religious movements responded to these measures, as well as how the laity made sense of plans laid by the church leaders in implementing the measures by the government. The section below interrogates responses to mandatory vaccination by the clergy and the laity. The discussion will conclude by discussing the transformations that government COVID-19 containment measures such as prohibiting gatherings, allowing up to fifty congregants and mandatory wearing of face masks had on RCC and RCZ religious activities. Furthermore, the section captures the differences that result from geographic locations of the churches under discussion.

The Word and COVID-19 Messaging

Through key informant interviews, it was established that almost all RCC and RCZ clergy were knowledgeable of the cause of the COVID-19 virus and mechanisms for reducing the spread of the virus. The clergy noted that they dedicated some time in their sermons to teach about the virus, share with their members the latest information on COVID-19 and encourage members to go for vaccination. Furthermore, the pastors and priests noted that as religious experts, they had to find a balance between the scientific information from doctors and eschatological positions informed by the Bible. One of the priests noted that in his sermons, he framed the COVID-19 pandemic "as one of the signs of the end times stated in the Bible". For this clergy, pandemics are God's way of bringing people back to God. In his explanation, China was the instrument for fulfilling the divine mandate. Members of RCZ and RCC communities corroborated that the clergy provided information on COVID-19, at times taking questions from members. During the total lockdown, the clergy continued to provide information through mobile phones on WhatsApp and Short Messages Services. The transformations in liturgy made in the wake of the pandemic shows the ability of religious leaders to respond to the reality on the ground. Sermons addressed pertinent issues facing members of the two churches, showing the flexibility of the gospel to speak to the everyday concerns of members. However, it was also indicated that the COVID-19 induced shift to online liturgy was exclusivist in that not all members could have access to gadgets for online liturgy. Access to the gadgets had gender inclinations, with men and boys having more access than women and girls.

Vaccination Uptake

Interviews with the RCZ clergy in Bikita showed an understanding of the COVID-19 pandemic, its causes and effects. The deacon interviewed indicated that COVID-19 was a disease caused by a virus. He stated that they were perplexed as to how it was transmitted. The deacon submitted that as a church, RCZ followed government measures in fighting the COVID-19 virus. The church complied with government directives to close the church in 2020. Furthermore, the churches had to customise government directives. He intoned:

> When the government relaxed rules on gatherings, we encouraged our members to practice social distancing, wearing of masks, sanitising members who came for church services and fumigating our premises after every gathering.

From the deacon's narrative, the church's official position was guided by government containment measures and directives. In rural areas, the pastor noted that there was laxity in the enforcement of COVID-19 regulations. However, the centralised administration of church governance restricted local clergy's ability to make decisions at a local level. The RCZ followed the decision to stop gatherings that were made by its leadership in Masvingo.

The pastor interviewed went on to indicate that members of the RCZ had mixed feelings on the closure of churches, especially in a rural setup where members of African Independent Churches continued to gather and conduct religious activities. To illustrate this, the pastor noted that:

People do not have the same understanding of the pandemic. One's understanding is determined by the level of education one has attained. We have different levels of education among our members. The more educated one is, the more COVID-19 understanding one becomes. We had less understanding among the less formally educated members.

At an institutional level, the RCZ encouraged its members to get vaccinated with the available vaccines. To set an example, the church's clergy were encouraged to be vaccinated earlier to minimise the risk of the virus. The clergy interacted with many people and vaccines were the only bulwark. Furthermore, some members of the clergy were old and at high risk of death from COVID-19. The leader of the RCC noted that the RCC national leaders were vaccinated publicly, as a way of encouraging the RCC members to get vaccinated. The decision to be vaccinated or publicly showing vaccination cards by the clergy were acts that aimed to reconfigure daily lives of their followers. These acts promoted vaccination, and shaped individual choices. It showed that religion co-exists with biomedicine in daily lives. At the time of the interview, the deacon had already received two jabs and a booster shot. He said:

As the RCZ we follow what the Ministry of Health and Child Care says. This is where the knowledge about the pandemic comes from. We have clinics around and that is where we get information from as a church. We get information from Environmental Health Technicians, radios and televisions.

The deacon's narrative illustrates that there are synergies between biomedical science and mainline religion, as the latter is accommodative of the former. The clergy acted as role models whose vaccination influenced their followers. In a focus group discussion, one member noted that:

We were largely guided by our church leadership, especially our pastor and church elders. We reasoned that these people were well-informed as they attended workshops and came back to teach us. When they encouraged us to get vaccinated, we followed suit because the leadership showed us the way.

The laity depended on the actions and decisions made by the clergy. Accepting vaccination and showing their followers vaccination cards dispelled misinformation, doubts and hesitancy in some of the members. This increased the number of people vaccinated. Furthermore, participants in the FDG noted that the local pastor in Bikita opened sermons by sharing information on COVID-19. The participants noted that this was important as it assisted members to have correct information about the vaccines and vaccinations.

In Masvingo urban, the RCZ pastors adhered to government regulations. Unvaccinated members were not allowed to attend church gatherings. It was noted that when churches were allowed to open, the deacons were responsible for checking the vaccination status of attendees before they entered the church.

Cases of members who were turned away were cited. However, this created some strife between those who denied the unvaccinated entry into the church. One RCC interviewee said:

> Barring unvaccinated members of the church at the gate created conflicts between the church leadership and the unvaccinated members. One unvaccinated member asked those who had attended the church how it was in heaven where they had gone. She further asked how Jesus was.

The above satirical sayings indicate how the unvaccinated felt when denied entry into the church. This left the church deeply divided between the vaccinated and the unvaccinated. Unhealthy relations ensued in the same church, a condition uncalled for in the church as the body of Christ where unity and unison are the major characteristics.

Factors such as fear of police and health inspectors, restricted access to public transport and forced unpaid leave for those who worked in the public sector may explain the high number of respondents who were vaccinated in Masvingo urban. In Bikita, respondents noted that the clergy encouraged them to get vaccinated. However, there were no measures in place to check and restrict participation in church activities for members that were unvaccinated. This partly explains the low vaccination numbers among the congregants that participated in the FGD. Furthermore, Bikita is a predominantly rural district, where inhabitants do not rely on public transport daily and police presence is low. Those employed in surrounding areas walk to their workplace. In such a setting, people could forgo vaccination, despite the church's encouragement for vaccination. The example discussed above sheds light on the shortfalls of religion in health messaging. There are discrepancies between religious beliefs and what transpires on the ground. In their everyday lives, Christians redefine, reinterpret and reconfigure statements that are made by the clergy. A focus on the everyday life of Christians helps researchers to study what Christians actually do and not what they claim to do (Ammerman 2013).

COVID-19 and the Search of a Cure

As illustrated above, mainline churches spearheaded the establishment of mission hospitals in colonial Zimbabwe (Zvobgo, 1996). Mission hospitals were part of a proselytising strategy for early mainline missionary churches. Conversion of local inhabitants brought with it access to mission schools and hospitals. From their inception, mainline churches embraced biomedical approaches to health and well-being. In postcolonial Zimbabwe, mainline churches such as the RCC and RCZ have continued to operate and fund health intervention approaches that are based on biomedicine. The rapid spread of the COVID-19 virus and the slowness in the development of vaccines brought a crisis for mainline churches. The biomedical approach that mainline churches depended on could not offer immediate solutions to the virus. In order to overcome these challenges, some of the clergy from the RCZ and RCC acknowledged that during the pandemic they resorted to the use of indigenous herbs and remedies. One of the clergies noted that "Steaming and indigenous herbs saved our lives. These remedies worked for me."

The existential challenges posed by the pandemic widened the choices that religious people had. Some of the clergy resorted to indigenous herbs and practices. In face of the limitations of biomedicine, the search for cure and treatment was found in indigenous remedies.

The clergy noted that – in their personal capacities – they encouraged members of their church to test for COVID-19, practice all preventive measures put in place by the government, continue with supplicatory prayers and use indigenous remedies as a preventive strategy. This is interesting in that faith leaders were encouraging their followers to seek assistance from different healthcare systems, namely religious, indigenous and medical institutions. The clergy promoted vaccination as well as indigenous remedies that are used in the treatment of fever and colds. The pandemic opened a portal that allowed us a glimpse of what an integrated healthcare system looks like. The pandemic created synergies and linkages between different actors providing healthcare. *Sangomas* and herbalists embraced some elements of biomedicine, requesting their clients to bring COVID-19 results from laboratories and clinics. Despite these collaborations and synergies, issues of power and hegemony remain.

The use of indigenous remedies by the clergy and the encouragement to make use of the same in private illustrate the subordinate position of indigenous medicine. The clergy noted that they would not publicly encourage the use of herbs during a sermon. One of the clergy noted that he feared being labelled "traditionalist" by members of his church. Birgit Meyer (1999) has shown that in Ghana, missionaries deployed the trope of the devil to subjugate the local worldview. Christianity represented God while local religions and systems were inspired by the devil and his agents. Indigenous religion had to be eradicated for all the power of the Christian God to prevail. This process of diabolisation, that is, framing indigenous worldviews as heathen, still informs most Christians' understanding of indigenous practice and herbs. The devil's power is at work. Thus, the clergy are ashamed to promote the use of indigenous herbs as it is a pointer to backsliding or sidestepping, as Premawardhana (2018) conceptualises it. When contacted by followers whose relatives were infected with the virus, the clergyman would advise his followers to use *Zumbani* and *mufandichimuka* (resurrection plant) among other local herbs. This was done in privacy. Members of the mainline churches noted that they used indigenous remedies as preventive measures. In one FGD, one participant noted that:

It was a matter of life and death, we had to use whatever would save us. Plants were made by God, they can't be evil ... They are at our disposal and we have to use them. It is even biblical to use herbs.

For this Christian, the use of available herbs that are known to cure is not a sin. For her, herbs are part of God's creation and must be used for the purpose of sustaining life. This narrative illustrates ways in which lived religion emerges from everyday praxis shaped within a milieu. Faced with existential challenges such as a pandemic and possible death, Christians find ways of redefining the boundaries of what falls under God's creation. This allows them to incorporate indigenous herbs into their everyday lives. The notion that indigenous herbs and remedies are evil has been popularised in recent years by Pentecostal movements that emphasise "a complete break with the past" (Meyer, 1998). The past – which implies both life before conversion and indigenous religion – is framed as machinations of the devil. In place of indigenous remedies, Pentecostal movements valorise faith and divine healing. However, it is not an anomaly for mainline churches to incorporate indigenous practices. Both churches, the RCC and RCZ, have transformed local practices such as mortuary rituals and *kurova guva*, incorporating them into religious ceremonies (see Gundani, 1994; Munikwa and Hendriks, 2011; Mubvumbi, 2016).

Religious Innovations and Power Dynamics in the Time of a Pandemic

The COVID-19 pandemic disrupted the rhythm of religious life that Christians in Zimbabwe had become accustomed to. When churches closed and religious activities were suspended, new ways of worshipping and constituting religious communities emerged. Church activities were transferred to online platforms. In both the RCC and RCZ, WhatsApp groups among church members were already functional before the pandemic. However, it was not a medium for conducting religious activities; it mainly served as a platform for relaying information on social events among members. During the lockdown that started in March 2020, both RCZ and RCC took sermons to WhatsApp groups and also as a medium for teaching followers about COVID-19. One of the members of the clergy from the RCC noted that ways of packaging sermons changed. For online sermons, the message had to be short, brief and straightforward in order for the sermon to be communicated effectively to a diverse audience.

Members of the RCZ noted that WhatsApp groups were used either to make church announcements or inform the members of the government's notices. Members of the RCZ divided themselves into smaller groups of fifteen people. Members in Bikita continued to meet in small numbers. Members noted that even those not vaccinated would attend small gatherings because excluding them was seen as spiritual violence and 'forcing members to backslide'.

The COVID-19 pandemic led to transformations in power dynamics. The clergy at the RCC noted that they stopped to attend funerals and perform mortuary rituals. However, for the purpose of the bereaved, close family members replaced the priests by performing prayers meant for the departed loved ones. Some of the RCC priests noted that the COVID-19 pandemic forced the church to rethink the importance of the family within Christianity. Family members had to stand in for the priest and pray for the sick and the dead and also led worship within the confines of the home. This revived the concept of the priesthood of all believers existent among most mainline Christian churches.

Conclusion

The chapter sought to examine the mainline Christian churches' response to COVID-19 vaccination in Masvingo urban and Bikita rural districts with specific reference to the Roman Catholic Church and the Reformed Church in Zimbabwe. In both the RCC and RCZ, the clergy provided information and communication through mobile phones on WhatsApp and Short Messages Services, which was a transformation in liturgy by religious leaders in response to the existential realities on the ground. Their sermons addressed pertinent issues facing members of the two churches, showing the flexibility of the gospel to speak to the everyday concerns of members. In terms of vaccination, members of the RCC and RCZ were encouraged to get vaccinated using the available vaccines to minimise the risk of the virus. The leaders were vaccinated publicly as a way of encouraging members to get vaccinated and to reconfigure daily the lives of their followers, which promoted vaccination and shaped individual choices. The study showed that religion co-exists with biomedicine in daily lives. In some contexts, the clergy noted that – in their personal capacities – they encouraged members of their church to test for COVID-19, practice all preventive measures put in place by the government, continue with supplicatory prayers and use indigenous remedies as a preventive strategy. This is interesting in that faith leaders were pragmatic by encouraging their followers to seek assistance from different healthcare systems, namely the religious, indigenous and medical institutions. In other words, the clergy promoted vaccination as well as indigenous remedies that are used in the treatment of fever and colds. The pandemic opened a portal for an integrated healthcare system. At the same time, religious innovations and power dynamics manifested during bereavement where close family members performed prayers meant for the departed loved ones in the absence of religious leaders, showing the priesthood of all believers in some mainline Christian churches under the shadow of the pandemic. The chapter concludes that, overall, the adherents of both the RCC and the RCZ in Masvingo and Bikita Districts responded positively towards the vaccination programme in Zimbabwe.

Note

1 This chapter evolved from the findings of a broader research project entitled: "African Spirituality, Health and Well-being in the Face of the COVID-19 Pandemic in Zimbabwe". The research project was generously supported by the Nagel Institute for the Study of World Christianity at Calvin College, USA under the theme: "Engaging African Realities".

References

Afrobarometer. 2017. *Zimbabweans Place Most Trust in Religious Leaders, NGOs and President Mugabe.* www.afrobarometer.org/articles/zimbabweans-place-most-trust-religious-leaders-ngos-and-president-mugabe/

American Anthropological Association. 2012. Statement on ethics: Principles of professional responsibilities. V. 2016. Arlington, VA: American Anthropological Association. Available: www.ethics.americananthro.org/category/statement/

Ammerman, N.T. 2013. *Sacred Stories, Spiritual Tribes: Finding Religion in Everyday Life.* Oxford: Oxford University Press.

Anthropology Southern Africa. 2005. Ethical guidelines and principles of conduct for anthropologists. *Anthropology Southern Africa,* 28(3&4), 142.

Appleby, S.R. 2000. *The Ambivalence of the Sacred: Religion, Violence and Reconciliation.* Lanham, MD: Rowman & Littlefield.

Boeije, H.R. 2010. *Analysis in Qualitative Research.* London: Sage Publications.

Bowa, M.A. 2022. The coronavirus pandemic and persons with disabilities: Towards a liberating reading of the Bible for Churches in Southern Africa. In F. Sibanda, T. Muyambo and E. Chitando (Eds), *Religion and the COVID-19 Pandemic in Southern Africa.* London and New York: Routledge, pp. 186–201.

Chennells, A.J. 1980. The Catholic Church in Zimbabwe. *Zambezia,* 8(2), 195–212.

Clandinin, D.J., and Connelly, F.M. 2000. *Narrative Inquiry: Experience and Story in Qualitative Research.* San Francisco, CA: Jossey-Bass.

Delamont, S., and Atkinson, P. 2018. The ethics of ethnography. In R. Iphonen and M. Tolich (Eds), *The Sage Handbook of Qualitative Research Ethics.* Thousand Oaks, CA: Sage, pp. 119–132.

Desplat, P. 2022. Doubting the Malagasy remedy. Rumours and suspicion during COVID-19 in Madagascar. *Slovenský národopis,* 70(2), 411–429. https://doi.org/10.31577/SN.2022.3.32

Gelfand, M. 1973. Medicine and the Christian Missions in Rhodesia, 1857–1930. In H.J.A. Dachs (Eds), *Christianity South of the Zambezi,* Vol. 1. Gwelo: Mambo Press, pp. 109–124.

Gundani, P. 1994. The Roman Catholic Church and the *kurova guva* ritual in Zimbabwe. *Zambezia,* XXI(ii), 123–146.

Igo, R. 2005. *Listening with Love: Pastoral Counselling – A Christian Response to People Living with HIV/AIDS.* Geneva: World Council of Churches.

Isichei, E.A. 1995. *A History of Christianity in Africa: From Antiquity to the Present.* Grand Rapids, MI: Eerdmans.

Kirby, B. Taru, J, Chimbidzikai, T. 2020. Pentecostals and the spiritual war against coronavirus in Africa. *The Conversation,* 30 April 2020.

Knibbe, K., and Kupari, H. 2020. Theorizing lived religion: Introduction. *Journal of Contemporary Religion,* 35(2), 157–176. https://doi.org/10.1080/13537903.2020.1759897

Kowalczyk, O., Roszkowski, K., Montane, X., Pawliszak. W., Tylkowski, B., and Bajek, A. 2020. Religion and faith perception in a pandemic of COVID-19. *Journal of Religion and Health,* 59, 2671–2677. https://doi.org/10.1007/s10943-020-01088-3

Meyer, B. 1998. 'Make a complete break with the past.' Memory and post-colonial modernity in Ghanaian Pentecostalist discourse. *Journal of Religion in Africa,* 28(3), 316–349.

Meyer, B. 1999. *Translating the Devil: Religion and Modernity among the Ewe in Ghana.* Edinburgh: Edinburgh University Press.

Mubvumbi, P.D. 2016. *Christianity and Traditional Religions of Zimbabwe: Contrasts and Similarities.* Bloomington, IN: WestBow Press.

Mundagowa, P.T., Tozivepi, S.N., Chiyaka, E.T., Mukora-Mutseyekwa, F., Makurumidze, R. 2022. Assessment of COVID-19 vaccine hesitancy among Zimbabweans: A rapid national survey. *PLoS ONE*, 17(4), e0266724. https://doi.org/10.1371/journal. pone.0266724

Munikwa, C. and Hendriks, H.J., 2011. The Binga outreach: Towards intercultural mission in the Reformed Church in Zimbabwe. *Dutch Reformed Theological Journal*, 52(3), 453–464. DOI:10.5952/52-3-55

Muyambo, T., Sande, N., and Tendere, J. 2022. 'Wash and Pray': The nexus of African Christianity and science in the context of COVID-19 in Zimbabwe. *Journal of Religion in Africa,* 52, 348–373.

Muyambo, T. and Tendere, J. 2023. Beyond the COVID-19 pandemic: Is rethinking the interface of religion and science possible in Zimbabwean context? In M. Manyonganise (Ed.), *Religion and Health in a COVID-19 Context: Experiences from Zimbabwe.* Bamberg: University Bamberg Press, pp. 285–304.

Nakkazi, E. 2020. Obstacles to COVID-19 control in East Africa. *The Lancet*, 20(6), 660.

Okyere-Manu, B. and Morgan, N. 2022. Exploring the ethics of *Ubuntu* in the era of COVID-19. In F. Sibanda, T. Muyambo, and E. Chitando (Eds), *Religion and the COVID-19 Pandemic in Sothern Africa.* London and New York: Routledge, pp. 25–36.

Premawardhana, D. 2018. *Faith in Flux: Pentecostalism and Mobility in Rural Mozambique.* Philadelphia, PA: University of Pennsylvania Press.

Pretorius, S.F. 1999. *A History of the Dutch Reformed Church in Zimbabwe with Special Reference to the Chinhoyi Congregation.* DPhil Thesis. Pretoria: University of South Africa.

Riessman, C.K. 2008. *Narrative Methods for the Human Sciences.* Thousand Oaks, CA: Sage.

Sibanda, F. 2017. Servant leadership and the paradox of Africa's [Under-]development Predicament, in M. Mawere, T.R. Mubaya, and J. Mukusha (Eds), *The African Conundrum: Rethinking the Trajectories of Historical, Cultural, Philosophical and Developmental Experiences of Africa.* Mankon, Bamenda: LangaaResearch & Publishing CIG, pp. 243–266.

World Health Organization. 2022. *COVID-19 Research and Innovation: Powering the World's Pandemic Response – Now and in the Future.* Geneva: WHO.

Zvobgo, C.J.M. 1996. *A History of Christian Missions in Zimbabwe, 1890–1939.* Gweru: Mambo Press.

6 'Can Anything Good Come Out of Nazareth?' (John 1:46)

The Relevance of the Apostolic Women's Empowerment Trust in the Context of COVID-19 Vaccination in Zimbabwe

Tobias Marevesa and Fortune Sibanda

Introduction

The coronavirus (COVID-19) pandemic brought in dark times, which resulted in significant loss to lives, livelihoods, social and physical connections. This complex global pandemic affected the usual ways of life as well as how people grappled with death, grief and loss in the context of COVID-19 (Pentaris, 2022). Thus, COVID-19 ignited traumatic experiences of unimaginable proportions without discrimination across the class, race, creed and gender divides. In Sub-Saharan Africa in face of this atmosphere of crisis, health risks and uncertainties brought about by COVID-19 pandemic, Zimbabwe rolled out a national vaccination programme in February 2021. Zimbabwe is among the African states and governments that introduced vaccination as the key control strategy to curb the spread and reduce the adverse effects of the COVID-19 pandemic and targeted vaccinating at least 60% of its eligible population to attain a herd immunity by December 2021 (Murewanhema et al., 2022). Yet, the landscape of COVID-19 vaccination in Zimbabwe was faced with an assortment of successes, challenges, threats and opportunities testified by vaccination hesitancy, acceptance and total rejection. The issue of COVID-19 vaccination in Zimbabwe brings the Apostolic Women's Empowerment Trust (AWET) to the fore. AWET is an inter-faith-based, non-governmental organisation mandated to promote the rights of adolescents and women issues and mainstreaming of gender in Apostolic Church activities (https://awet.org.zw/about-us/).

This chapter focuses on the relevance of AWET in the context of COVID-19 vaccination in Zimbabwe. The chapter posits that AWET, a faith-based organisation (FBO) which is advocating for the vaccination of women in Apostolic churches, is breaking new ground by convincing the once-sceptical congregants of the Apostolic churches (particularly women) in Zimbabwe to get vaccinated against the backdrop of death, dying and bereavement in the context of COVID-19 pandemic. Important insights can be gained by engaging and closely looking at the positive responses of the Apostolic women groups as people living on the margins in the context of vaccination in Zimbabwe.

DOI: 10.4324/9781003388630-6

The chapter underscores that "invisibility" and lack of social recognition of Apostolic women living on the margins in a patriarchal society are important markers for their minority status and marginalisation, but did not necessarily render them as helpless victims without agency. Instead, research has shown that the margins are "spaces of resistance" such that even the most vulnerable groups possess the ability to respond to processes of marginalisation (Hammer, 2009). Therefore, given that "to act, a group must first be visible" (Hammer, 2009: n.p.), the story of AWET's intervention is a positive one. We seek to demonstrate that action and the agency of Apostolic women through AWET's information, education and communication strategies catapulted the visibility of Apostolic women in the context of positive vaccination uptake in Zimbabwe. This is a critical under-documented and under-studied trend that can serve as a model for others facing vaccine hesitancy. In fact, the vaccine acceptance among some of the Apostolic women is a surprising new twist and deviation from their well-known traditional reputation of resistance to modern healthcare system, including vaccination (Maguranyanga, 2011; Ntali, 2023). Arising from this, there is an underlying question based on John 1:46: "Can anything good come out of the Apostolic women?" Before exploring the Apostolic women responses to vaccination in Zimbabwe, we first present the theoretical framework and research methodology.

Theoretical Framework and Research Methodology

The chapter is a qualitative study informed by insights from the RARE leadership model as a theoretical framework in the context of COVID-19 vaccination in Zimbabwe. A RARE leadership model is premised on being Responsible, Accountable, Relevant and Ethical (Ngambi, 2014; Ely & Thomas, 2001). This model incorporates diversity and combines integration and learning. RARE leadership is informed by responsible behaviour among citizens and all stakeholders. Responsible leadership is a catalyst for change through engaging with current realities and persuasions (Ngambi, 2014). Accountable leadership fosters connectivity with the people. It is accountable to itself and to all stakeholders by taking ownership of decisions and actions. In addition to being responsible and accountable, leadership must be relevant. Relevant leadership is engaging in that it is contextual and in touch with the environment. Therefore, it is flexible, innovative and adaptable. RARE leadership must be ethical. Ethical leadership maintains integrity, which is demonstrated by being authentic (Ngambi, 2014). The RARE leadership model is useful for the study as AWET readily intervened to facilitate the collaboration between Apostolic members and the formal health providers through positive engagement, dialogue, and information, education and communication strategies in the context of COVID-19 vaccination. Therefore, components of RARE leadership can be applied at individual level, in families, communities, organisations and the nation at large. The "choice to die" (see Maguranyanga, 2011: 49) under the conviction of faith is an endemic position of ultra-conservative Apostolic group, which undermines modern healthcare, including vaccination. This is a position that AWET has dedicated itself to transforming by spreading positive messages and information on health, gender, rights to health, particularly of women and children against the backdrop of toxic leadership (of the ultra-conservative male apostolic members), which is irresponsible, unethical, immoral, self-centred, irrelevant, "emotionally illiterate, unfit and shallow" (Ngambi, 2014: 115).

In terms of methodology, the study reviewed existing literature and documentary analysis of the print and electronic media. In addition, the research utilised a biblical hermeneutical approach, which brought selected biblical scripture under focus. This is relevant because the Bible in the Zimbabwean context is one of the most popular texts, invoked in day-to-day lives of many (Chitando et al., 2013). The Bible appealed to the "men of God" (including the ultra-conservative male apostolic church leaders) to entrench their male leadership and decisions as well as in providing solace to those experiencing death, loss and grief in times of COVID-19 pandemic, by giving assurance that it shall be well. On this basis, exerting scriptures under scrutiny was useful to understand the Apostolic church communities' response in the context of COVID-19 vaccination. As some of the women and men of the Apostolic churches acceded to the vaccination and the information, education and communication programmes championed by AWET, it brings John 1:46 to the fore raising the question: "Can anything good come from the women and men of the Apostolic churches?" We now turn to a brief overview of COVID-19 pandemic.

COVID-19 Pandemic: A Historical Overview

This section explores a brief historical background of COVID-19 pandemic in Zimbabwe in order to situate the health emergency in context. The outbreak of COVID-19 pandemic in December 2019 brought a lot of suffering to humankind which claimed many lives globally, and Zimbabwe was not an exception. Therefore, COVID-19 pandemic became one of the most disturbing diseases to humankind in the contemporary times. Since December 2019, this disease has received much scholarly and scientific attention due to its devastating impact on humanity. According to a number of scholars such as Sibanda et al. (2022); Myers (2020); Verma (2020); Rachman (2020), the whole world led by World Health Organisation (WHO) grappled with the public health emergency caused by novel COVID-19 disease, which sparked a mirage of conspiracy theories. Some of these conspiracy theories created fear, misinformation and lack of understanding on health matters, which culminated in vaccination hesitancy and rejection. Another dimension to conspiracy theories resulted in an open confrontation between two major international giants, which are United States of America and China, on the genesis of coronavirus disease (Shanapinda, 2020; GMT Media, 2020; Myers, 2020; Rachman, 2020; Verma, 2020).

As the coronavirus disease escalated, WHO announced a raft of mitigatory measures to be undertaken by countries across the globe. In this way, COVID-19 vaccination became one of the best public health strategies to limit the spread of the infectious disease, reduce morbidity and usher in a return to normal life activities (Murewanhema et al., 2022). Zimbabwe was among the few African countries which had an aggressive vaccination programme in order to reach a 60% herd immunity so as to allow all the sectors of the economy to function to full capacity. The government through the Ministry of Health and Child Care (MOHCC), rolled out the vaccination programme in February 2021 and as of January 2022, about 21.4% of the eligible population had been fully vaccinated (Murewanhema et al., 2022). As the disease continued to rage, there was both vaccine compliance and vaccine hesitancy among the people. In Zimbabwe, there were underlying factors, which were associated with COVID-19 vaccine intentions such as knowledge, attitudes and behaviour (McAbee et al., 2021). Religion has been listed among the factors that influence the patterns in vaccine intentions and motivations. A case in point is the conservative Apostolic churches' stance, which regarded vaccines as dangerous, a cause of disease and death. Constituting about one third of the population, the Apostolic churches had a track record of low vaccination rates among children and for other adult vaccination interventions as compared to other religious groups (McAbee et al., 2021; Kriss et al., 2016). This was important in gauging the high probability of hesitancy among the Apostolic church members to take up a new vaccine such as that for COVID-19 pandemic. In order to better appreciate the relevance of AWET in addressing the problem of COVID-19 vaccine hesitancy among some members of the Apostolic churches, we begin with an exegesis John 1:46.

Re-reading John 1:46 in Light of Zimbabwean Experiences during COVID-19

The verse in question reads as follows: "And Nathanael said to him, 'Can anything good come out of Nazareth?' Philip said to him, 'Come and see'" (John 1:46, The King James Version). To start with, it is important to note that the Gospel of John is different from the synoptic Gospels which are Mark, Matthew and Luke. This means that the themes and purposes are also different from the synoptic Gospels. The Gospel of John was written by John the beloved disciple who is believed to have been one of Jesus' disciples. However, this is contested by a number of scholars such as Fuller (1971); Gundry (2003); Bock (2007). Nevertheless, this debate goes beyond the purview of this study. According to Gundry (2003), the major focus of the Apostle John in writing his Gospel was to encourage his audience/readership to believe in Jesus for their eternal life. This theme resonates well with the experiences of death, loss and grief in Zimbabwe in the context of COVID-19 pandemic. Related to the above major theme in the Gospel of John, is the reason or purpose of writing. The purpose of writing was to demonstrate that Jesus was both God and human. This resulted in the notion of a higher Christology where Jesus is perceived as deity who existed before the world was created. In fact, He was a creating agent (Ehrman, 2009). The humanity of Jesus and his death was questioned by the Gnostics who were the heretics of early Christianity (Bock, 2007). The heretics argue that the material and immaterial will never come together. With this view, this movement rejected the resurrection of Jesus, this is why at the beginning of the Gospel of John there is a phrase "the word was with God" (Culpepper, 1983).

What also emerges in this chapter is the theme of faith, which is revealed in the initial ministry of Jesus, including in John 1:46. This verse is situated in the context of perceiving Jesus as a Lamb of God waiting to be sacrificed as a ransom for humanity. The immediate context was when Jesus was in the process of calling His disciples (Counet, 2001). It is against this background that Philip saw Nathanael and told him that he found Jesus of Nazareth but Nathanael answered saying, "Can anything good come out of Nazareth?" The question is: What was the meaning and implication of Nathanael's question? Generally, where one is coming from determines the social status of that person. Similarly, it is possible that Nathanael, a Galilean rabbinic teacher, was informed by the fact that Nazareth was regarded as a miserable place, one which was despised even by its neighbours, including the Galileans. According to Bock (2007), this inclination was not novel in the first century and particularly in Israel. People would be judged and ranked in society basing on whether they grew up in places such as Samaria, Judea or Galilee (Acts 2:7). Therefore, those who grew up in urban areas gained more respect than those from the rural areas. Even in Zimbabwe, those who come from the affluent suburbs are more respected than people who stay in high density suburbs. By the same token, the choice of a religion dove-tails with class and status, just as "the package of a religion affects people's choice of it" (Bourdillon, 1993: 85). Indeed, there are some contrasting socio-economic conditions between "churches for the rich" (Togarasei, 2010: 19) patronised by a class of black elite and those churches (read Apostolic churches), which meet under trees, lacking affluence and respectability. In this case, Nazareth, where Jesus grew up, was regarded as remote and rustic, which made people from there to be despised. No one could ever have imagined that any good thing, or person, the Messiah, could spring from it. Similarly, one can situate the low, obscured and despised status of Apostolic churches in the context of their uptake of COVID-19 vaccines in Zimbabwe.

Nathanael's initial objection and prejudice did not only emanate from the obscurity of Nazareth, but was also based on the oracle that the Messiah was to be born in Bethlehem (Micah 5:2). Yet, Nathanael was a professional, honest and upright person. Philip invited Nathanael so that he would discover Jesus alone in Nazareth a place where they could not expect to see the Messiah. It was a good way of convincing Nathanael to prove for himself that Jesus the Son of God and King of Israel was from Nazareth. This was a place which was least expected to be associated with Jesus because of its wickedness, meanness and obscurity. In a similar way, the same question can be asked in the contemporary context, thus: Can anything good come from Africa or Zimbabwe in particular in relation to COVID-19 vaccination? Can any good thing or person come from the Apostolic churches in the context of COVID-19 vaccination? Can the government and church leadership support and console those who will be mourning their beloved after succumbing to the COVID-19 pandemic? Can the government of Zimbabwe and the non-governmental organisations such as AWET be able to establish trauma centres in order to manage the level of stress after the loss of a beloved relative? Can AWET establish networks and introduce awareness programs that provide correct and up-to-date information on COVID-19 vaccines? These and many other questions are the subject of the next section that focuses on the activities of AWET in the context of COVID-19 vaccination in Zimbabwe.

AWET and the Advocacy for COVID-19 Vaccination in Apostolic Churches

As an inter-faith-based, non-governmental organisation formed in 2016 with a mandate to advance the rights of adolescents and women in Apostolic churches, AWET is strategically positioned to mobilise women of faith in order to tackle existential challenges they face in their day-to-day lives. The Apostolic faith community is a heterogeneous group with different religious teachings, doctrine and regulations. This plurality of beliefs, practices, values and perceptions have an over-arching influence on their decisions concerning social issues such as early child marriage and education, as well as diverse health-related decisions on the uptake of modern healthcare services and vaccination (https://awet. org.zw/about-us/). Prior to the onset of COVID-19, Maguranyanga (2011) studied Apostolic faith communities and formulated three categories, namely, (a) ultra-conservative Apostolic groups; (b) semi-conservative groups; and (c) liberal Apostolic groups. The categorisation was done on the basis of the extent to which the groups perceived the uptake modern healthcare services, immunisation and their preparedness to change their beliefs, teachings and practices to match with emerging trends and new ways of looking at reality. It can be argued that AWET sought to register change not only among Apostolic churches, but also on how society viewed the Apostolic faith community. This goal is clearly expressed on their website where it is said that "AWET intends to change the negative perceptions society holds about the Apostolic community through dealing with contemporary issues facing the Apostolic community whilst being sensitive to the members' expectations" (https://awet.org.zw/about-us/). On this basis, AWET's strategy has won the trust of the Apostolic faith community, which resulted in their behaviour change towards COVID-19 vaccination.

In line with the above, AWET is making use of a team of Volunteers and Behaviour Change Facilitators (BCFs) spread across the ten provinces of Zimbabwe. Through the intervention of AWET, dialogues with women of diverse Apostolic churches were held by the BCFs. The Apostolic position of shunning medical interventions, including vaccination, began to soften amidst COVID-19 due to the effective strategies adopted by AWET (Ntali, 2023). AWET exploited the opportunities of collaborating with UNICEF and the

Ministry of Health and Child Care to hold dialogue with interfaith and community leaders, as well as youth networks across the country in order to get the support for COVID-19 rollout and recovery through the provision of correct and up-to-date information on COVID-19 vaccines (Maiden, 2021; Nyathi, 2021). Therefore, enticing key stakeholders such as faith leaders and other members is critical because it can unlock the jigsaw puzzle that has been a barrier to the uptake of essential health services, including vaccination.

In addition, through the use of BCFs, AWET scored success among male and female Apostolic members as they embraced COVID-19 vaccination. For instance, one elderly member of the Johanne Marange Apostolic Church in Hurungwe District of Mashonaland West testified that she had no regrets for embracing COVID-19 prevention measures and receiving the vaccine. In her words, she said: "Our church doctrine says we don't go to the hospital when [...] sick or get vaccinated, with COVID-19 it is a new ball game altogether and I have to take matters into my own hands ... After we were taught about the dangers of COVID-19 I took the decision to get vaccinated because my life is my responsibility" (Nyathi, 2021). Along the same lines, the woman elder emphatically stated: "I chose to be vaccinated against COVID-19 because is a matter of life and death for me and my family" (Nyathi, 2021). What is critical to note is that this particular woman Apostolic elder from Hurungwe was one of the beneficiaries of AWET's COVID-19 awareness programmes to address vaccine hesitancy across the country. In addition, there is an extent to which the woman elder displayed RARE leadership qualities as she considered the needs and fears of her family at a point "when the right to health and the right to religion conflict" (Stone et al., 2009). This shows that the efforts of AWET on the problem of vaccine hesitancy is bearing positive results.

The agency and resilience of women Apostles are also useful indicators of their leadership qualities in their engagement with contextual existential realities that combined risk, innovation and learning from the BCFs. The significant behaviour change registered among some of the Apostolic members that AWET interacted with, demonstrates a shift from widespread misinformation and the long-held conservative religious beliefs. This is evident through an Apostolic church woman elder who said, thus: "At my church I am seeing a lot of people embracing the vaccines because they now understand that their lives and those of their loved ones depend on them getting COVID-19 vaccines [...] No pastor or elder will chase me from the church because I got the vaccine, it is now a matter between me and God" (Nyathi, 2021). This shows the empathetic attitude that is emerging among some of the Apostolic members in the context of COVID-19 vaccination. Ntali (2023) also refers to a similar situation of hope that countered vaccine hesitancy. In the words of one woman, it was stated: "Personally, I had fears, because growing up, we were of the belief that taking vaccines was getting the biblical mark of the beast. I am happy that our church leaders who had not been tolerating immunisation are now encouraging us to take our children to clinics.

Among some of the transformed male Apostolic counterparts, similar narratives have been recorded where they warmed up to COVID-19 vaccines. For instance, a 73-year-old male leader of Johanne Marange Church in Hurungwe, with over sixty years as a member, said he voluntarily got vaccinated after attending COVID-19 awareness programmes conducted by AWET (Nyathi, 2021). Reasoning from a standpoint consistent with RARE leadership, the elder argued that when religious leaders led by example in terms of getting vaccinated, the adherents were likely to follow suit. He testified that "Some believed that the vaccines cause impotence or will drain their energy and make it difficult for them to do their work in the fields, but it's been two months since I was vaccinated nothing happened to me" (Nyathi, 2021). What is evident is that through the efforts of AWET, something good is emerging from the Apostles in the context of embracing modern medical services.

Imagining Goodness through RARE-Grief Leadership during Troubled Times: Critical Reflections

Having looked at the efforts of AWET in awareness campaigns for a positive inclination towards vaccination, it is critical to situate this in the context of RARE and grief leadership in the context of Apostolic church responses to COVID-19 vaccination. This is significant because over the years, members of the Apostolic churches viewed vaccines as dangerous and a cause of disease and death such that COVID-19 vaccination becomes a litmus test for the leadership patterns in families, churches and the nation at large. In other words, COVID-19 pandemic vaccination as well as the post-traumatic stress after the death of people who succumbed to the coronavirus disease can be used to gauge whether anything good (positive) can be realised from members of the Apostolic churches. In fact, the outbreak of COVID-19 pandemic challenged leaders across the world in terms of preparedness to combat the disease and the adoption of critical measures such as vaccination. In addition, both RARE and grief leadership entail being empathetic to the realities of death, dying and loss. Over the years, "stupid deaths" (See Paul Farmers' phrase cited in Redfield, 2020; Sibanda, 2022: 229) were experienced in Apostolic churches due to a history of low vaccination rates for childhood and adult vaccination programs on the basis of ultra-conservative attitudes and behaviours. Therefore, at this stage with AWET's influence over interfaith leaders (including Apostolic members) across Zimbabwe to support COVID-19 vaccine rollout, we can re-imagine goodness through RARE and grief leadership during troubled times. This can be appreciated alongside the reactions of the bereaved after the loss of a loved one and the role which the leader plays in supporting and consoling those mourning (Centre for the Study of Traumatic Stress, 2020). It was critical for leaders to deal with the post traumatic events or death of people who died from COVID-19. During pandemics, leaders need to be there for the bereaved and those who are affected by the pandemics. As such, church and community leaders needed to be able to identify when grief and anxiety turned into mourning and also encourage communities to warm up towards government interventions to take up the new vaccine as the way forward.

As people responded to interventions in health emergencies, there were steps which RARE and grief leaders had to follow if they were to lead by example. First, they had to communicate effectively when there was a crisis or pandemic in a particular community where special skills, principles and concept are required. According to the Centre for the Study of Traumatic Stress (2020), church and community leaders should be able to learn the said skills or to find assistance from the crisis communication specialists. This is so because distress and worry may spread into the church and communities, which are affected by a health emergency such as COVID-19, which may result in the rumour, misinformation and 'conspirational thinking' that distort what is transpiring in a particular community. The loss of human life may amplify these effects. Therefore, church and community leaders should be able to handle and share grief by communicating hope and manage gossip and give moral support to others. This is what AWET offered through the awareness campaign programs among the Apostolic churches in the 52 Districts of Zimbabwe, which were spear-headed by BCFs. Strategically, the BCFs were recruited to work in wards they stayed, so as to reach out on their families, neighbours and other church or community members armed with life-saving information that dispelled myths and disinformation about vaccines (Nyathi, 2021).

The second aspect which church and community leaders need to bear in mind when there is a pandemic is the immediate response to the situation and being visible to either the bereaved family or to the infected person. According to the National Child Traumatic Stress Network (2020), when-ever there is a pandemic, leaders of the church and communities should make public announcements to show that they are in solidarity with those in crisis. Such an approach is empowering to the infected and affected. AWET was a champion of providing targeted information, education and communica-tion strategies that transformed some members of the Apostolic churches to be open to modern medicine. According to Robbins (2022), where necessary, AWET advised women in Apostolic churches to go against church rules if it meant helping and saving the lives of their children. The third element which leaders of the church and community should be equipped with is being able to conceptualise that traumatised people react differently about the loss of the beloved one, work mate, member of the community among others (American Academy of Child and Adolescent Psychiatry, 2020). People vary in the way they handle grief, some may be fine with time, while others' instant responses to grief may take longer than usual and this may affect their work and families. In the context of COVID-19 pandemic, there were many people who died. This resulted in grief symptoms which included: withdrawal from friends and relatives, waves of sadness and "intrusive images of the traumatic event and lost loved ones" (Centre for the Study of Traumatic Stress, 2020: 2). In light of this, the role of the RARE and grief leader became significant in order to avert the signs and symptoms of traumatic grief. In addition, provision of correct and up to date information on COVID-19 vaccines, it was possible for some Apostolic members to embrace the vaccination programme in Zimbabwe. In light of the above argument, RARE and grief leadership required leaders to encourage calmness, collective healing and recovery, hope, assertiveness among other things to the affected families, churches and communities. It was also imperative for church and community leaders to interact with parents and children due to the pandemic. In a situation where a parent or both parents had succumbed to COVID-19, going back to school brought calmness in children, but became stressful for parents when they are left alone (Kerr et al., 2021). AWET was strategically positioned to accompany Apostolic parents and children to respond to the effects of COVID-19 and played a key role in mobilising the conservatives within the Apostolic community to embrace COVID-19 vaccines.

Conclusion

The chapter has demonstrated that notwithstanding the 'ambivalence of the sacred', vaccination acceptance among some Apostolic members is a good indicator of AWET's positive engagement to promote human flourishing amidst a health emergency in Zimbabwe. Through the use of BCFs, AWET encouraged Apostolic, interfaith and community leaders to embrace the COVID-19 vaccination programme in Zimbabwe. Given that over the years, some members of the Apostolic churches viewed vaccines as dangerous and a cause of disease and death, the fact that AWET's intervention made some Apostolic members to change their mind set is something good coming out of Nazareth (the Apostolic adherents). In this way, the provision of targeted information, education and communication strategies on COVID-19 vaccination was instrumental in promoting health-care seeking behaviour among the Apostolic Church members. Of interest to note is that women Apostolic members were empowered to the extent that they confidently expressed their agency and embraced COVID-19 vaccination without fear. In other words, the "invisibility" and lack of social recognition of Apostolic women living on the margins in a patriarchal society are important markers for their minority status and marginalisation, but this did not necessarily render them as helpless victims without agency. Instead, in the context of this chapter the margins are "spaces of resistance" such that even the most vulnerable groups (Apostolic women) possess the ability to respond to processes of marginalisation. Therefore, pertaining to the question: 'Can any good thing or person come from the Apostolic churches in the context of COVID-19 vaccination?', it can be concluded that vaccination acceptance among some Apostolic members is a good indicator of AWET's positive engagement to promote human flourishing amidst a health emergency in Zimbabwe. Through AWET, we can re-imagine goodness, RARE and grief leadership among some Apostolic members during the troubled times of COVID-19 pandemic.

References

American Academy of Child and Adolescent Psychiatry Annual Meeting. 2020. https://pro.psycom.net/american-academy-of-child-and-adolescent-psychiatry.com

Bock, D. 2007. *Acts: Baker Exegetical Commentary on the New Testament.* Grand Rapids, MI: Baker Publishing Group.

Bourdillon, M.F.C. 1993. *Where are the Ancestors? Changing Culture in Zimbabwe.* Harare: University of Zimbabwe Publications.

Center for the Study of Traumatic Stress. 2020. Advancing psychological health and resilience through trauma research, education, and consultation. *Uniformed Services University*, https://ceterforstudyoftraumaticstress.com

Chitando, E., Gunda, R.M., & Kugler, J. 2013. Introduction in E. Chitando, R.M. Gunda & J. Kugler (Eds), *Prophets, Profits and the Bible in Zimbabwe.* Bamberg: University of Bamberg Press, pp. 9–27.

Counet, P.C. 2001. *John, a Postmodern Gospel: Introduction to Deconstructive Exegesis Applied to the Fourth Gospel.* Leiden: Brill.

Culpepper, R.A. 1983. *Anatomy of the Fourth Gospel: A Study in Literary Design.* Philadelphia, PA: Fortress Press.

Ehrman, B.D. 2009. *A Brief Introduction to the New Testament.* Oxford: Oxford University Press.

Ely, R.J. & Thomas, D.A. 2001. Cultural diversity at work: The effects of diversity perspectives on work group processes and outcomes. *Administrative Science Quarterly*, 462, 229–273.

Fuller, R.H. 1971. *Critical Introduction to the New Testament.* London: Gerald Duckworth.

GMT Media 2020. The geopolitical battle for the COVID 19, *China News,* 4 April

Gundry, R.H. 2003. *A Survey of the New Testament* (4th edition). Grand Rapids, MI: Zondervan.

Hammer, P.J. 2009. Introduction: Living on the Margins: Minorities and Borderlines in Cambodia and South East Asia. In P.J. Hammer (Ed.), *Living on the Margins: Minorities and Borderlines in Cambodia and Southeast Asia*, Wayne State University Law School Legal Studies Research Paper Series No. 09-07. https://awet.org.zw/about-us/

Kerr, M.L., Rasmussen, H.F., Fanning, K.A., & Braaten, S.M. 2021. Parenting during COVID-19: A study of parents' experiences across gender and income levels, *Fam Relat.*, 70(5), 1327–1342. Available at: https://doi:10.1111/fare.12571

Kriss, J.L., Goodson, J., Machekanyanga, Z., Shibeshi, M.E., Daniel, F., Masresha, B., & Kaiser, R. 2016. Vaccine receipt and vaccine card availability among children of the apostolic faith: Analysis from the 2010–2011 Zimbabwe demographic and health survey, *Pan Afr. Med. J.*, 24(47). Available at: https://doi:10.11604/pamj.2016.24.47.8663

MacAbee, L., Tapera, O., & Kanyangarara, M. 2021. Factors associated with COVID-19 vaccine intentions in Eastern Zimbabwe: A cross-sectional study, *Vaccines*, 9(10) https://doi.org/10.3390/vaccines9101109

Maguranyanga, B. 2011. Apostolic religion, health and utilization of maternal and child health services in Zimbabwe Available at: www.unicef.org/zimbabwe/media/1006/file/Apostolic%20Religion,%20Health%20and%20Utilization%20of%20Maternal%20and%20Child%20Health%20Services%20in%20Zimbabwe.pdf

Maiden, J. 2021. Zimbabwe's religious leaders increase efforts to tackle COVID-19 and support vaccines. Available at: www.unicef.org/zimbabwe/press-releases/zimbabwes-religious-leaders-increase-efforts-tackle-covid-19-and-support-vaccines

Murewanhema, G., Musuka, G., Denhere, K., Chingombe, I., Mapingure, M.P., & Dzinamarira, T. 2022. The landscape of COVID-19 vaccination in Zimbabwe: A narrative review and analysis of the strengths, weaknesses, opportunities and threats of the programme. *Vaccines*, 10(262) https://doi.org/10.3390/vaccines10020262

Myers, S.I. 2020. China spins the tale that the US army started the coronavirus epidemic Available at: www.nytimes.com/2020/03/13/world/asia/coronavirus-china-conspiracy-theory.html. Accessed 10 October 2020.

The National Child Traumatic Stress Network. 2020. *Child and Family Traumatic Stress Intervention*, www.nctsn.org

Ngambi, H. 2014. RARE Leadership: An alternative leadership application for Africa In K. Kondlo (Ed.), *Perspectives on Thought Leadership for Africa's Renewal*. Pretoria: Africa Institute of South Africa.

Ntali, E. 2023. How an Apostolic Woman's group helped Zimbabwe counter vaccine hesitancy. Available at: www.gavi.org/vaccineswork/

Nyathi, K. 2021. Religious groups warm up to COVID-19 vaccines in Zimbabwe. Available at: www.unicef.org/zimbabwe/stories/religious-groups-warm-covid-19-vaccines-zimbabwe

Pentaris, P. 2022. Introduction: Capturing the beginning of a long journey of loss, trauma and grief. In P. Pentaris (Ed.), *Death, Grief and Loss in the Context of COVID-19*. London: Routledge, pp. 1–13.

Rachman, G. 2020. How the outbreak is changing global politics Available at: www.ft.com/content/fd8bfd8a-5a25-11ea-abe5-8e03987b7b20

Redfield, P. 2020. COVID-19: The danger of a single threat. Retrieved from https://culanth.org/fieldsights/the-danger-of-a-single-threat

Robbins, J. 2022. Women in Zimbabwe protect children with secret vaccinations. Available at: https://learningenglish.voanews.com/a/6760623.html

Shanapinda, S. 2020. No, 5G radiation doesn't cause or spread the coronavirus. Saying it does is destructive. La Trobe University, 7 April.

Sibanda, F. 2022. Repositioning the agency of Rastafari in the context of COVID-19 Crisis in Zimbabwe and Malawi. In F. Sibanda, T. Muyambo & E. Chitando (Eds), *Religion and the COVID-19 Pandemic in Southern Africa*. London: Routledge, pp. 213–231.

Sibanda, F., Muyambo, T., & Chitando, E. (Eds). 2022. *Religion and the COVID-19 Pandemic in Southern Africa*. London: Routledge.

Stone, L., Gable, L., & Gingerich, T. 2009. When the Right to Health and the Right to Religion Conflict in Wayne State University Law School Legal Studies Research Paper Series No. 09-09 Available at: www.ssrn.com/link/Wayne-State-U-LEG.html

Togarasei, L. 2010. Churches for the rich? Pentecostalism and elitism. In L. Togarasei and E. Chitando (Eds), *Faith in the City: The Role and Place of Religion in Harare*. Uppsala: Swedish Science Press, pp. 19–39.

Verma, R. 2020. China's diplomacy and changing the COVID-19 narrative. *International Journal*, DOI: 10.1177/002020930054 pp.1–11.

7 Muslim Responses to COVID-19 Vaccination in Zimbabwe

A Focus on Mberengwa *ummah*

Edmore Dube

Introduction

Muslim immunization in Mberengwa, as elsewhere, is theologically guided by the infallible second source of the *Shariah* (Muslim law), the *Sunnah* (tradition) of the Prophet Muhammad. The central tradition is the proclamation by Muhammad that "To remove a harmful object from the road is an act of benefaction" (Al-Bukhari, 1996, as cited by Al-Khayat, 2004: 23). The physical act of removing objects from the environment is generalized to include all environmental health pollutants, including viruses for which immunization may be legally mandatory according to the *Shariah*. This chapter analyses the Mberengwa *ummah*'s (Muslim community) overall response to COVID-19 immunization with respect to the stated formal theological position. The analysis, however, shows that the response itself, though positive, has been based on a mosaic of reasons rather than a homogeneous theological position. Sheikhs and imams have consistently advocated for positive responses based on the national Muslim position to back immunization with their inter-religious partners. Praxis has shown that those with official duties have publicly taken doses to encourage their followers, both at national and local Mberengwa *ummah* levels. In that regard those compelled by their duties to take doses of the vaccine with little or no resort have been among the first to take the jabs. The Muslim legal or theological position has not resulted in spontaneous responses though it has been an invaluable safeguard, in terms of offering relevant justification. Some Muslims retained reservations for vaccines coming from China and India, where Muslim populations are maltreated and live in fear of decimation. That conspiracy theory has been neutralized by Muslims availing themselves for vaccination in public places where recipients were not grouped along faith lines. It was therefore difficult to target Muslims in the mixed vaccination groupings in schools, clinics and other public places. This has especially been impractical due to the comparatively small numbers of Muslims in the area covered by fieldwork. That there are twenty-one centers in the district has been due to distance rather than numbers of Muslims per se.

This research intends to delineate and explicate the Muslim responses to government calls for COVID-19 nationwide vaccination in Zimbabwe, with

DOI: 10.4324/9781003388630-7

special reference to the Mberengwa *ummah*. First, it analyses the operational framework; assessing whether Muslims set out exclusive models to fight COVID-19 as a separate entity. In that regard, it is important to evaluate their responses to overtures by other religious entities, government and the World Health Organization (WHO) to join in a monolithic approach to combat the virus through vaccination. The research employs documentary analysis to evaluate Muslim praxis at national level. This is followed by presentation of results of fieldwork among the Muslims of Mberengwa. Their motivation for immunization is analyzed both in context and in relation to the official position. Digressions from the theological framework are analyzed in terms of the dominant discourse theory as a contextual praxis variable. This is followed by an overall conclusion.

Institutional and Theological Approaches to Vaccination Mobilization

The government of Zimbabwe, like the World Health Organization (WHO), values leadership of faith communities as important in health promotion (Dube, 2022: 202). The government therefore gives religious leaders the latitude to inculcate the values necessary for the acceptance of official government health policies. It was particularly important with respect to the immunization for COVID-19, "a sickness of solitude" (Winiger, 2020: 252). Immunization was offered as the only way for the reopening of the world, and normalizing relations. UNICEF is cognizant of the fact that "faith leaders are critical partners in addressing many known barriers to the uptake of health and other essential services, including vaccines" (Maiden, 2021: 1). Religious leaders apply their sacred scriptures and traditions in ways acceptable to faith communities, in ways capable of steering communities out of pandemics and epidemics. The Quran is "revered for its overall guidance on health and disease control", particularly Surah 17:82 that refers to healing, legitimizing "all forms of surveillance meant to forestall sickness including vaccinations and lockdowns" (Dube, 2022: 203). Health is seen as both an honor to humanity and a human right (Surah 17:70) conferred onto the children of Adam by God (Rahman & Mahmud, 2014: 2). Health being a divine right makes it surpass economic enterprises. Religious leaders therefore stress the tradition of Muhammad which states that: "Wealth is of no harm to a God-fearing person, but to the God-fearing, health is better than wealth" (Ibn Majah et al., as cited by Al-Khayat, 2004: 14). Sheikhs and imams use the *hadith* (tradition) as a call for immunization, stating that health is divinely willed by God and therefore must be prioritized.

For viral diseases including COVID-19, vaccination bestows health on the people of God making it inevitable for all health-loving submitters. For that reason the Supreme Council of Islamic Affairs worked closely with the Zimbabwe COVID-19 Taskforce (Moyo, 2020), ensuring that government policies on immunization reached Muslims on time. It is interesting how Muslim leadership interrogates tradition for the salvation of the community. One good example is in the interpretation of a *hadith* exhorting the community to "keep away from a leper [one with a contagious disease] as one keeps away from a lion" (Consorti, 2020: 10). Though its straightforward interpretation is with respect to lockdowns and social distancing, religious leaders also take it to mean that immunization stays one clear of 'leprosy'. Religious leaders teach that disease is stalled by immunization which is taken as divinely willed, collapsing barriers in the smooth uptake of preventive and curative medicines. Religious leaders affect behavioral change leading to the embracing of government immunization.

Muslim authorities joined an interfaith partnership on COVID–19 immunization convened by UNICEF and Ministries of Primary and Secondary Education and Health and Child Care in association with Apostolic Women Empowerment Trust (AWET). The idea was to use the three-day workshop to harness the attention of religious leaders to support the rollout of COVID-19 vaccines (Maiden, 2021). The major religions represented included Islam, African Indigenous Religions and Christianity. These "were represented by the Zimbabwe Council of Churches, Evangelical Fellowship of Zimbabwe, Zimbabwe Catholic Bishops Conference, Seventh Day Adventist, The Supreme Council of Islamic Affairs in Zimbabwe and Zimbabwe National Association of Traditional Healers and Dare reMweya neVadzimu" (Maiden, 2021: 1). Muslim leaders were among 850 interfaith and community leaders mobilized by AWET and UNICEF's Global Faith for Positive Change Initiative to engage communities for the purposes of influencing positive attitudes toward immunization. The project that aimed at reaching out to at least five million Zimbabweans also emphasized nutrition, education and child protection. The multi-religious grouping was to target conspiracy theories spreading false anti-vaccination information responsible for the initial rampant vaccine hesitancy. Muslims were willing participants in this capacity building workshop aimed at addressing religious sensitivities, with the aim of providing fresh insights into health and healing. Leaders could then use the deed and trusted connections with their communities to move their communities forward by influencing behavioral and cultural changes in tandem with the new survival skills.

Leading by Example: National Muslim Leadership

Sheikh Ismael Duwa committed himself to lead by example. As the president of the Supreme Council of Zimbabwe, he took the first dose of the vaccine and went public about it to encourage the whole Zimbabwe *ummah* to follow his example and get vaccinated. In fact, his encouragement went beyond the *ummah* itself to generality of the Zimbabweans: "I am sharing my vaccination experience to Islamic followers and Zimbabweans at large to prove that these vaccines are safe and taking them is how we can protect our children, families and communities from this pandemic" (Maiden 2021: 1). He became a religious model for the promotion of good attitudes toward vaccination by demonstrating that the exercise was bereft of faith-related impediments and the religious fraternity could participate in the program with free conscience. Like his fellow inter-religionists he focused on official information from UNICEF and the Ministry of Health and Child Care. There have been claims that religious leaders joined the vaccination bandwagon to escape proscription from houses of worship where they get stipends, but Sheikh Duwa says they are in it for its own merits to save humanity. For that reason he was first among Muslims to get the dose and lead the rest on (Moyo, 2021). With him Muslim sheikhs and imams across the nation took the lead in vaccination and show-casing their dosages to their co-religionists and congregants.

The Ministry of Health and Child Care (MoHCC) is especially grateful to such religious leadership because "Zimbabwe continues to experience a disease burden of preventable diseases such as HIV and AIDS, tuberculosis, malaria, diarrheal diseases, and other vaccine-preventable diseases" (MoHCC and UNICEF, 2016: 13). Lessons have been learnt from West Africa with respect to Ebola vaccines:

> Evidence from the roll-out of the Ebola vaccines in West Africa suggests that the physical presence of the vaccine drives the involvement of national leadership, which trickles down to local communities. The field deployment of the experimental Ebola vaccines combined with an innovative social mobilisation and community engagement strategy overcame vaccine hesitancy in this instance.
>
> (Mudombo et al., 2021: 1)

Community involvement was one single cog that drove away vaccine hesitancy. More emphasis was placed on community leadership including religious *gurus* to drive the program forward on the basis of grassroots upwards mobility. There was clear emphasis on culturally and religious relevant knowledge. Such lessons from Ebola and subsequently from HIV and AIDS provided bases of mobilization by UNICEF and the MoHCC. In East Africa, for example, Muslim faithfuls wanted assurance from their leadership and government on the efficacy, side effects and absence of alternatives before they could embrace the COVID-19 vaccines (Tulloch, 2021). There was need for relevant knowledge and praxis by the leadership to make the rest take cue (Dereje et al., 2021). Their greatest fear surrounded the possibility of vaccines having ingredients prohibited by Islamic law (UNICEF ESARO C4D, 2020). The Zimbabwe *ummah* was in agreement with the Ethiopian *ummah* which authorized Muslim associations to release "statements to recommend immunization for COVID-19 for eligible individuals, assuring that the vaccines do not contain any human or animal ingredients" (Tulloch, 2021: 16). The Islamic Medical Association of South Africa went further by declaring vaccination obligatory in terms of Islamic statutes placing health ahead of all enterprises (Islamic Medical Association, 2021). Such positions compelled leadership to lead by example.

In Tandem with National Leadership: Mberengwa *Ummah* Praxis

Field research reveals that the Mberengwa Muslim community is relatively new. It owes its lease of life to the new inclusive approach by the government, which has seen the introduction of a new curriculum designed for Primary and Secondary schools. Armed with a new democratic constitution of 2013, the government of Zimbabwe decided to facilitate a new approach to religious pluralism. The first serious step was the opening up of the study of religions, seen in the introduction of the Family and Religious Studies (FRS) syllabus in 2017 (Zivave and Muzambi, 2022). For the first time the nomenclature of the religious studies syllabus was revolutionary. In the past names were changed but the content remained the same –Christocentric. But from 2017 inclusion became a reality both in theory and praxis. That led to the mandatory inclusive teaching of Islam, Judaism, Christianity and African Indigenous Religions (AIR). Muslims and Jews seized the opportunity to penetrate Remba communities they had been in contact with for quite some time. Their discussions pertained to their possible common 'Abrahamic' origins (Dube, 2018). Sheikh Zhou[1] describes the Mberengwa *ummah* as a fast-growing community of twenty-one centres. Seven of these (Ragonya, Mponjani, Zebra, Makereni, Gwai, Machingwe and Ghaha) have built mosques and the rest (fourteen) are tree-shed prayer centres. He admits though that the number of centers is dictated more by the spatial nature of the believers rather than their numerical implications. Though the Muslims are a cosmopolitan group of believers from various tribes, the seven sheikhs in charge of one mosque and two tree-shed centres each, are all Remba, both local and from other places like Gutu and Buhera.

The fact that the *ummah* is new has a bearing on its position on government programs. Sheikh Remba[2] maintains that Muslim prosperity at the moment lies in government protection as a relatively 'new faith' in the area. Many Christians and traditional believers are still skeptical about the plausibility of Islam as a true religion leading people to salvation. Respondents noted with concern that they were negatively reviled as "Christian apostates"[3], and "clear candidates for terrorism"[4]. Both criticisms sent the *ummah* into proof mode. Muslims set out to prove that they were not terrorists by working closely with the ruling Zimbabwe African National Union Patriotic Front (ZANU-PF). Though the seven sheikhs do not play any active roles in politics, as neutral mediators of various political persuasions that their followers might legally choose, they discourage their members from open opposition politics. Their central message is centered on the preservation of their nascent *ummah,* as not a threat to the establishment. For that reason they closely follow government programs and projects. Such programs include water provision and various vaccinations. They provide community boreholes wherever they build mosques. Zhou[5] contended that "close Muslim compliance with government vaccination programs, in particular secures the *ummah* as a close partner of government". This eliminates any chance of them being counted among terrorists and saboteurs.

Interviewed Muslims were eager to prove beyond reasonable doubt that they had been vaccinated for COVID-19. Proof of vaccination cards was often emphasized with no prompting whatsoever. Children in the vaccination bracket (twelve years and above) were invited to contribute verbally that they had been vaccinated with the encouragement of their parents. Some of them, however, noted that they would not have volunteered on their own to get vaccinated because of misinformation peddled by some groups pertaining to dangers associated with vaccination. Such misinformation was readily available on WhatsApp and other social platforms, as well as oràl discussions at school and in play centers. They noted that both their sheikhs and parents led by example which encouraged them. They were also aware that national Muslim leadership was also in support of the program and had been vaccinated prior to their sheikhs, imams and parents. Their sheikhs and imams had been workshopped and made aware that the vaccines had nothing *haram* (illegal by Muslim law) in them. One vaccinated student still doubted vaccines from India which was fighting Muslims in Kashmir on the borders of India and Pakistan. He thought Indians might take aim at Muslims. He was only pacified by the fact that Muslims were not vaccinated at mosques where he feared Muslim culling. Instead they were vaccinated at the high school where the population of Muslims was insignificant and difficult to target. In fact, a single dose of vaccine covered two recipients at random. In that regard no one would take chances hoping to harm a Muslim in the process. Some were also comforted by the enduring relations tying India and China to Zimbabwe. These would make it difficult for these countries to transfer their domestic conflicts to Zimbabwe. That would estrange their relations and cut the two Asian giants from coveted Zimbabwe raw materials.

Muslims were confident that none among them had suffered apparent side effects to date. Abdullah[6] was jubilant that both men and women had successfully set aside claims that vaccines resulted in infertility. Vaccinated married women had given birth to healthy children in the aftermath of vaccination. He counted no less than seven healthy deliveries, just off hand. That further bolstered the *ummah*'s commitment to vaccination, as conspiracy theories were tumbling one after another to the advantage of not just Muslim citizens.

Muslim Vaccination and Problems of the Dominant Discourse

Results of fieldwork in Mberengwa show that though Muslims may have been theologically prepared for vaccination, there were certainly other dominant pressures that forced them to act in certain extra compliant ways. Those pressures are discussed here as "dominant discourses". The expression itself emanates from the field of media criticism, and is attributed to two theorists of communication, Michel Foucault (1980) and Stuart Hall (1997) (Front Row Crew Forum, 2013). The dominant discourse itself is created by the powerful, making it the acceptable way of saying or conceiving something due excessive repetition orally, literally and behaviorally. In other words, it is the spoken, written or expected behavioral response to particular issues of importance to a particular community. Fleming (2019: 1) puts it succinctly as follows: "dominant discourse is a way of speaking or behaving on any given topic – it is the language and actions that appear most prevalently within a given society. These behaviors and patterns of speech and writing reflect the ideologies of those who have the most power in the society." The power dynamics in this definition are very important when discussing a dominant discourse.

The dominant discourse "embodies socialization by the dominant or decision-making group. Dominant discourse gives us the prevailing 'accepted' rules of everyday living as practiced by our decision-makers. Dominant discourse rarely includes the perspective of the Other, the non-power holding Other" (Front Row Crew Forum, 2013: 1). Its exclusive 'othering' of the supposed non-compliant is the subject of the post modernism and the critical theory which question compartmentalization and divisions within specific groupings within individual communities. The questioning is based on the fact that the dominant discourse may develop into propaganda that tends to limits civil liberties of some groups within the same community. In the 1930s it actually resulted in the Jewish Holocaust in which over six million Jews are alleged to have died at Nazi German gas chambers. The Jews were accused of taking over businesses leaving the indigenous German population descending into acute poverty. Some readers may be familiar with Operation Dudula in South Africa, a xenophobic movement against 'illegal' African immigration. Operation Dudula especially targets Zimbabweans and to some extent Mozambicans for taking over menial jobs at a lower labour cost than South Africans. The dominant discourse cascaded by the operation has to do with the expulsion of African immigrants, as a way of returning livelihoods to indigenous South Africans.

The argument here is that, as elsewhere, the othering of Muslims as potential terrorists in Mberengwa has the potential of developing into physical violence. Its short-term result has been to make the nascent Muslim *ummah* extra compliant. The question is whether it will always have the same effect. This is particularly because the discourse makes painful allegations regarding interaction between people of different religious persuasions. The foregoing has shown that the tendency of the dominant discourse is highlighting a particular issue and making people believe it. Two issues were prominent in the Mberengwa *ummah*. One was that Muslims were potential terrorists/saboteurs, and the other was that they were outright Christian apostates. Though both were advanced by Christians, the first one was very political and Muslim leadership was worried about such labeling. Such labeling made the *ummah* afraid of the state rather than Christians propagators. This is because the state approach to any alleged saboteurs has been vindictive and severe (Ndlovu-Gatsheni, 2017; Raftopoulos and Savage, 2005). The allegations limited Muslim civil liberties to openly fraternize with political persuasions of their choices. Open association with opposition political outfits might be interpreted as a precursor for open terrorism to sabotage government programs, leading to regime change.

The narrative around "regime change" is used by the ruling elite to inhibit political opposition and to proscribe any members deemed to have potential to challenge the government even within legal boundaries (Tarusarira, 2016). To avoid such reading Muslims have been positively ready to prove their compliance with government vaccination programs. This has been clear at both institutional and family levels.

Rezaei et al. (2019) maintain that the tendency is worse off when propagated by electronic and print media rather than being dominated by the oral perspective as witnessed in Mberengwa. Media, especially online newspapers, has been misappropriated by the powerful to propagate negative perceptions of Muslims since the 9/11 bombing of the United States' twin towers of the World Trade Center by al-Qaeda terrorists. The emergence of the "so-called Islamic terrorist groups, has turned the focus largely on Islam and Muslims" (Rezaei et al., 2019: 55). The Muslims in Mberengwa have not escaped the noose, albeit on a micro scale. This is coupled by the fact that Zimbabwe mass media is not overtly against Muslim faith. This is probably because such Muslim nations as Iran, Dubai, Kuwait and Malaysia, among others, have been our political all-weather friends for years. Otherwise the media has a tendency of positive presentation of the powerful and negative presentation of the Other. This is not to say that oral presentation does not do the same. Christians in Mberengwa presented themselves as enduring faithful monotheists, and Muslims as fickle apostates. This, however, would be different if the media in all its modes was seized with the issue of selectively portraying Muslims in the negative. Modern media is more incisive in "public's consensus management, distortion of data, manipulation of the news, [and] brainwashing individuals" (Rezaei et al., 2019: 56). Such a scenario limits the chances of self-actualization of the Other. From the foregoing, Muslims in Mberengwa represent the Other despite tacit constitutional and political support. That Muslims have tended to identify with the ruling/powerful makes them darling friends of the ruling party which tolerates praise, but negates any criticism as a regime change agenda sponsored by outsiders (Zimbabwe Catholic Bishops Conference, 2020). Muslims are therefore between the rock (ruling elite) and the hard place (competing religious persuasions). To survive in this context Muslims have decided to identify with the former, by openly supporting vaccination together with their families. In this regard, it could be not an exaggeration to say that for Muslims in Mberengwa, COVID-19 vaccination acceptance is a vaccination of expedience. Meanwhile Christians, as fervent supporters of a dominant discourse based on the application of the Judeo-Christian template, have remained seized with criticism of local Muslims. Christians are critical of religious persuasions not in tandem with the Biblical Judeo-Christian template (Dube, 2017). The template judges religions based on their agreement with Biblical presentation of salvation, which Muslims criticize as corrupted.

It is important not to blame those who accuse Muslims of potential terrorism and recession into paganism. They were themselves cognitively under the control of the powerful. The said control manifests itself in cognition in order not only to restrict freedom but also to exercise a huge impact on public opinion. Today, this control is indeed largely in the form of cognitive control being enacted by persuasion, dissimulation or manipulation as strategic means to manipulate and alternate public opinion for the sake of own interest.

(Rezaei et al., 2019: 56)

The cognitive takeover has made non-Muslims take for granted that Muslims are fundamentalists, aggressive terrorists, intolerant and violent. This narrative has been used to inhibit Muslim evangelism in Mberengwa. This new narrative is despite the fact that for centuries Muslims have been viewed in the Western media as ruthless slavers, anachronistic and ignorant (Esposito, 1992). Of course the concepts of anachronism and ignorance still survive in claims of regression into paganism or apostasy for which they have been accused in Mberengwa. The Mberengwa Muslims, like their counterparts in the various parts of the global village, "have attempted to clarify their worldview by distinguishing themselves from the extremist groups who in reality do not even remotely represent the 1.4 billion Muslims in the world, the majority of Muslims are bearing the brunt of these isolated terrorist acts" (Rezaei et al., 2019: 56). Innocent Mberengwa Muslims bear the brunt of labeling being fronted by Western media and local Christians using the Judeo-Christian template.

Conclusion

Muslim response to the government-led COVID19 vaccination program was in tandem with both Muslim theological underpinnings and contextual demands for compliance and survival. Theologically, vaccination was acceptable on the basis of the *hadith* rendering the ridding of the environment of pollutants as divinely ordained. Pollutants were read to include viruses for which vaccination was taken as mandatory. Muslim scholars at national level offered assurance that vaccines were safe. They were free of anything prohibited by the *Shariah*. To prove this point beyond doubt they went public about their own vaccination, and inducted those below them to do the same. They also made synergies with other religions for a formidable interreligious campaign meant to reach five of the ten million citizens targeted by government.

At the grassroots the dominant discourse enhanced compliance in a manner that can be called 'progress by compulsion'. This is despite the operational framework hinged on the *Shariah,* which was already in place. The dominant discourse bent on othering Muslims, tended to reduce Islam to violence, aggression and terrorism. This claim by Christians was meant to thwart Muslim evangelization. The Christian reading scaffold by the Judeo-Christian template tended to dismiss all religious persuasions not in tandem with the Biblical rendering of salvation. To escape the noose of proscription by government, Muslims increased their compliance with the demands for vaccination and were ready to publicize their proof at the slightest prompting. They desisted from publicly fraternizing with opposition political parties in order to receive favorable ratings from the ruling elite. They were prepared to sacrifice their civil liberties regarding freedom of association, as a way of earning protection for their nascent Mberengwa *ummah.* Association with the opposition might earn them the terrorism and regime change tag not favorable for their existence. Their idea was not just to do what was right, but to be seen doing it.

In the end Muslims celebrated the safety guaranteed by the way government carried out vaccination in public places. That approach dealt blows to conspiracy theories surrounding vaccination as a way of culling Muslims by Chinese and Indians. It was extremely difficult to target Muslims in public considering their small numbers. Results also showed that claims of causing infertility were fallacious. Vaccinated couples were blessed with healthy babies. The practical disapproval of conspiracy theories gave further impetus to the vaccination drive. By the time vaccination included twelve-year-olds, Muslims had stopped worrying about conspiracy theories. Praxis was clearly the best way of burying conspiracy theories.

Notes

1 Sheikh Zhou, V. Interviewed in Mposi chiefdom of Mberengwa district, 2022.
2 Sheikh Remba, T. Interviewed in Mposi chiefdom of Mberengwa district, 2022.
3 Aisha, P. Interviewed in Mposi chiefdom of Mberengwa district, 2022.
4 Taibu, M. Interviewed in Mposi chiefdom of Mberengwa district, 2022.
5 Sheikh Zhou, V. Interviewed in Mposi chiefdom of Mberengwa district, 2022.
6 Abdullah. Interviewed in Mposi chiefdom of Mberengwa district, 2022.

References

Al-Bukhari, M. 1996. *Sahih.* Riyadh: Darussalam.
Al-Khayat, M.H. 2004. Health as a human right in Islam. *WHO Regional Office for the Eastern Mediterranean.* Cairo: Harmony.
Consorti, P. 2020. Introduction. In P. Consorti, Pierluigi (Ed.), *Law, Religion and Covid-19 Emergency.* Pisa: DiReSom, pp. 7–11.
Dereje, N., Tesfaye, A., Tamene, B., Alemeshet, D., Abe, H., Tesfa, N., Gedion, S., Biruk, T., and Lakew, Y. 2021. COVID-19 vaccine hesitancy in Addis Ababa, Ethiopia: A mixed-methods study [Preprint]. *Public and Global Health,* accessed May 7, 2022, from https://doi.org/10.1101/2021.02.25.21252443
Dube, E. 2017. The Great Zimbabwe monuments and challenges in African heritage management. In M.C. Green, R.I.J. Hackett, L. Hansen, and F. Venter (Eds), *Religious Pluralism, Heritage and Social Development in Africa.* Stellenbosch: African Sun Media, pp. 221–237.
Dube, E. 2018. Religions and insecurities: Heritage contestations and religious praxes in Mberengwa and Masvingo, Zimbabwe. In A. Nhemachena & M. Mawere (Eds), *Thinking Security in an Emergent New World Order: Retracing the Contours for Africa's Future.* Bamenda: Langaa Research and Publishing, pp. 237–258.
Dube, E. 2022. The influence of health perceptions on Zimbabwe Muslim responses to COVID-19 restrictions over Ramadan, pilgrimages and funeral rites in 2020.

In F. Sibanda, T. Muyambo, and E. Chitando (Eds), *Religion and the COVID-19 Pandemic in Southern Africa.* London: Routledge, pp. 202–212. DOI: 10.4324/9781003241096-14.

Esposito, J.L. 1992. *The Islamic Threat: Myth or Reality?* London: Oxford University Press.

Fleming, E. 2019. What does dominant discourse mean? *SidmartinBio: Wide Base of Knowledge*, accessed May 10, 2022, from www.sidmartinbio.org/what-does-dominant-discourse-mean/

Foucault, M. 1980. 'Truth and Power.' *Power/Knowledge: Selected Interviews and Other Writings 1972–1977.* New York: Vintage Books.

Front Row Crew Forum. 2013. Dominant discourses and dis-empowerment. Accessed May 8, 2022, from https://forum.frontrowcrew.com/discussion/9339/dominant-discourses-and-dis-empowerment

Hall, S. 1997. *Representation: Cultural Representations and Signifying Practices.* London: Sage Publications & Open University.

The Herald. 2013. *Sikombela declared national monument.* Published August 28, 2013. www.herald.co.zw/sikombela-declared-national-monument/

Islamic Medical Association. 2021. *Position Statement of the Islamic Medical Association of South Africa [IMASA]–COVID-19 Vaccines–IMA SA*, accessed February 28, 2022, from https://ima-sa.co.za/position-statement-of-the-islamic-medical-association-of-south-africa-imasa-covid-19-vaccines/

Maiden, J. 2021. Zimbabwe's religious leaders increase efforts to tackle COVID-19 and support vaccines. *UNICEF Zimbabwe,* 5 May, accessed May 7, 2022, from www.unicef.org/zimbabwe/press-releases/zimbabwes-religious-leaders-increase-efforts-tackle-covid-19-and-support-vaccines

Moyo, J. 2020. Zimbabwe: Villagers cancel ritual of meeting dead spirits. *AA World-Africa*, April 21, 2020, viewed May 31, 2021, from www.aa.com.tr/en/africa/zimbabwe-villagers-cancel-ritual-of-meeting-dead-spirits-/1812480

Moyo, J. 2021. Once-skeptical congregants in Zimbabwe scramble for COVID vaccines, Anadolu Agency Website, 11 September, accessed January 10, 2022, from www.aa.com.tr/en/latest-on-coronavirus-outbreak/once-skeptical-congregants-in-zimbabwe-scramble-for-covid-vaccines/2361834

Ministry of Health and Child Welfare Zimbabwe & UNICEF. 2016. *Factors Influencing Vaccine Hesitancy and Immunization Coverage in Zimbabwe: A Rapid Assessment.* www.unicef.org/zimbabwe/media/356/file/Factors%20Influencing%20Vaccine%20Hesitancy%20and%20Immunization%20Coverage%20in%20Zimbabwe.pdf. Accessed 17 June 2023.

Ndlovu-Gatsheni, S.J. (Ed.). 2017. *Joshua Mqabuko Nkomo of Zimbabwe. African Histories and Modernities.* Palgrave Macmillan.

Raftopoulos, B. and Savage, T. 2005. (Eds). *Zimbabwe: Injustice and Political Reconciliation.* Harare: Weaver Press.

Rahman, A.A. and Mahmud, A. 2014. A review of the Islamic approach in public health practices. *International Journal of Public Health and Clinical Sciences*, 1(2), 1–13.

Rezaei, S., Kobari, K., and Salami. A. 2019. The portrayal of Islam and Muslims in Western Media: A critical discourse analysis. *Cultura. International Journal of Philosophy of Culture and Axiology*, 16(1), 55–73.

Tarusarira, J. 2016. An emergent consciousness of the role of Christianity on Zimbabwe's political field: A case of non-doctrinal religio-political actors. *Journal for the Study of Religion*, 29(2), 56–68.

Tulloch, O. 2021. 'Data synthesis: COVID-19 vaccine perceptions in Africa. *Social and Behavioural Science.* March 2020–March 2021, pp. 1–35, accessed January 5, 2022, from https://opendocs.ids.ac.uk/opendocs/bitstream/handle/20.500.12413/16580/Data%20Synthesis_Covid19%20Vaccine%20Perceptions%20Africa_Social_Behavioural%20Science%20Data%20Mar%202020-Mar%202021.pdf?sequence=3&isAllowed=y

UNICEF ESARO C4D. 2020. *Digital and Social Media Monitor on Immunization in Eastern and Southern Africa,* Rep Nr 2 (December 1–31, 2020) (No. 2). UNICEF ESARO.

Winiger, F. 2020. More than an intensive care phenomenon: Religious communities and the WHO guidelines for Ebola and Covid-19. *Spiritual Care,* 9(3), 245–255. https://doi.org/10.1515/spircare-2020-0066

ZCBC. 2020. *The March Is Not Ended.* Harare: Social Communications Department.

Zivave, W. and Muzambi, P. 2022. Suspicions, fears and misgivings around the family and religious studies syllabus: Lessons for Zimbabwe. In E. Dube and P. Muzambi (Eds), *Religious Practice in a Plural Milieu: Identity, Gender, Justice and the Environment.* Johannesburg: UNISA Press, pp. 6–21.

8 Migrant Communities and COVID-19 Vaccination at Tongogara Refugee Camp in Zimbabwe

Wisdom Sibanda

Introduction

This chapter seeks to explore the responses of women refugees of the Johanne Marange Apostolic Church (JMAC) to the mandatory vaccination programme introduced by the host government against the backdrop of religious beliefs and individual standpoints at the Tongogara Refugee Camp (TRC) in Chipinge, Zimbabwe. Whereas there is an abundance of literature linking religion and vaccination hesitancy on the global scale during the COVID-19 pandemic, there is scant literature on the responses of refugee women to COVID-19 vaccination. It is within this context that this chapter interrogates the relationship between religion and women refugee responses to COVID-19 vaccination in a refugee camp in Zimbabwe. Notwithstanding the fact that the government's priority is to attain herd immunity, without leaving anyone behind, vaccination hesitancy and general apathy toward inoculation remain a thorn in the side for the United Nations High Commissioner for Refugees (UNHCR) and its partners in the camp.

There has been a tendency to overlook the role played by women in advocating cultural and religious campaigns at community level as they are often left out of decision making and planning meetings (Bulle, 1999). In most societies, women have primary responsibility for management of household welfare and health (Ananga, 2015), yet their needs, priorities and voices are often missing from policies designed to protect and assist them. The relevance of refugee women in community health activities had not been widely acknowledged in previous studies which were largely gender neutral (Skider, 2010; Arabi, 2019; Wangdah et al., 2015), hence it then became essential that an investigation be conducted from a women-specific perspective that seeks to establish how and to what extent the Johanne Marange Apostolic sect refugee women are responding to the government-initiated vaccination programs in TRC. There is also a cultural and religious assumption that men are ideal leaders, given the malevolence and domination at household level based on the postulation that women are second-class citizens who cannot make their own decisions (Puri et al., 2020). Women also suffer the burden of health compromises as the need to look after the house and care for the sick rests on their shoulders. Thus, these

DOI: 10.4324/9781003388630-8

gender inequalities at the societal level, as well as harmful social norms that discriminate against women and girls, lead to gender based violence (GBV) exacerbated by emergencies (Peterman et al., 2020). This makes the Feminist Political Ecology (FPE) approach to research an appropriate framework to this study as it gives precedence to women while looking at their relationship with men against the backdrop of religion. Before considering the theoretical framework and research methodology, the identity of the study participants is covered first.

JMAC Women at Tongogara Refugee Camp: An Overview

It is strategic to provide some historical background on women refugees belonging to Johanne Marange Apostolic Church at TRC. It is essential to situate their membership in the wider context of the Church itself. Notably, the JMAC was founded by Johanne Momberume Marange as a separatist religious movement from the United Methodist Church in Manicaland province around 1932. As noted by Sibanda, Makahamadze and Maposa (2008), the founder saw a vision and pronounced oracles to people of his community and ultimately the movement spread to other Southern African countries such as Malawi, Mozambique, the Democratic Republic of Congo, Angola, and Zambia, among others. This list of countries to which the movement has spread resonates with the countries of origin of the women refugee participants selected from seven major countries present in the camp (Democratic Republic of Congo, Rwanda, Burundi, Somalia, Ethiopia, Eritrea, and Mozambique). The Church holds its Annual Paschal Festivals in Marange attended by local and international members from Africa and beyond. It is important to note that some of the women were members of the JMAC even before they had come to settle in Zimbabwe as refugees. Yet others joined the Church at TRC due to their social condition with the hope that it would take away their sorrow and memories of losing their loved ones due to war in their original countries. In addition, there is quite a good number of women refugees in the camp, with the biggest numbers being from the DRC, Mozambique, Rwanda, and Burundi. Their religiosity is partly evidenced by some of them joining others for their annual festival in Bocha, Marange area after getting permission from the Department of Social Welfare. Finally, the women are in the majority of membership in the JMAC partly because they operated in polygamous frameworks and pursued self-reliance economic activities in the camp such as trading homemade artifacts to supplement the material and financial handouts from the UNHCR, the government, and local NGOs.

Theoretical Framework and Research Methodology

Theoretically, the study is informed by the Feminist Political Ecology framework to research and the appropriation of religion to the vaccination response by Johanne Marange Apostolic sect refugee women at TRC. The research is rooted in a FPE perspective that connects gender in vaccination hesitancy by women and theories of religion that bring unequal power relations between men and women, whereby men dominate/exploit women (Wilson et al., 2018). Since this chapter focuses on the pathways theorized to have a direct relationship with COVID-19 vaccination hesitancy, issues such as inability of women to temporarily escape abusive partners, virus-specific sources of violence and general response, remain topical (Kabonesa et al., 2020). The framework resonates well with the focus of this chapter as its intent on addressing the environmental crisis, though not specifically "religious", offers some challenging perspectives for reflecting on traditional Christian doctrines of creation and redemption (Sundberg, n.d.). If it is Christianity's anthropocentric bias which is responsible for the consequent subjection and domination of nature, it is imperative for Christian theology to re-examine the foundation of these doctrines (Jeneen, 2011). Hence related to philosophy of religion, feminist standpoint epistemology involves thinking from the perspective of women who have been oppressed by specific monotheistic religious beliefs. Anderson et al. (2019) challenge both the privileged model of God as a disembodied person and the related model of reason as neutral, objective, and free of bias and desire.

From a historical, political, and ecological perspective shaping our understanding of nature, religion, humanity, and identity, Bauman (2014) collapses the boundaries separating male from female, biology from machine, human from more than human, and religion from science. He encourages readers to embrace cosmopolitanism and the inherent fluctuations of an open, evolving global community. Through the use of a FPE framework to illustrate the gendered power dynamics that intercede the knowledge, valuation, and use of indigenous knowledge and religion, this study describes how women's everyday practices, traditions, and resistance strategies are being deployed to promote religious knowledge (Guy-Antaki et al., 2016; Starke, 2016). The interdependencies between women and men alongside gender differences position women's relationship with nature, instead of grounding women's relationship with the "material, historical, socio-cultural, and political realities of specific places" (Sulley, 2018). It therefore entails that gender intersects with class, age, and ethnicity to influence the relationships people establish with nature and the way they use natural resources (Adams et al., 2018; Sundberg, n.d.). FPE assists in giving women a voice to speak about their situation in their own words to challenge simplistic analyses of the victimization of women or their valorization as symbols of resistance (Beuchler et al., 2015). Such methodologies combine political engagement, participatory approaches, and critical analysis relevant to everyday lives (Rocheleau, 2008; Clement et al., 2019). Thus, the theoretical framework is justified by the way women negotiate their marginal positionality by creating opportunities to continue their religious practices coupled with health knowledge. Hence, the need to close the gap on religion and vaccination hesitancy and apathy by Johanne Marange Apostolic refugee women in TRC, has been the reason for using this framework.

Methodology

The study is expected to contribute scientific knowledge on how migrant communities respond to the mandatory COVID-19 vaccination program being implemented in TRC, providing valuable feedback on how it impacts their health and socio-cultural well-being. It will also proffer significant policy recommendations that will contribute to the provision of administering the jab and shed light on how women groups can contribute to the attainment of total vaccination in the camp. This is a qualitative research that focuses on women's experiences in TRC as they grapple with an opportunity to get vaccinated at the expense of their religious beliefs. The section will give an outline of the data collection methods adopted and the data analysis, as well as the research method to the study.

Data Collection and Analysis

The research method revealed how women refugees grapple with an opportunity to access the COVID-19 vaccine at the sympathy of their religious beliefs in TRC. All interviews and focus group discussions (FGDs) were conducted in confidentiality, and the names of the respondents were withheld by mutual consent. For accountability and to ensure the reliability of the results, verification of the findings was done by triangulation between different types of sources that include the key informants, participant interviewees, and FGD participants. Data was coded according to emerging themes that include accessibility, hesitancy to vaccination, gender equality, and gender-based violence. A thematic approach to data analysis was also adopted which entailed sifting of the collected data according to the emerging themes. A FPE approach to data analysis was also applied as it gave a gendered perspective to the analyzed data. The reading of transcripts was done several times (on average ten times) in order to formulate the themes from the coded data. Data was also obtained from relevant literature on vaccine hesitancy and religion, and the FPE theoretical framework. The interviews usually lasted 45 to 90 minutes, with the proceedings being recorded, noted, and transcribed for analysis.

Qualitative Research: The Use of Interview Guides for Data Collection

The study is based on field research undertaken in TRC between August 2019 and December 2021. A pilot study to test the interview questions was conducted in September 2018, as the researcher was still gathering information on the topic, with the final guide being approved by the Ethics Committee of the University of the Free State in July 2019. Along with secondary data, information was collected through sixty-five household interviews conducted in the nine residential sections and five in-depth interviews with key informants, local NGOs (World Vision and Terres Des Homes), and government representatives (Department of Social Welfare, Department of Public Works and Department of Public Health). A total of eight Focus Group Discussions (FGDs) were conducted with sixty-eight participants selected from seven major countries present in the camp (Democratic Republic of Congo, Rwanda, Burundi, Somalia, Ethiopia, Eritrea, and Mozambique). In-depth interviewing was done with key informants such as the Camp Administrator, Engineer, and three NGO staff members. The study had to use purposive sampling to select households according to country of origin and to get equal representation from all sections.

Research Questions

As a qualitative research that endeavors to explore the extent to which the Johanne Marange Apostolic group refugee women access and respond to the COVID-19 vaccination program in TRC, this study gave priority to women's direct experiences. The study aims to respond to two key research questions and to contextualize the findings based on FPE framework and literature on women's access and response to the vaccination exercise against the backdrop of religion and individual standpoint. The two research questions are:

1. What is the response of women refugees to the rollout of the mandatory COVID-19 vaccination program against the backdrop of religion in TRC?
2. How did gender inequality impact on women's religious beliefs and need for moral freedom in the face of COVID-19 vaccination in the TRC?

General Overview: Responses to COVID-19 Vaccination

This section will give a general overview of refugee responses to COVID-19 vaccination worldwide and then home in on the Zimbabwean scenario where TRC is the case study. Refugees are people who have been forced to leave their home country and cross national borders in search of safety. Refugees often leave their homes to escape war, famine, or persecution (UNHCR, 2020). A person becomes a refugee after formally applying for asylum and being granted refugee status (Saiffe et al., 2021). There are approximately 25 million refugees worldwide, most of whom are women and children (UNHCR, 2021). The World Health Organization (WHO) has promised to assist governments who host refugees to ensure they access COVID-19 vaccines like nationals, eliminating the xenophobic discourse around migrants and infectious disease that alienates them from health systems (Owens, 2021). In the midst of public health crises, the needs of vulnerable populations such as refugees have been neglected or overlooked (Gautham et al., 2021), thereby exposing them to the social and economic disparities brought about by the pandemic. However, the vaccination campaigns have been met with some positive and negative outcomes surrounding hesitancy and misinformation on the effects/impacts of the jab by some religious sectors. Chief among those peddling such malignant information are the Muslims, and some Protestant Churches around the world who believe that the vaccine has some preservatives from pork which is not acceptable in their religions (Sachedina et al., 2020).

Vaccine hesitancy can drive outbreaks of vaccine-preventable diseases leading to slower vaccination rates that hinder the attainment and sustainability of herd immunity (Peterman et al., 2020). The anxiety in vaccination hesitancy is revealed in religiosity; studies have shown that religious teachings give priority to prayers over medicine, thus resulting in vaccination hesitancy among devotees (Garcia et al., 2021; Lucia et al., 2020). This is coupled with the lack of appropriate knowledge of the available vaccines, thus making devotees accept alternative approaches such as use of holy water and prayers to treat diseases, fearing vaccination may lead to the death of their children (Griffiths, 2021). In the case of other religious beliefs such as Islam, vaccines with pork derivatives are prohibited (Grabenstein et al., 2021; Garcia et al., 2021). Research has revealed that the 2003–2004 polio vaccine boycott in Nigeria, resistance toward the oral cholera vaccination in Mozambique, and continued objections to routine childhood vaccinations by members of the Apostolic group in Zimbabwe all illustrate the negative public health impact of vaccine hesitancy (Ekwebelem et al., 2021; McAbee et al., 2021). Dhama et al. (2021) opine that resistance to vaccination is one of the major threats that directly impacts global health as it challenges the ability to eradicate infectious diseases and achieve significant herd immunity through vaccination.

The COVID-19 pandemic threatens the health and well-being of refugees by exacerbating the existing social disparities that these populations face (Turner-Musa et al., 2020). The unique challenges that refugee communities face in the midst of global health crises require specifically targeted culturally sensitive interventions (Haq et al., 2020). Such information is required to plan and implement effective response efforts as COVID-19 and its related developments such as lockdowns and mandatory vaccination are being imposed. Studies have shown that vaccination campaigns were effective for infectious, emerging, and lethal pathogens. This was the case with the Spanish flu epidemic of 1918 (Card and Ladaria, 2020; Garcia et al., 2021). While attempts are being made to stop the coronavirus from spreading, the vaccine is the only way to stop the ongoing pandemic (Caserotti et al., 2021; Garcia et al., 2021). However, not everyone wants to get vaccinated as some people are reluctant to be vaccinated and could delay or forego COVID-19 vaccination completely. Such actions are not circumscribed to any specific country, community, or religion, but are a global phenomenon (Lucia et al., 2020). Lebano et al. (2020) opine that discrimination, fear, and lack of trust in authorities means several thousand migrants do not engage in health systems, an important concern during a global pandemic. Around the world, migrants, asylum seekers, and refugees are among the social groups most affected by the pandemic (Graffith et al., 2021), disproportionately suffering from the perceived danger of vaccines, the associated risks and seriousness of the illness, affects vaccination complacency (Larson et al., 2011). Astonishingly, it is to be noted that the success of various clinical trials to elucidate the effectiveness of vaccine against COVID-19 has led to significant complacency by lowering the expected risk and seriousness of illness (Dhama et al., 2021; Finney Rutten et al., 2021).

Tongogara Refugee Camp: An Overview

Tongogara Refugee Camp (TRC) is situated in the South Western part of Chipinge District in Zimbabwe. The camp was established in 1981 to house over 60,000 Mozambican refugees fleeing the Mozambique National Resistance (RENAMO) insurgency. Their stay in TRC was until the Mozambique Liberation Front (FRELIMO) and RENAMO ceasefire in 1992 when they returned to Mozambique leading to the camps' final shutdown in May 1995 (UNHCR/WFP, 2014). The political tensions in the Great Lakes Region caused the camp to be reopened in 1998. Today the camp hosts over 16,000 refugees from Ethiopia, Somalia, Eritrea, South Sudan, Burundi, Rwanda, Democratic Republic of Congo, and lately Mozambique. People of different social, cultural, and religious backgrounds have been grouped together in the camp. The camp is run by the United Nations Humanitarian Commission for Refugees (UNHCR), an arm of the United Nations, together with the Department of Social Welfare (DSW), who represent the host Government, Zimbabwe (UNHCR/WFP 2014). The camp is divided into nine residential sections. Initially refugees were settled according to their country of origin, but with the continued influx they are now settled as they come.

A game reserve and Sabi River border the camp to the west where predators, poaching game, are prevalent to the south, the camp is bordered by Taguta Farm (the owner of Johanne Marange Apostolic Church), hence the influx of refugees seeking divine intervention. A number of researchers have carried out research on vaccination and immunization in refugee settings, but little has been done in the area of women access to vaccination (Dhama et al., 2021; Soares et al., 2021; Finney Rutten et al., 2021; MacDonald, 2015, Dala et al., 2015; Gautham et al., 2021), in Zimbabwe.

Although vaccines have a long history and have been demonstrated as an effective way to combat outbreaks and the only efficient and reliable method for disease prevention (Garcia et al., 2021), some religious leaders still fear being vaccinated. However, there are no studies in Zimbabwe, specifically from TRC, addressing the response of migrant communities on the impact of vaccination against the pandemic as regards religion. This chapter will therefore endeavor to explore the responses of the Johanne Marange Apostolic group women refugees, a predominant religion among the refugees from Mozambique and DRC in the camp. This is despite the fact that the refugee camp is a cosmopolitan society that brings together people of various cultures and religious backgrounds. Interestingly, with their diverse cultural and religious context, they have grouped under the Johanne Marange Apostolic church by default. The desire to get protection from the evil spirits and the trauma of the past haunting them, has led to the need to join the church. The group has gained prominence ahead of other Christian doctrines because Noah Taguta, the leader of the Johanne Marange Apostolic group, owns a farm that borders the camp to the south. The church of white garments, as they are affectionately known, does not discriminate on ethnic grounds but welcomes converts from all over the world.

Women in the Johanne Marange Apostolic Church are guided by their Church's doctrines in their way of living, and this case study incognizant of the high vaccination hesitancy rates of mothers, analyzed and revealed that women's knowledge, attitude, and perception toward vaccination is guided by their husbands. Loyalty to your husband is viewed as respect while others take it to be suppression. Men in the sect are sexually dominant over their wives as they determine their day-to-day lives to the extent that women suffer to please them at the expense of their health. Thus, religion has effected the infringement of women's human rights in the camp as they are denied the chance to be vaccinated against the deadly pandemic, hence the need to revise the Church's doctrines. It is imperative to note that the government, UNHCR, and civil society organizations (CSOs) are working hard to ensure that refugees in camps are safe from COVID-19 by further scaling up water and sanitation activities. However, despite efforts to provide refugees with extra soap to reinforce personal hygiene practices, while enticing them to get vaccinated, this is usually diverted by men for personal gain, thereby fueling gender-based violence in the camp.

Response of Women Refugees to Vaccination

In TRC, most immediate religious rulings were sought regarding attending services which are usually open-air and the holding of mass congregational prayers by the Johanne Marange church. Findings also show that the leading religious authorities, together with law enforcement agents, supported the lockdown policies and advised people to keep away from religious institutions and observe strict rules against spreading the virus. Even the annual pilgrimage or *gungano* in Bocha, Marange area was cancelled due to the pandemic. The church has a long history of abstinence from immunization and vaccination. However, acceptance of vaccination by the Johanne Marange apostolic group is uncertain. Research findings show that this group is suspicious of the efficacy or potential side effects of the vaccines. They believe that Johanne Marange, or *Mutumwa*, will reveal the solution to the vaccine through his prophets in the camp. One church leader in the camp has this to say:

> As apostolic groups we shun vaccinations programs because of our religious beliefs. Our religion has diverse beliefs but as for the pandemic, we are awaiting a revelation from God's Messiah, Johanne, as to whether we should be vaccinated or not. We have survived so many pandemics that include measles, but our God has seen us through. It is religious folly to believe that the virus has a medical cure. Only God has the answer to this pandemic. We have avoided social and religious gatherings in keeping with

the mandatory social distancing and covering of the face outside the shrine. When in the holy ground, there is no need for masking-up or social distancing as one will be in the presence of God.

[Interview Participant]

The controversy surrounding the COVID-19 vaccine has been significant, with conspiracy theories abounding. Such theories include the apocalyptic theory that the COVID-19 vaccine is the "mark of the beast", a sign of the end times and a symbol of alignment with the Antichrist (Sachedina, 2021). They associate the vaccine and the pandemic with the Bible which they do not believe in, as they claim Johanne never read the Bible. This fear has driven some members of the Apostolic group to shun vaccination as they might be "corrupted". This has led to hesitancy and resistance among members of the Johanne Marange group in the camp as they remain unmoved. Most members fear the vaccine as they associate it with satanism. Even the camp health department cannot convince them to be vaccinated unless one of their leaders is given the nod from Johanne Marange.

Research has revealed that such Apostolic groups that infuse traditional beliefs into a Pentecostal doctrine are among the most skeptical in Zimbabwe when it comes to COVID-19 vaccines, as they strongly mistrust modern medicine. The group adheres to a doctrine that demands followers avoid medicines and medical care and instead seek healing through their faith. Many followers put faith in prayer, holy water, and anointed stones to ward off disease or cure illnesses. The congregants believe that they are protected by the Holy Spirit, but have at least acknowledged soap and masks as a defense against the coronavirus. However, convincing them to also get vaccinated is a mammoth task. The contrast in attitudes displayed by the Johanne Marange Apostolic group members shows that the solution to the vaccination hesitancy is not homogenous in convincing hesitant religious citizens to get vaccinated. As one leader of the Johanne Marange retorts:

We are agreeing that the Holy Spirit may not be enough to deal with the virus. We are really considering vaccines since others are doing the same but still waiting for a revelation from the messiah. However, our members have always been suspicious of injections. But with social distancing, sanitizing, and masking up, we might get maximum protection. With the supply of soap, buckets, sanitizers, and masks, we will be free from the pandemic.

[Interview Participant]

Reviewed literature shows that the rollout of COVID-19 vaccine has seen religious actors playing a crucial role in maximizing access to healthcare for communities globally (Birdsall, 2021). Religious actors play both positive and negative roles when it comes to supporting public health guidance during the pandemic. There is a lot of misinformation associated with vaccination and religion as efforts to convey messages about health and vaccination has been a much more positive role . Faith-based advocacy for COVID-19 vaccination is important, especially since members of some religious communities are resistant to vaccination (Clarke, 2021; Hodge et al., 2021). There are some very specific religiously linked concerns about what the vaccines are made of and the process, as politics and fear shape vaccine hesitancy . However, advocacy on the part of religious leaders can help build trust in COVID-19 vaccination as well as support equity in vaccine distribution. Faith engagement in the COVID-19 pandemic is not without its challenges, since the health crisis has contributed to forms of social and religious exclusion. The COVID-19 vaccination tended to deepen women's fears that comes with patriarchy with a deepening inclination to be more nuanced about religious differences. One woman congregant had this to say:

> As women we are by our husbands when it comes to vaccination. Our church doctrine says we don't go to the hospital when we are sick or get vaccinated. After we were taught about the dangers of COVID-19 I took the decision to get vaccinated because my life is my responsibility. We don't participate in the vaccination programs because we are against the use of patent medicine but holy water, stones, and cross artifacts made from reeds. Our church leaders can cure COVID-19. They pray and sprinkle water on people with the disease and they are healed.

As a way to combat the spread of the deadly virus, interfaith leaders, under the banner of the Apostolic Women's Empowerment Trust (AWET), formed the COVID-19 awareness programmes targeting interfaith leaders to address vaccine hesitancy across the country. Research shows that interfaith and community leaders are helping shift negative perceptions about the COVID-19 vaccines that have been attributed to widespread misinformation and long-held religious beliefs. This will drastically reduce the spread of the virus through taking the jab. However, debate on some religious reasons for not getting the COVID-19 vaccine has seen very few religions documenting doctrinal reasons for not believing in immunizations . According to the Vanderbilt University Medical Center research in the USA, some Christians and other people of faith are citing their religion as a reason why they won't get the COVID-19 vaccine (Feldman, 2021). There are many religious arguments for and against the COVID-19 vaccination. Some members decline vaccination on the basis that it interferes with divine providence. Yet others within the faith accept immunization as a gift from God to be used with gratitude. These have brought about mixed reactions on vaccination. In Zimbabwe, the Johanne Marange group, though not documented, declines immunization citing doctrinal reasons.

Research has shown that gender-based violence precipitated by the social religious beliefs rooted in gender-inequitable norms or power dynamics, has contributed to the refusal of vaccination by some women. Some women suffer violence once they want to be vaccinated. Such violations may be physical, emotional, psychological, or sexual and may include sexual violence, intimate partner violence, and other forms of sexual abuse and exploitation (Vahedi et al., 2021). Although persons of any gender can experience these violations, women and girls in fragile settings are disproportionately affected (Freedman, 2016). It was noted that patriarchy was the driving force behind the perpetuation and high prevalence of GBV as some refugee women had to seek permission from their husbands for them to get vaccinated (Landis, 2020). According to the Johanne Marange church doctrine, women lack decision-making power over their own bodies and health, hindering their ability to choose whether to get the COVID-19 vaccine or not. This may increase family tensions and risks of exposure to intimate partner violation (IPV), denial of resources, and other forms of GBV (McAbee et al., 2021. They also have restricted decision-making power as well as limited access to and control over resources needed for advancing their health, including information about vaccines and vaccine safety (Kabonesa et al., 2020). Refugee women are also at risk of experiencing sexual harassment and other forms of gender-based violence when seeking healing services from their church leaders when they are sick. This was the case in Jordan, where refugee women experience similar challenges to access vaccination centers due to gender inequality, patriarchal system, and harmful traditional practices (Al-Qerem et al., 2021). Women also reported incidents of denial of resources, opportunity, and services mainly perpetrated by their husbands and male relatives, due to their religious beliefs that discriminate against women (Fisher et al., 2020).

Research findings show that some churches in the TRC have taken steps to address hesitancy among their congregants. Reports from staff from the local Non Governmental Organization in the camp show that plans were underway to use a mass messaging platform to send text messages to the cellphones of followers to adhere to the government directive to get vaccinated and avoid gatherings. As some churches in the camp were breaking the lockdown measures restricting meetings, efforts were being made to dispel misinformation pertaining to vaccination. This became a trend for the majority of the "white garment" Apostolic groups in TRC as some refugees sought divine intervention for their mounting social problems. As one study participant retorted:

> There is a need for messaging aligned around reiterating for the refugee population that the vaccine is safe, that it's been tested. The ingredients are safe for use in humans and will not make you magnetic as purported. The vaccine is not satanic. Convincing members of the white garment is a tall order as they are defiant, relying on prayer and water for healing against the pandemic. They claim that they can heal coronavirus through praying and sprinkling of water on people with the disease. What apostolic sects are doing is medically unproven, and they put their worshippers, especially women, in danger of infections from COVID-19.
>
> [Interview Participant]

Findings reveal that the major problem they encountered in trying to convince women church congregants to be vaccinated is stigmatization. Although some female church members are willing to get vaccinated, they hesitated doing so because they feared being ostracized by their peers and leaders. Such scenes led to the feeling of advising the UNHCR and the government not to consider the door-to-door campaign strategy to vaccination as this might have led to chaos in the home. However, as a way of avoiding stigmatization, findings show that some women would visit the clinic and get vaccinated and keep it to themselves as it was their secret. It was also noted that some of the leaders of the Apostolic group present in the camp repeatedly criticized the wearing of face masks, limits on in-person gatherings, and COVID-19 vaccines. Findings also reveal that they considered their places of worship as mask-free areas. As one congregant stated:

> We are forced to remove our masks or never to enter the place of worship wearing one. Our church leaders discourage us from getting the jab, purporting that they celebrate faith over fear. The call for mandatory vaccination by the host government has been met with resistance by our church leaders who are leading the anti-vaccination campaign in the camp. A lot of negative information is being circulated by these churches against vaccination on the pretext that it is satanic.
>
> [Interview Participant]

Research shows that the anti-vaccination campaigns by some of the leaders of the "white garments" in the camp led to low vaccination rates. Reports from the local health center show that there was reluctance to get vaccinated among some within the refugee population due to religious beliefs, apathy, and hesitancy. It was also noted that the vulnerable and the defenseless were among those who were resisting vaccination on the guise of religion. Securing the protection for the world's most vulnerable has been at the heart of the UNHCR as refugee families have already been through so much, displaced from their places and people they love (UNHCR, 2020). However, many still suffered some level of neglect as they were being denied access to the vaccine in the guise of religious guidance or teaching. Access to a vaccine for these families would mean not just survival but a chance at normalcy for them to move freely. As the local Environmental Health Technician from World Vision reported:

> As an organization, we are committed to supporting the fair and equitable global rollout of WHO-endorsed vaccines and we are partnering with government, faith leaders, and community health workers in combatting the spread of COVID-19 in TRC. However, there is a high degree of apathy being instigated by some members of the Johanne Marange Apostolic group leaders. They are misinforming their followers pertaining to the vaccination. A lot of negatives have been said about the effects of taking the jab. This is

a blow to the programme, as efforts by the government and WHO to have the people of concern vaccinated is met with resistance.

It was noted that many of the leaders of Johanne Marange Apostolic sect remained resolute and steadfast in their belief in eternal life, believing that living on this earth is but a blip on the screen, hence there was no need to be so scared of anything, including those deaths that could be deemed untimely. They believe that God controls everything and criticize some churches who justify the use of vaccines.

Critical Reflections

The research findings have shown that there is scant information regarding knowledge, attitudes, and practices surrounding vaccines. Research evidence shows a semblance of historic mistrust of vaccines in the Johanne Marange Apostolic group refugee women communities. As a way of overcoming these and associated barriers, information and data are desperately needed in real time for migrant communities to adhere to the call for vaccination to avoid infection. Once this community is educated on the efficacy of the vaccine and its impact on human health, there is a probability of a high uptake of the jab. There is a need to find ways of reaching out to these churches with the vaccination message to encourage them to comply with WHO and government regulations to be vaccinated, for COVID-19 and other concerns. The lack of correct information on the COVID-19 vaccine, as well as beliefs and practices in refugee communities, associated with lack of vaccination intent, are tantamount to low vaccination uptake. The absence of information education campaign material at church level in multiple languages indicating the importance of taking the jab and other factors associated with COVID-19 vaccine, has also led to such resistance. Health education in these churches targeting the safety and efficacy of the vaccine will mostly have a positive impact on vaccine intentions and eventual uptake, especially if the messaging comes from their church leaders.

There is also the feeling that migrant populations are not homogeneous, and communities vary greatly in their experience with, and attitudes toward, vaccination. The common barriers to vaccination faced by migrant communities include cultural factors, differing understanding and beliefs of disease processes, and healthcare utilization challenges (Thomas et al., 2021). However, different arguments and explanations against vaccine avoidance have been arrayed. Chief among these include safety concerns, confusion over protection levels, perceived risk and fears, poor health literacy, lack of awareness about the virus, misinformation or lack of accurate knowledge about the vaccines. Women refugees, being the guardians of the home, were concerned about the safety of the vaccines when administered to the elderly as they doubted the efficacies of the vaccines compared to the healing water they get from the church leaders. The anti-vaccine myths and confusing messages about some severe side effects of the vaccines that were being peddled by the church leaders were a way of avoiding vaccination. The distortions regarding the origin of the vaccine and the allegation of the use of pork (regarded as polluting) in preserving the vaccine led to negative responses from most refugee women of the Apostolic groups. Further, there is under-representation of church members in researches relating to health. This has led to a mistrust and suspicion of medical companies that produce vaccines. It was also argued that the political and economic intentions that were perceived to be driving the pandemic or vaccine preparation contributed to vaccine hesitancy as the inflationary environment in the country did not favor a pandemic such as COVID-19 (Garcia et al., 2021). Collectively, these factors can erode the beliefs and trust that are important in the acceptance of COVID-19 vaccination (MacAbee et al., 2021; MacDonald et al., 2015). This was evidenced by the resistance encountered when World Vision officials were dealing with refugee women from the Johanne Marange Apostolic group.

Conclusion and Recommendations

The chapter, therefore, concludes that debates regarding appropriate knowledge of the efficacy and effectiveness of COVID-19 vaccines coupled with the doctrine of the church (Johanne Marange Apostolic group) had an impact on the uptake of COVID-19 vaccines among some refugee women at TRC. To counter this, there is a need for a multisectoral approach that involves partnership between various stakeholders, such as government, private companies, religious groups, and other agencies, to leverage the knowledge, expertise, and resources, to enhance the creation of longstanding public trust of vaccines. Creativity engaging with religious ideologies, gender dynamics, the challenges wrought by the refugee status and more effective use of communication strategies can contribute toward building greater public trust in outreaches by health personnel.

References

Adams, E.A., Sambu, D., and Smiley, S.L. 2018. Urban water supply in Sub-Saharan Africa: Historical and emerging policies and institutional arrangements. *International Journal of Water Resources Development*, 1–24. https://doi.org/10.1080/07900 627.2017.1423282

Al-Qerem, W.A. and Jarab, A.S. 2021. COVID-19 vaccination acceptance and its associated factors among a Middle Eastern population. *Front Public Health*, 10(9), 632914. DOI:10.3389/fpubh.2021.632914. PMID: 33643995; PMCID: PMC7902782.

Ananga, E. 2015. *The Role of Community Participation in Water Production and Management: Lessons From Sustainable Aid in Africa*. International Sponsored Water Schemes in Kisumu, Kenya, University of South Florida.

Arabi, M. 2019. Water, sanitation and hygiene in the Minawao refugee camp, Far North Cameroon. *International Journal of Resource and Environmental Management*, 4(1), 1–25.

Bauman, C.W., McGraw, A.P., Bartels, D.M., and Warren, C. 2014. Revisiting external validity: Concerns about trolley problems and other sacrificial dilemmas in moral psychology. *Social and Personality Psychology Compass*, 8(9), 536–554.

Beuchler, S. and Hanson, A. 2015. *Women, Water, and Global Environmental Change. Routledge International Studies of Women and Place*. Berkeley, CA: University of California Press.

Birdsall, C., Halaunova, A., and van de Kamp, L. 2021. Sensing urban values: Reassessing urban cultures and histories amidst redevelopment agendas. *Space and Culture*, 24(3), 348–358.

Bulle, S. 1999. *Issues and Results of Community Participation in Urban Environment: Comparative Analysis of Nine Projects on Waste Management, ENDA/WASTE, UWEP Working Document 11*. Nieuwehaven, Netherlands. www.waste.nl

Campbell, M., Hilton, J.D.X., and Anderson J.R. 2019. A systematic review of the relationship between religion and attitudes toward transgender and gender-variant people. *International Journal of Transgender Health*, 20(1), 21–38 https://doi.org/10.1080/15532739.2018.1545149

Card, L.F and Ladaria, S.I. 2020. *Note of the Congregation for the Doctrine of the Faith on the Morality of Using Some Anti-Covid-19 Vaccines*.

Caserotti, M., Girardi, P., Rubaltelli, E., Tasso, A., Lotto, L., and Gavaruzzi, T. 2021. Associations of COVID-19 risk perception with vaccine hesitancy over time for Italian residents. *Soc Sci Med*, 272, 113688. DOI:10.1016/j.socscimed.113688.

Clarke, S.K., Kumar, G.S., Sutton, J., et al. 2021. Potential impact of COVID-19 on recently resettled refugee populations in the United States and Canada: perspectives of refugee healthcare providers. *J Immgr Minor Health*, 23, 184–189. [PMC free article] [PubMed] [Google Scholar]

Clement, F., Harcourt, W. Josh, D., and Sato, C. 2019. A feminist political ecology of the commons and the communing (Editorial to the Special feature). *International Journal of the Commons*, 13(1), 1–15. http://doi.org/10.18352/ijc.972

Dhama, K., Sharun, K., Tiwari, R., Dhawan, M., Emran, T.B., Rabaan, A.A., and Alhumaid, S. 2021. COVID-19 vaccine hesitancy: Reasons and solutions to achieve a successful global vaccination campaign to tackle the ongoing pandemic. *Human Vaccines & Immunotherapeutics*, 17(10), 3495–3499. DOI: 10.1080/21645515.2021.1926183

Ekwebelem, O.C., Yunusa, I., Onyeaka, H., Ekwebelem, N.C., and Nnorom-Dike, O. 2021. COVID-19 vaccine rollout: Will it affect the rates of vaccine hesitancy in Africa? *Public Health*, 197, e18–e19. www.ncbi.nlm.nih.gov/pmc/articles/PMC7843135/

Feldman, J.M. and Bassett, M.T. 2021. Variation in COVID-19 mortality in the US by race and ethnicity and educational attainment. *JAMA*, 1(4), 1–10.

Finney Rutten, L.J., Zhu, X., Leppin, A.L., Ridgeway, J.L., Swift, M.D., Griffin, J.M., St Sauver, J.L., Virk, A., and Jacobson, R.M. 2021. Evidence-based strategies for clinical organizations to address COVID-19 vaccine hesitancy. *Mayo Clin Proc*, 96, 699–707. DOI:10.1016/j. mayocp.12.024

Fisher, K., Bloomstone, S., et. al. 2020. Attitudes toward a potential SARS-CoV-2 vaccine: A survey of US adults. *Ann Intern Med*, 173, 924–973.

Freedman, J. 2016. Sexual and gender-based violence against refugee women: A hidden aspect of the refugee "crisis", *Reproductive Health Matters*, 18–26.

Garcia, B.W. et al. 2021. *Multiple SARS-CoV-2 variants escape neutralization by vaccine-induced humoral immunity: Cellpress*, https://doi.org/10.1016/j.cell.2021.03.013

Gautham, I., Albert, S., Koroma, A., and Banu, S. 2021. Impact of COVID-19 on an urban refugee population, *Health Equity*, 5(1), 718–723. DOI: 10.1089/heq.2020.0148.

Grabenstein, J.D. 2013.What the world's religions teach, applied to vaccines and immune globulins. *Vaccine*, 31(16): 2011–2023.

Griffith, J., Marani, H., and Monkman, H. 2021. COVID-19 vaccine hesitancy in Canada: Content analysis of Tweets using the theoretical domains framework. *J Med Internet Res*, 23(4), e26874. DOI:10.2196/26874. PMID:33769946; PMCID:PMC8045776.

Haq, C., Hostetter, I., Zavala, L., et al. 2020. Immigrant health and changes to the public-charge rule: Family physicians' response. *Ann of Family Med*, 458–460. [PMC free article] [PubMed] [Google Scholar]

Hodge, J.G. and Carey, E. 2021. Charting the legality of religious-based exemptions to COVID-19 vaccinations. Berkeley Center for Religion, Peace and World Affairs.

Jeneen, H. 2011. *Encyclopedia of Cultures and Daily Life*. University of Philadelphia Press. p. 232. ISBN 9781414448916. US Druze settled in small towns and kept a low profile, joining Protestant churches (usually Presbyterian or Methodist) and often Americanizing their names.

Kabonesa, C. and Kindi, F.I. 2020, Assessing the relationship between gender-based violence and COVID-19 pandemic in Uganda. Conrad Adenauer Stiftung.

Landis, D. 2020. Gender based violence (GBV) and Covid-19: The complexities of responding to "the shadow pandemic". A Policy Brief.

Larson, J.J., Cooper, L.D., et.al. 2011. *Addressing the Vaccine Confidence Gap*. https://pubmed.ncbi.nlm.nih.gov/21664679/

Lebano, A., et al. 2020. Migrants' and refugees' health status and healthcare in Europe: A scoping literature review. *BMC Public Health*, 20(1039), 1–22.

Lucia, V.C., Kelekar, A., and Afonso, N.M. 2021. COVID-19 vaccine hesitancy among medical students. *Journal of Public Health*, 43(3): 445–449.

MacDonald, N.E. 2015. SAGE working group on vaccine hesitancy. Vaccine hesitancy: Definition, scope and determinants. *Vaccine* [Internet], 33(34), 4161–4164. DOI:10.1016/j.vaccine.2015.04.036

McAbee, L., Tapera, O., and Kanyangarara, M. 2021. Factors associated with COVID-19 vaccine intentions in Eastern Zimbabwe: A cross-sectional study. *Vaccines (Basel)*, 29(9). https://doi.org/10.3390/vaccines9101109

Owens, R. 2021. *Know Your Bugs: A Collaborative Evaluation of a Community Health Education Module That Aims to be Accessible to Adults with Learning Disabilities*. Open University (United Kingdom).

Peterman, A., Potts, A., O'Donnell, M., et al. 2020. *Pandemics and Violence Against Women and Children. Working Paper 528*. Washington, DC: Center for Global Development. https://plato.stanford.edu/entries/feminist-power/

Rochelaeu, D.E. 2008. Political ecology in the key of policy: From chains of explanation to webs of relation. *Geoforum*, 39, 716–727. https://pdf.sciencedirectassets.com/271790/

Sachedina, A. 2021. *Religion, Bioethics, and COVID-19 Vaccination: Muslim Views*. Berkeley Center for Religion, Peace and World Affairs.

Sibanda, F., Makahamadze, T., and Maposa, R.S. 2008. 'Hawks and Doves': The Impact of Operation Murambatsvina on Johanne Marange Apostolic Church in Zimbabwe. *Exchange*, 37, 68–85.

Skider, A.H.M.K. 2010. *Access to Water and Sanitation in Refugee Settings: Success and Setbacks in Bangladesh*. Dhaka, Bangladesh: Institute of Water and Flood Management, Bangladesh University of Engineering and Technology.

Soares, P., Rocha, J.V., Moniz, M., Gama, A., Laires, P.A., Pedro, A.R., Dias, S., Leite, A., and Nunes, C. 2021. Factors associated with COVID-19 vaccine hesitancy. *Vaccines*, 9, 300. DOI:10.3390/vaccines9030300

Sulley, R. 2018. *Re-Conceptualising Gender and Urban Water Inequality Applying a Critical Feminist Approach to Water Inequality in Dhaka*. London: Bartlett Development Planning Unit, University of London. www.ucl.ac.uk/bartlett/deve lopment/sites/bartlett/files/wp195_sulley.pdf

Sundberg, J. n.d. Feminist political ecology. Forthcoming in *The International Encyclopedia of Geography*, Wiley- Blackwell & Association of American Geographers, Editor-in-Chief D. Richardson.

Thomas, C.M., Osterholm, M.T., and Stauffer, W.M. 2021. Critical considerations for COVID-19 vaccination of refugees, immigrants, and migrants. *The American Journal of Tropical Medicine and Hygiene*. Official Journal of the American Society of Tropical Medicine and Hygiene.

Turner-Musa, J., Ajayi, O., and Kemp, L. 2020. Examining social determinants of health, stigma, and COVID-19 disparities. *Healthcare*, 8, 168. [PMC free article] [PubMed] [Google Scholar]

UNHCR/WFP. 2014. *Zimbabwe – UNHCR/WFP Joint Assessment Mission Report: Tongogara Refugee Camp*. www.wfp.org/publications/zimbabwe-unhcr-wfp-joint-ass essment-mission-tongogara-refugee-camp-september-2014

United Nations High Commissioner for Refugees (UNHCR). 2020. *Global Focus*. Available online at: http://reporting.unhcr.org/node/2544?y=2020#year

United Nations High Commissioner for Refugees (UNHCR). 2021. *UNHCR Zimbabwe fact sheet, September 2021*. Geneva: UNHCR.

Wangdah, J., Lytsy, P., Martensson, L., et al. 2015. Health literacy and refugees' experiences of the health examination of asylum seekers: A Swedish cross-sectional study. *BMC Public Health*, 15, 1162.

Wilson, L., Rubens-Augustson, T., Murphy, M., Jardine, C., Crowcroft, N., Hui, C., and Wilson, K. 2018. Barriers to immunization among newcomers: A systematic review. *Vaccine*, 36, 1055–1062. [PubMed] [Google Scholar].

9 COVID-19 Vaccination in Zimbabwe

Sites and Scenes of Power Contestations through the Lenses of Spirituality and Uncertainty

Tarsisio M. Nyatsanza

Introduction

Epidemics are not new in the history of human existence. Responses to the epidemics have ranged from non-action, deliberate suppression, border controls, quarantine and sometimes selective vaccination based on chosen criteria by the political establishments through their governmental institutions. Ranger and Slack (1996) argue that the common thread in epidemics is that not only are they contagious, but also rapidly lead to a high rate of mortality. Pandemics invariably tend to inflict a shock effect. To that extent, the shock reaction invariably occurs on a global level across all cultures. This has the effect of reshaping religious, social and political as well as medical assumptions and attitudes. The same argument is also reiterated by Dry and Leach (2010), Hays (2005), McNeill (1998) and Showalter (1997).

In this chapter, the emergence, spread and impact of COVID-19 will be examined in discursive ways. The main focus of this chapter is the COVID-19 pandemic and Zimbabwe's[1] response to it, with particular reference to vaccine uptake in the wake of vaccine hesitancy (Kabakama et al., 2022). It follows that the struggle to come to terms with COVID-19 has led to medical pluralism which dictates choices and their accompanying meanings. This chapter will also demonstrate how the existing metrics of interrogating the dynamics of COVID-19 in Zimbabwe resonates with those used with regards to HIV and AIDS and other pandemics. Extensive work on the "hierarchy of resorts" through deconstructing monolithic medicine policy and practices and the creation of multiple medical responses to complex health issues has already been well-documented by Hsu (2008), Lane & Millar (1987), Rao (2006) and Schwartz (1969). The reflections and contests over COVID-19 vaccination (Dzinamarira et al., 2021; Garcia and Yap, 2021; Maketo and Mutizwa, 2021; McAbee et al., 2021; Kabakama et al., 2022) must be located in this broader context. As various studies confirmed with special reference to Zimbabwe (Murewanhema & Mutsigiri-Murewanhema, 2021; Murewanhema et al., 2022), many factors affected COVID-19 vaccine uptake.

DOI: 10.4324/9781003388630-9

Background and Context

In the Zimbabwean case, religion played a pivotal role in framing the responses to the COVID-19 pandemic (Chirombe et al., 2020; Tom, 2021; Sibanda et al., 2022). Prior to the COVID-19 pandemic, a number of the Mapostori/Apostolic faith groups and other non-faith groups had already set a precedent of the refusal of their children to be vaccinated against any form of disease, let alone allow their believers to seek any form of medicine – traditional or Western. For particular Mapostori groups, the only acceptable form of treatment and 'vaccination' is the use of water, eggs, stones, oil and other items of *muteuro* (rituals which also sometimes involve some forms of libation) which would be the designated prayer portions to be used as instructed by the designated church leadership.

For the traditional medicine adherents, their perceptions were grounded on different rationalities that were based on discourses of ancestral cosmologies of causation of disease and how to appease the spirits, witchcraft, as well as other cosmogonic heuristic paradigms. Some versions of traditional religions in Zimbabwe continued to claim and perpetuate the narrative that they could cure COVID-19, thereby militating against the local and global public health messaging that vaccination was medically proven to significantly reduce chances of transmission. It goes without saying that the tenets of some faith-based organisations in Zimbabwe have some medical prohibitions. A case in point are the Jehovah's Witnesses who refuse blood transfusion, potentially creating medical risks for their members in general, as well as more recently in relation to the issues to do with the COVID-19 vaccination, especially for young children (Will, 2022).

One of the critical issues is the interface between human rights, freedom of religion and the resistance and/or acceptance of vaccinations in respect of COVID-19 (Mugari & Obioha, 2021). This has been, and continues to be, paradoxical in terms of the World Health Organization and the local Zimbabwean public health guidelines. As the paradox persists, and having no easy solution in sight in terms of COVID-19 vaccinations and managing the pandemic, it definitely calls into question how more subtle and negotiated strategies need to be generated in order to strike a plausible balance among all the stakeholders.

COVID-19 is no exception to the above characterisations. Regrettably, most Western anthropologists have previously tended to negatively depict and interpret African people's ways of constructing their own worldviews. This often leads to using biased and misaligned Euro-centric Western frameworks. Evidence of this is replete in the early and other writings of Douglas (2013), Ross (2002), Mead (1995) and Evans-Pritchard (1937) just to name a few. Some of their views are broadly based on ethnographic writings of missionaries, colonialists, explorers, hunters and traders who had visited Africa and often lacked a robust understanding of the issues they were writing about. In the same vein, there were also some enthusiastic, albeit not so well-informed, recipients of the skewed narratives of the Western returnees from Africa who provided these armchair enthusiasts with information that was regarded to be authentic – yet the research writings published were not only superficial but not verified, controversial and lacked academic rigour and substantiated evidence. In between those theoretical layers, one would find some non-African medical professionals whose views on African experiences of disease, health and well-being were based on treading more astutely when dealing with the data gathered from their respondents and research sites. Such authors include the likes of Aschwanden (1989) and Gelfand (1988).

More recently, with the rise of African academia and critique, the above constructs were disrupted and equally problematised in order to provide more robust and nuanced understandings of the role and functions of spirituality and how it interplays with uncertainty as a way of trying to connect between the known and the unknown. Notable proponents of these revisionary initiatives include African philosophers and African anthropologists such as Nyamnjoh (2012), Mafeje (2001), Hountondji (1996), Chavunduka (1994), Appiah (1993), Mudimbe (1988) and Serequeberhan (1994). Not only did they de-create but they continue to re-create the efficacy of spirituality and uncertainty as coherent and sustainable constituents of grounding pandemics including COVID-19 as super complex occurrences in Africa.

Others have relied on eclectic approaches regarding the COVID-19 pandemic which essentially resembles the typology that Luedke and West (2006: 1) describe. Within that typology, they argued that:

> medical practitioners in south-eastern Africa … are brokers between different cultures, between the rural and urban, local and global, between places of daily life and spaces of potentialities. They appear to derive their therapeutic powers precisely from this movement and straddling of boundaries. Rather than invoking a clearly bounded culture concept with a culturally adept healer in its centre, the notion of 'medical landscapes' implies social processes, relatedness and movements between foregrounds and backgrounds, and across boundaries. It thus promises to provide a theoretical framing for future studies on theme that until recently has remained central to medical anthropology, the study of medical pluralism.

A unique feature of COVID-19, in Africa and indeed elsewhere, was its indiscriminate nature across all categories of society – rich and poor, male and female, young and old – and this simply added to the chaotic scenes and sites of the power contestations as stated in the UN document 'Everyone Included: Social Impact of COVID-19'.[2]

The difference between COVID-19, which was not selective of any social group, and the other pandemics is that in respect of the previous pandemics, there is a perennial label of otherness which depicts them as diseases of the poor, the powerless and the disenfranchised (Hotez et al., 2006). Nonetheless, the impact of inequality later became clear when more poor and marginalised people in the Global North died than those who had greater access to resources (Chitando et al., 2023: 1).

However, the old challenge of the 'big brother' syndrome is once again disproportionately associating the COVID-19 pandemic with the perceived poor African and other low-income countries. This is done in a bid to try and resolve the vagaries of the pandemic. This scenario very much resembles how the West dominates in controlling world affairs while the 'rest' are incessantly made to wait until a solution is promulgated by the 'big brothers' of the West. Vaccination in Zimbabwe therefore becomes one of those strands of contestations of power despite its potential efficacy. These contestations of power have been profiled by Edward Said's theoretical insights on Orientalism (Said, 1979). This very much resonates with Stuart Hall's (1992) critique of the social construct of the 'West and the Rest'.

Conceptual Framework

There are, however, many resemblances between COVID-19 and the HIV and AIDS scourge that continue to burden the African continent but Zimbabwe as well in many ways. Some of the characteristics that are common to both pandemics are bewilderment, angst, the unprecedented nature of the occurrence, fear of the unknown regarding the pandemics' future, lack of a predictable sequence of events and the generation of conspiracy theories when attempting to explain their existence. All these dimensions were relevant in attitudes towards COVID-19 vaccines by religious groups in Zimbabwe and Africa.

Although in Zimbabwe and Africa, the observable physical and experienced components of COVID-19 were morbidity, death and recovery, this chapter will argue that there is also a strong spiritual dimension and so the whole idea of vaccination as a biomedical technology and its acceptance or denial creates a new epidemiological fulcrum in terms of how it relates to the spiritual dimensions. This has a ripple effect of the profound feeling of uncertainty that underpins the socio-cultural aetiology of the illness. This chapter is equally foregrounded against the background that both individuals and communities in Zimbabwe and indeed in Africa resorted to the metaphysical realms with spirituality and uncertainty as heuristic lenses of engaging with the perplexities of the COVID-19 pandemic. The challenges of COVID-19 led to a deep Zimbabwean spirituality that precipitated a sense of awe that militated against any single or simple explanation of its existence. Spirituality, therefore, presents itself as a way of expressing one's relationship with the superior terrestrial and extra-terrestrial beings. It also provides the much-needed spaces for reflecting on and searching for profound religious understandings of the meanings of COVID-19 within the indigenous Zimbabwean cosmological and existential encounters.

Methodology

Unknown to the world, COVID-19 just appeared on the surface of the earth like a bombshell. The most harrowing thing was the lightning speed, the devastation, the rapture and pyscho-social emotional distress that it brought with it. Such baggage was just too ghastly to contemplate. Worse still, for Africa and Zimbabwe in particular whose health infrastructure and livelihoods were already fragile, and the human rights record is highly controversial, the consequences were excruciating. The methodology is developed against the backdrop of the controversial and lack of clear policy positions of the political establishment that have been compounded by the constant conspiracy theories with regards to the management of COVID-19 on multiple dimensions in Zimbabwe. In order to interrogate some of the moments and representations, this chapter will rely on a hybrid methodological tool that comprises the fusion of narrative analysis and a postcolonial heuristic lens.

Narratives depict the cultural terrains that mark the people's social geographies of life experiences. The origins of narratives are associated with Aristotle in his explanation of the Greek tragedy in his classical book *Poetics* (2006). The idea was then developed in the Chicago School studies based on the particular people's histories, life experiences, a range of social and other structural factors like their physical environments. Sometimes narratives can be selective depending on the purpose and the audience. More recently, narratives have been popularised as tools that do political work through the analysis of the language in terms of the how and why events are storied (Riessman, 2008).

Alongside the narratives is the postcolonial heuristic lens which serves as part of the hybrid tool that not only recognises the complexity of the COVID-19 pandemic, but also analyses it in order to make sense of the messy phenomena (Law, 2004) under investigation. The term 'postcolonial' denotes the struggle against European domination through colonisation and the emergence of new political and cultural actors in the later part of the twentieth century with the impact of reshaping the power distribution on the world stage. In other words, the term postcolonial means a whole range of practices and perspectives in relation to power issues that have shaped the world. It is an active engagement to change the legacies of colonialism and the Western/Euro-centric dominance of the colonised spaces (Schwarz, 2000). Thus, this hybrid tool is useful in analysing the interstices of power which clarify how the various contours of the COVID-19 pandemic are constructed and what they represent in the different domains.

Spirituality and COVID-19 in Zimbabwe

Human existence in Africa and indeed in Zimbabwe is not just a purely mundane experience but one which is guided by spirituality and constituted by various complex layers, perceptions and multiple configurations within the terrestrial and extra-terrestrial. Spirituality with the Zimbabwean context is inextricably linked with their ontology and metaphysics. Through colonisation, trade and globalisation, African spirituality expanded beyond the realms of African Traditional Religion(s) (Idowu, 1973) and has increasingly interacted with other religions – most notably, Christianity, Islam, Buddhism, Hinduism, Confucianism, Taoism and others. To this end, spirituality transcends the African physical bodies – from conception, birth and adulthood – into the land of the living dead via the unbroken linkages of the various rites of passage (Mazama, 2002).

While spirituality within the Zimbabwean context provides a template and logic of the cycle and trajectories of birth to death and thereafter, COVID-19 raptured this worldview by engraining phenomenon of uncertainty within the totality of the indigenous African life experience to such an extent that the values, expectations, norms and vision of life and its concomitant benefits have been shattered. Not only have the socio-cultural barometers of human hope and happiness plummeted to unimaginable levels; the volume edited by Michael Peters and Tina Besley (2021) indicates that the economist Robert Shiller has in fact identified at least two simultaneous COVID-19 pandemics: one which is essentially health related and the other economic. The health may be interpreted as the biomedical clinical human condition, while the economic constitutes issues of trade, tourism, international education, travel and retail. The resultant effect of these two levels of the pandemic have not only affected how the emerging and even the unknown social formations and relationships are unfolding, but they are also necessitating the formation of new cultural realities for the post COVID-19 Zimbabwe and indeed beyond.

Closely related to unexpected developments emerging out of the pandemic is the observation that although this chapter specifically focuses on COVID-19 in Zimbabwe, there are some important developments which have been thrown up by the pandemic. Vaccinations against COVID-19 not only throw up the problematics of the clinical biomedical aspects to heterogenous populations like Zimbabwe, but they also seek to interrogate individual and collective human rights in terms of access to the acceptance or resistance of the COVID-19 vaccine irrespective of one's social standing in Zimbabwe. Once again issues of age, gender and religious contexts underpin and lurk behind this perennial controversy. There are, however, some examples within the last few decades that have indicated that, for example, Europe has increasingly been seen as more secularised than ever before. One such example is that the levels of church attendance and congregants has drastically dwindled. Surprisingly, COVID-19 has led a phenomenal resurgence of keeping the faith across all religious groups and none. This is rather interesting considering that full places of worship had become synonymous with poor Africa and Asia. If the article by Harriet Sherwood in *The Guardian* (2020) is anything to go by, then certainly, spirituality has been rekindled as a global human experience.

Within the context of the HIV/AIDS pandemic, Chitando and Klagba (2013) have also highlighted different kinds of healing which are constitutive of the spirituality that African people resort to in terms of their health and well-being. These range from African traditional medicine, Western biomedical healing, prayers from traditional mainstream churches to African Independent and Pentecostal healing. Underlying these initiatives is a deep sense of spirituality and the uncertainty of which option provides the best solution to the medical challenges.

Uncertainty: Scenes and Sites of Power Contestations in the COVID-19 Context

Lest we fall into the same trap like the colonial anthropologists who tended to lump Africa as one homogenous polity with uniform experiences in all respects, we are cognisant that 'Africa' (within which Zimbabwe is to be located) is very much a socio-political-historical-economic construct that was designed to serve the interests of the perpetrators. There is ample historical evidence to demonstrate how this construct was developed and applied in a sample of Mazrui's writings (Mazrui, 1980, 2004, 2009). Notwithstanding that, there is also a unique peculiarity about Africa as a continent, especially in her victimhood at the hands of the perpetrators. It is important to recognise that despite the later influences of colonialism, missionary activities of which Christianity, Islam and other imposed religions, African Traditional Religions and its cognates of which Zimbabwe has different permutations, continue to provide the basis for defining and understanding spirituality and uncertainty in Africa. It is therefore imperative to note that when COVID-19 emerged, the impact of the precolonial, colonial and postcolonial persisted. Some selected examples of these will be highlighted in the paragraphs below.

The COVID-19 pandemic brought with it critical epistemological questions insofar as it has been problematic to verify the truth of what actually transpired. The aura of scepticism persists and continues to evoke all sorts of individual and collective emotional, psychosocial and medical pressure and discomfort. The persistent doubt is part of what has created a theatrical arena of the pandemic which I refer to as sites and scenes of power contestations. There are many competing conspiracy and scientific theories, none of which have managed to create a permanent fulcrum. In Zimbabwe, the issues range from the views and perceptions of traditional to political to religious and medical authorities. It is differentially crafted and interpreted by male and female, young and old, urbanites and rural dwellers let alone from one geographical country jurisdiction to another. Of particular significance is how uncertainty is addressed from the religious realm. Chitando (2009) aptly engages with this phenomenon within the context of African lives. It is worth noting that as I have discussed throughout this chapter, Zimbabweans and Africans are not only deeply religious but they are very much spiritual beings. This idea runs through Mbiti's (1990) writing and most of the Africanist religionists on the continent and elsewhere (Magesa, 2014).

Typical examples of the above include constant and conflicting messages by, for example, the late former Tanzanian President John Magafuli who not only dismissed the virus but insisted that it was 'the devil's tool' and encouraged his people to go to places of worship without observing social distancing. He emphasised the spiritual aspect in terms of prayer rather than the bio-medical physical condition of COVID-19. In Madagascar, President Andry Rajoelina tried against all odds to claim a cure for the pandemic, only to be rubbished by the 'big brothers' in the West. In Nigeria, the National Institute of Pharmaceutical Research and Development's Director General Obi Adigwe argued that their analysis of the 'Madagascar cure' demonstrated no efficacy with regards to treating COVID-19.[3]

In Zimbabwe, on the other hand, the prevalent discourse was a curious silence about the testing, prevalence and the comprehensive statistics of the mortalities, equipment and related issues. Not only that, the earlier media briefings in Zimbabwe described COVID-19 as a 'returnees' pandemic', a per-ception that seems to suggest that it was a returnees' issue and those who had been in the country despite not having been tested for their status were nonetheless free of the disease! In the context of COVID-19 vaccination and religious beliefs, Zimbabwe presents a classic example of the myriad of issues that have emerged. These include hesitancy, ignorance and sometimes various levels of religious fanaticism which will need to be further investigated for the benefit of the health and well-being of the Zimbabwean populace and beyond.

A number of the Western countries have not been left out in the creation and propelling myths that feed into the feelings of uncertainty for many black people, including in Zimbabwe. As the pandemic escalated in Europe, Western media was awash with the troubling and increasingly dominant construct of racialising COVID-19 as a Black and Ethnic Minority (poor people's) pan-demic despite the indubitable evidence of the 'developed' rich white Westerners having been hit hardest. Equally, news of some of the African black leadership playing into that trap and trivialising the reality of the pandemic was not only politically and medically worrying but further problematised the subversion of the postcolonial project. These perspectives tended to ignore the fact that the historical legacy of exclusionary policies of equal economic access and better livelihoods for all are the primary reasons that make Black people more vul-nerable rather than simply the colour of their skin. These and other factors put together generate uncertainty which leads to the multiple hierarchy of resort that I have discussed in the other section of this chapter.

Discussion and Analysis

One way of interrogating how spirituality and uncertainty are core components of the COVID-19 discourse in Zimbabwe and Africa is to examine how templates of disaster management criteria have been resorted to as a response to the pandemic. Inasmuch as COVID-19 was a disaster, it is worth noting that sometimes the existing disaster management criteria are not inclusive enough insofar as they fail to encompass the sensing of spirituality and uncertainty as core phenomena in dealing with issues of dire need in the Global South, including Zimbabwe.

On a broader level, Roy (2020), for example, depicts the origins and initial reactions to COVID-19 in India grounded within sociopolitical and religious discourses in a way that mirrors in multiple dimensions almost a template which the rest of the global world would utilise as a convenient heuristic lens. Not only does it resort to the imagination and limitations of medical sciences, his arguments equally evoke emotions and resonate with other feelings of what pandemics do to humanity. The construction of otherness and scapegoating are clear and repetitive themes that justify skewed analysis of what pandemics are understood to mean and how the mystical solutions may be obtained both terrestrially and extra-terrestrially. Roy's (2020) framing of COVID-19 as a portal succinctly summarises what humanity in one part of an economically polarised jurisdiction engaged with the devastating pandemic. The polarity is almost unbelievable insofar as there is extreme "wealth, development and cutting-edge biomedical evidence" on one hand and indescribable poverty and anguish within the same geo-physical space (Massey, 1996).

In terms of COVID-19, there did not seem to be any ubiquitous and unanimous standards for controlling the spread or providing curative prescriptions. What existed were the contestable recommendations of using masks, maintaining social distancing and/or staying in quarantine. All these had a bearing on the popularity or otherwise of vaccines. The latter in themselves seemed to cut across the cultural fabric of the Zimbabwean and African beliefs and practices that characterise the much adhered to traditional and current ways of relating and interacting with each other in a dignified *ubuntu* fashion. Masks naturally obfuscate one's facial appearance and are not in tandem with normal practice unless if one has a facial injury or toothache. Both social distancing and quarantine presented problematic expectations among the Zimbabwean individuals and communities. Social distancing entails not only a geo-physical separation but an emotional and more fundamental descriptor of negative perceptions of the other. Quarantine on the other hand implies that the quarantined should not be publicly seen to be part of the family and community and as such would be essentially un-African. This is why, for example, individuals with mental health issues would normally be accommodated by the extended family in order to protect them from any form of ostracization or ridicule. Therefore, the point is that resorting to the COVID-19 requirements of social distancing and quarantine somehow implied imposing a rather new and uncomfortable type of spirituality which is alien and consequently arose feelings of anxiety, individual and collective guilt, thereby raising critical questions of moral and cultural abrogation. *Ubuntu* is therefore an indispensable source and product of African spirituality (Masango, 2006; Mazama, 2002; Olupona, 2000).

Conspiracy theories are prevalent all over the world. They exist in both scientific and popular domains. The acceptance of, rejection or hesitancy of

COVID-19 vaccines was equally shrouded in conspiracy theories (Humbe, 2022). One key underlying factor of conspiracy theories is the negativity, arousing fear and ascribing of blame and the attempt "to explain the cause of an event as a secret, deceptive plot by a covert alliance" (Rödlach, 2006). Rödlach goes on to argue that conspiracy theories are part of "a broad cross-cultural category of origin narratives". There is substantial evidence to demonstrate that in Zimbabwe and Africa (and indeed elsewhere), pandemics significantly draw on conspiracy theories to explain the complex, the unknown and the unexpected. Conspiracy in this instance is being used not in the sense of crafting spurious explanations but discursive attempts to develop profound understandings of complex realities using 'non-traditional' approaches in the form of cultural traditions, collective wisdom, reflective narratives and other locally generated hermeneutical tools.

Conspiracy theories broadly represent the practice of ascribing blame for negative occurrences to some evil. Conspiracy theories are not in themselves wholly unrelated to the reality that they will be seeking to explain but they are often self-justifying rather than seeking to subject themselves to the laws of rationality and objectivity source. The racist conspiracy theory is also premised on the missionary and colonial collusion which, in the wider scheme of themes, white supremacy discourses have always tended to be suspicious. In Sub-Saharan Africa in particular, there are equally other cultural myths and conspiracy theories which have been associated with undermining social progress in terms of seeking progress to pandemic challenges (Nyatsanza, 2015; Nyatsanza & Wood, 2017; Rödlach, 2006). This was played out in the responses to COVID-19 vaccines in Zimbabwe, with some religious people and others questioning whether the Global North, which has a long history of exploiting Africans, could be trusted to provide life-saving vaccines to the same people they have exploited throughout history.

In spite of the global public health guidelines regarding restrictions on physical proximity, public worship and rituals across the various religions and none, Zimbabweans recalibrated ways of ensuring that they either used online worship, prayer and reflection or in terms of culturally-based activities like celebrating births, visiting the sick members of the family, funerals and burials, connectedness was ensured through the deeply held beliefs in the functionality of the spiritual dimension. The resonance and levels of engagement through alternative communicative arrangements outside the realm of direct physical contact are critical testimony of how Zimbabwean indigenous spirituality is being sustained and expressed. This connectivity and functionality of the people's spirituality is being exercised at the terrestrial levels where individuals and communities live in different geo-locations in the same country or with diasporic relations. Much more critical is that it is also strongly recognised that the spiritual dimension is being discerned and mediated through communion of the faith adherents, Allah, God, the ancestors and the wider family as the case may be. Even in these 'new normal' circumstances, spirituality still remains authentic among the African people. For some, it was this same spirituality that had to be invested in, and not the COVID-19 vaccines that were being promoted in Zimbabwe and Africa.

Recommendations

One of the observations that one can derive from the above conversations is that COVID-19, including the accompanying vaccines, has provided both possibilities and multiple spaces to challenge reductionist and uni-linear approaches to pandemics. Instead, it serves to challenge the primacy of science in the traditional sense of the word. The possibilities and spaces should provide opportunities for interdisciplinary approaches that, among other things, recognise the meaning and recognition of spirituality and uncertainty as core issues of COVID-19 and indeed other pandemics in Zimbabwe, Africa and beyond. Paul Gibbs (2020) makes this point very clear in his analysis of the limitations of the prevailing engagements with the COVID-19 global pandemic.

One of the worrying developments regarding COVID-19 in Zimbabwe and Africa related to the fragmented efforts which in the main were country-based. Although South Africa as the then Chair of the African Union made an initial step at the onset of the pandemic to coordinate a continent-wide response with the help of local input and the Global North, the management of the pandemic, including vaccine distribution and access, remained fragmented and patchy. In order to ensure a better outcome for all, it was imperative that a collaborative and participatory approach needed to be put in place. While there were (and are) other kinds of setbacks across the African continent, good leadership, a clearer vision and genuine cooperation need to be seriously considered in order to deal with a pandemic of the magnitude of COVID-19.

A key resource that Zimbabwe has is the ability to mobilise itself through *ubuntu* in order to systematically harness and defend Zimbabwean spirituality as a legitimate metric through which to-be-defined aspects of COVID-19 can be observed, analysed and be better understood. Given that Zimbabweans and Africans are indeed inherently spiritual, that in itself should be a guiding force for the analysis, de-constructing and reconstructing the metaphysics of a pandemic that ravaged all its citizens irrespective of social status.

Conclusion

The COVID-19 pandemic raised a plethora of issues, including vaccine uptake, which Zimbabwe grappled with in its search for a sustainable solution. This chapter has sought to demonstrate how it has created power contestations through the lenses of spirituality and uncertainty. Zimbabwe's (and Africa's) unique socio-cultural, historical and health policy frameworks should seriously consider developing a hybridised approach that seeks to combine both local wisdom and tradition and the WHO guidelines in order to deal with a pandemic which is at its very core sometimes distorted by certain notions of spirituality and uncertainty.

Notes

1 While the chapter focuses on Zimbabwe, its ideological commitment to Pan Africanism allows it to use 'Zimbabwe' and 'Africa' interchangeably.
2 www.un.org/development/desa/dspd/everyone-included-covid-19.html
3 www.aa.com.tr/en/africa/nigeria-madagascars-herbal-drink-cannot-cure-covid-19/ 1915948 (accessed 20 July 2020).

References

Appiah, A. 1993. *In my father's house: Africa in the philosophy of culture*. Oxford: Oxford University Press.
Aschwanden, H. 1989. *Karanga mythology: An analysis of the consciousness of the Karangi in Zimbabwe* (Vol. 5). Gweru: Mambo Press.
Chavunduka, G.L. 1994. *Traditional medicine in modern Zimbabwe*. Harare: University of Zimbabwe Publications.
Chirombe, T., Benza, S., Munetsi, E., & Zirima, H. 2020. Coping mechanisms adopted by people during the Covid-19 lockdown in Zimbabwe. *Business Excellence and Management, 10*(1), 33–45.
Chitando, E. 2009. Deliverance and sanctified passports: Prophetic activities amidst uncertainty in Harare. In L. Haram and C. Bawa Yamba (Eds), *Dealing with uncertainty in contemporary African lives*. Uppsala: Nordic Africa Institute, 29–47.
Chitando, E., & Klagba, C. (Eds). 2013. *In the Name of Jesus! Healing in the age of HIV*. Geneva: World Council of Churches.
Chitando, E., Maseno, L., and Tarusarira, J. 2023. Introduction: Religion and inequality in Africa. In E. Chitando, L. Maseno, and J. Tarusarira (Eds), *Religion and inequality in Africa*. London: Bloomsbury Academic, 1–20.
Douglas, M. 2013. *Evans-Pritchard*. London: Routledge.
Dry, S., & Leach, M. (Eds). 2010. *Epidemics: Science, governance and social justice.* London: Routledge.
Dzinamarira, T., Nachipo, B., Phiri, B., & Musuka, G. 2021. COVID-19 vaccine rollout in South Africa and Zimbabwe: Urgent need to address community preparedness, fears and hesitancy. *Vaccines, 9*(3), 250.
Evans-Pritchard, E.E. 1937. *Witchcraft, oracles and magic among the Azande* (Vol. *12*). London: Oxford.
Garcia, L.L., & Yap, J.F.C. 2021. The role of religiosity in COVID-19 vaccine hesitancy. *Journal of Public Health, 43*(3), e529–e530.
Gelfand, M. 1988. *Godly medicine in Zimbabwe: A history of its medical missions.* Gweru: Mambo Press.
Gibbs, P. 2020. *What might the pandemic have done to and for Higher Education? European Distance and E-Learning Network Conference Proceedings*. www.eden-onl ine.org/proc-2485/index.php/PROC/article/view/1798 (accessed 15 June 2023).
Hall, S. 1992. *The West and the rest in formations of modernity: Formations of Modernity.* Oxford: Polity Press in association with Blackwell Publishers Ltd and The Open University.

Hays, J.N. 2005. *Epidemics and pandemics: Their impacts on human history*. Santa Barbara, CA: Abc-clio.

Hotez, P., Ottesen, E., Fenwick, A., & Molyneux, D. 2006. The neglected tropical diseases: The ancient afflictions of stigma and poverty and the prospects for their control and elimination. In *Hot topics in infection and immunity in children III* (pp. 23–33). Boston, MA: Springer.

Hountondji, P.J. 1996. *African philosophy: Myth and reality*. Bloomington, IN: Indiana University Press.

Hsu, E. 2008. Medical pluralism. *Tobacco Control, 11*(1), 1–2.

Humbe, B.P. 2022. Living with COVID-19 in Zimbabwe: A religious and scientific healing response. In F. Sibanda et al. (Eds), *Religion and the COVID-19 pandemic in Southern Africa* (pp. 72–88). London: Routledge.

Idowu, E.B. 1973. *African traditional religion: A definition*. London: SCM Press.

Kabakama, S., Konje, E.T., Dinga, J.N., Kishamawe, C., Morhason-Bello, I., Hayombe, P., ... & Dzinamarira, T. 2022. Commentary on COVID-19 Vaccine Hesitancy in sub-Saharan Africa. *Tropical Medicine and Infectious Disease, 7*(7), 130.

Lane, S.D., & Millar, M.I. 1987. *The"Hierarchy of Resort" reexamined: Status and class differentials as determinants of therapy for eye disease in the Egyptian delta*. Urban Anthropology and Studies of Cultural Systems and World Economic Development, 151–182.

Law, J. 2004. *After method: Mess in social science research*. London: Routledge.

Luedke, T.J., & West, H.G. (Eds). 2006. *Borders and healers: Brokering therapeutic resources in Southeast Africa*. Bloomington, IN: Indiana University Press.

Mafeje, A. 2001. *Anthropology in post-Independence Africa: End of an era and the problem of self-redefination [sic]* (Vol. 1). Heinrich Böll Foundation.

Magesa, L. 2014. *What is not sacred?: African spirituality*. New York: Orbis Books.

Maketo, J.P., & Mutizwa, B. 2021. Dynamics and trends in vaccine procurement and distribution in Zimbabwe. *International Journal of Humanities, Management and Social Science, 4*(2), 62–75.

Masango, M.J. 2006. African spirituality that shapes the concept of Ubuntu. *Verbum et Ecclesia*, 27(3), 930–943.

Massey, D.S. 1996. The age of extremes: Concentrated affluence and poverty in the twenty-first century. *Demography, 33*(4), 395–412.

Mazama, M.A. 2002. Afrocentricity and African spirituality. *Journal of Black Studies, 33*(2), 218–234.

Mazrui, A.A. 1980. *The African condition: A political diagnosis*. Cambridge University Press.

Mazrui, A.A. 2004. *Power, politics, and the African condition* (Vol. 3). Africa World Press.

Mazrui, A.A. 2009. "Who are the Africans?" In J. Adibe (Ed.), *Who is an African? Identity, citizenship and the making of the Africa-Nation*. London: Adonis & Abbey. 29–34.

Mbiti, J.S. 1990. *African religions & philosophy*. Heinemann.

McAbee, L., Tapera, O., & Kanyangarara, M. 2021. Factors associated with COVID-19 vaccine intentions in eastern Zimbabwe: a cross-sectional study. *Vaccines, 9*(10), 1109.

McNeill, W. 1998. *Plagues and peoples*. London: Doubleday.

Mead, M. 1995. Visual anthropology in a discipline of words. *Principles of visual anthropology, 3*, 3–12.

Mudimbe, V.Y. 1988. *The invention of Africa: Gnosis, philosophy, and the order of knowledge*. Bloomington, IN: Indiana University Press.

Mugari, I., & Obioha, E.E. 2021. African beliefs and citizens' disposition towards COVID-19 vaccines: The belief guided choices. *African Journal of Governance & Development*, *10*(1.1), 277–293.

Murewanhema, G., & Mutsigiri-Murewanhema, F. 2021. Drivers of the third wave of COVID-19 in Zimbabwe and challenges for control: Perspectives and recommendations. *The Pan African Medical Journal*, *40*(46), 1–7.

Murewanhema, G., Musuka, G., Denhere, K., Chingombe, I., Mapingure, M.P., & Dzinamarira, T. 2022. The landscape of COVID-19 vaccination in Zimbabwe: a narrative review and analysis of the strengths, weaknesses, opportunities and threats of the programme. *Vaccines*, *10*(2), 262.

Nyamnjoh, F.B. 2012. Blinded by sight: Divining the future of anthropology in Africa. *Africa Spectrum*, *47*(2–3), 63–92.

Nyatsanza, T.M. 2015. *Developing a transformative approach to HIV/AIDS education: An analysis of Scotland and Zimbabwe* (Doctoral dissertation, University of Glasgow).

Nyatsanza, T., & Wood, L. 2017. Problematizing official narratives of HIV and AIDS education in Scotland and Zimbabwe. *SAHARA-J: Journal of Social Aspects of HIV/AIDS*, *14*(1), 185–192.

Olupona, J.K. 2000. *African spirituality: Forms, meanings, and expressions.* New York: Crossroad Publishing.

Peters, M.A. and Besley, T. (Eds). 2021. *Pandemic Education and Viral Politics.* London: Routledge.

Ranger, T.O., & Slack, P. 1996. *Epidemics and Ideas: Essays on the Historical Perception of Pestilence.* Cambridge: Cambridge University Press.

Rao, D. 2006. Choice of medicine and hierarchy of resort to different health alternatives among Asian Indian migrants in a metropolitan city in the USA. *Ethnicity and Health*, *11*(02), 153–167.

Riessman, C.K. 2008. *Narrative methods for the human sciences.* London: Sage.

Rödlach, A. 2006. *Witches, Westerners, and HIV: AIDS and cultures of blame in Africa.* Left Coast Press.

Ross, A.C. 2002. *David Livingstone: Mission and empire.* A&C Black.

Roy, A. 2020. The pandemic is a portal. *Financial Times*, *3*, www.ft.com/content/10d8f 5e8-74eb-11ea95fe-fcd274e920ca (accessed 15 July 2020)

Said, E.W. 1979. *Orientalism.* Vintage.

Schwartz, L.R. 1969. The hierarchy of resort in curative practices: The Admiralty Islands, Melanesia. *Journal of Health and Social Behavior*, *10*(3), 201–209.

Schwarz, B. 2000. Actually existing postcolonialism. *Radical Philosophy*, *104*, 16–24.

Serequeberhan, T. 1994. *The hermeneutics of African philosophy: Horizon and discourse.* Psychology Press.

Showalter, E. 1997. *Hystories: Hysterical epidemics and modern culture.* Columbia University Press.

Sibanda, F. et al. (Eds). 2022. *Religion and the COVID-19 Pandemic in Southern Africa* (p. 270). Taylor & Francis.

Tom, T. 2021. COVID-19, lockdown and peasants in Zimbabwe. *The Journal of Peasant Studies*, *48*(5), 934–954.

Will, J.F. 2022. Covid-19: Medical decisions, mandates, and high-risk minors. *Hastings Center Report*, *52*(3), 4–5.

10 African Indigenous Churches' Response to the COVID-19 Vaccination Rollout in Zimbabwe

A Case of the Johanne Marange Apostolic Church

Henerieta Mgovo

Introduction

COVID-19 is an infectious disease caused by the coronavirus, also known as severe acute respiratory syndrome coronavirus 2 (SARS-CoV-2), which was first identified in Wuhan City, China. It affects people differently as evidenced in the variety of symptoms and the recovery periods and processes. On 11 March 2020, the viral disease became a global pandemic as declared by the World Health Organization (WHO, 2020a). The World Health Organization (WHO, 2020b) laid down stipulations and regulations pertaining to the prevention and containment of the pandemic, which were supposed to be followed by all the countries of the world. On 27 March 2020, the government of Zimbabwe, led by Emmerson Mnangagwa, stated that the country was going on a total lockdown for three weeks and all non-essential activities should stop forthwith. Along with the lockdown, there were several containment measures such as social distancing, wearing of masks, use of alcohol-based sanitisers and washing of hands using running water and, ultimately and after relaxing the lockdown measures, the rolling out of the COVID-19 vaccine. As much as individuals and religious institutions were affected by the COVID-19 containment measures, the chapter explores how the COVID-19 vaccination programme affected the doctrine and beliefs of the Johanne Marange Apostolic Church, an African Indigenous Church which operates in Zimbabwe. This Church was chosen because of its fundamental beliefs which differ from the mainstream churches and Pentecostal churches in the country (Musoni and Chitando, 2022). The prevalence of the unprecedented pandemic and the rollout of the vaccine had an impact on the customised existence of the Johanne Marange Church. The purpose of the study was to highlight the inimical effects of COVID-19 vaccination programme on the members of the Johanne Apostolic Marange Church. How was the Johanne Apostolic Marange Church doctrine affected by the COVID-19 vaccination programme? The research was limited to members of the Johanne Marange Apostolic Church who reside at Mataga Growth Point in Mberengwa in Zimbabwe.

DOI: 10.4324/9781003388630-10

Background to the Study

The outbreak of COVID-19 in March 2020 from Wuhan, China, came as a surprise to the world and it affected all the wider social systems of life. World Health Organization (2020) laid down the regulations which were supposed to be followed in order to curb and minimise the spreading of the infectious disease. Some of the regulations which were stipulated by the World Health Organization included social distancing, wearing of face masks and wearing Personal Protective Equipment (PPEs), among others (WHO, 2020b). The rules and regulations affected the churches because most of the church doctrines which are practiced within a church service require the people to collectively sit together and the procurement of the Personal Protective Equipment among most of the congregants was a challenge because they are very expensive. Hence, church attendance was very much compromised. Only the vaccinated people in Zimbabwe were allowed to attend church services. However, the procured vaccines such as Sinovac and Sinopharm require only those who are 75 years and below to be vaccinated while in Zimbabwe about 45% of the church attenders are above 75. This means that the elderly who usually devote their late years on religion and morality are barred from attending church services and this was an effect which was caused by the prevalence of COVID-19 on church operations. Musoni and Chitando (2022) highlight that the churches in Africa suffered a lot because most African countries are low income countries and the church leadership survive from the tithes which are paid by the congregants. Therefore, a lot of papers have been written with regards to how COVID-19 affected the Western-based churches but very few has been written on AICs and in particular Zimbabwe.

African Initiated Churches in the Context of COVID-19

Ohlmann et al. (2016) described AICs as churches which were founded by Africans. Most African Initiated Churches follow the African norms, values and beliefs. Most AICs believe in the traditional healing processes which are different from the mainstream churches which are present in African communities. Some of the African Initiated Churches which are prevalent in Zimbabwe include the Johanne Marange Apostolic Church led by Noah Taguta, the African Apostolic Church led by Paul Mwazha and the Zion Christian Church led by Nehemiah Mutendi to mention a few.

The Johanne Marange Apostolic Church was formed in 1932 by the prominent cleric Johanne Marange who named the church after himself and it was well established and formulated on the need to ask spiritual intervention during the colonial period and leaders who have emerged have kept the same tradition kept by Marange. Spitzeck (2018) notes that most AICs are reluctant on infrastructural development as they prefer conducting their church gatherings in forests and bushes and they usually remove their shoes when they enter their designated praying place.

Congregants of the Johanne Marange Apostolic Church believe diseases and illnesses do not need to be treated scientifically through vaccination but they need to be exorcised through the power of the Holy Spirit. By banning churches from gathering, it meant that the congregants were no longer allowed to meet with their leaders. This was a stumbling block and a hurdle to the members of the Johanne Marange Apostolic Church because they believe that being granted permission to worship and pray openly and in numbers would help eradicate the pandemic. At some stage, the government allowed certain percentage membership physical church services attendance, and deployed police to monitor compliance. The proximity of the law enforcement agents meant that this was a blow to the Johanne Marange Apostolic Church. As if that was not enough, the government came up with the pronunciation that only fifty people were allowed to be in church attendance at any particular time and, for the Johanne Marange Apostolic Church with multitudes of followers who, according to the church doctrines, must be assembled at once at the shrine so as to make sure that the Holy Spirit descends on them, the fifty-people-at-a-time rule was not accepted at all. Nyangoni (2021) in the Standard 8 July 2021 reiterates that the announcement by the government that churches were being allowed to operate as long as they had 100 fully-vaccinated people (Xinhua Net, 2021) was yet another challenge to members of the Johanne Marange Apostolic Church. The government statutory instrument on limited numbers asserted and accentuated that only churches whose members had been fully vaccinated were the ones who would gather.

Furthermore, the ways of integration of most African Initiated Churches are based on the collectivistic approach to life, the concept of African communalism (*Hunhu/Ubuntu*). In African culture, there is a shared desire to maintain group harmony and persons tend to toe the line to remove the risk of being ostracised by the collective group (Triandis, 2012). The regulations of COVID-19 harped on individualism and social distancing which is a taboo within most African Initiated Churches because they believe that individualism promotes marginalisation of the other congregants.

Moreover, Musoni and Chitando (2022) posited that all the iconic celebrations of the African Initiated Churches were disrupted by the emergence of COVID-19 and this was a challenge as well experienced by the church leaders as they felt disgruntled by the government's decision of implementing a lockdown when they initially stated that the salvation towards the eradication of the pandemic lies within the church.

The impact of the pandemic was also psychological as statistics in Zimbabwe reveal that the majority of the congregants in the Johanne Marange Apostolic Church are the elderly and with some conspiracy theories alluding that the novel coronavirus is targeting the elderly. This had a psychological impact on the existence and operation of the church.

The emergence of the pandemic was problematic to the operations and beliefs of the Johanne Marange Apostolic Church as the rules and regulations stipulated by the World Health Organization defied the norms, values and beliefs of the church. The total lockdown introduced by the government on the churches was yet another problem because many of the African Initiated Churches do not believe in the use of scientific medicines as helpful in the face of a pandemic, but rather being given the opportunity to pray. Despite the government's call for a total lockdown, most of the African Initiated Churches congregants continued going to church and gathered in large numbers. The law enforcement agents would give them a torrid time and this was also yet another challenge which the members were exposed to due to COVID-19. Therefore, it can be alluded that the church has faced psychological, cultural and social challenges due to the prevalence of the COVID-19 pandemic.

Effects of Lockdowns on African Initiated Churches' Attendance

In Africa, most AICs prefer the physical church attendance congregants because the online services are only attended by a handful who have the resources to attend such services. Apparently, African Christians are used to church services in which the leader of the church physically touches congregants as he or she prays for them. Muyambo (2022) says lack of physical attendance of the congregants affected the spiritual growth of the congregations and this hugely affected the church because the church is there to cater for the well-being of its people. For example, it can be related that in Zimbabwe, when the pandemic broke out the first thing which was banned were the churches and this was oxymoronic since the ancient times the church has been known to be the house of deliverance.

Spiritually, African initiated churches were affected by the inevitability of the pandemic because they believe in the exorcism of most diseases. Most of the African initiated churches including the Paul Mwazha Church and the Johana Masowe Apostolic Church believe that true healing and eradication of diseases comes in the house of the Lord. Masondo (2014) alludes that most indigenous churches do not allow their congregants to visit the hospitals as they claim that the holy trinity will cure them. This was an effect to the AICs including the Johanne Marange Apostolic Church because the congregants were indoctrinated to the fact that the Holy Spirit will take care of any health problem they will experience. The problem which affected the churches, in particular the Johanne Marange Apostolic Church was that the government on the other hand is implementing stiff measures for those who would have not been vaccinated and attended hospitalisation and the churches for deliverance were closed. Thus, the spirituality levels of the churches and their congregants was greatly affected because of the directives which were made by the government over the vaccination programme within the country as the congregants were left confused over which trajectory to follow. This is one of the significant spiritual factors which affected AICs. Pillay (2017) notes that a church is an institution which consists of the clergyman and the congregants, hence any problem which affects the church can be explained with regards to the congregants.

The spiritual effects which were realised in the AICs is that the explanations which were given on COVID-19 were Biblical while the responsible authorities were giving a biological perspective on the prevalence of COVID-19.

Methodology

The research used the qualitative research method and was limited with regards to attaining a greater sample size. The etiology of the unprecedented pandemic meant that the researcher had limited physical contact with the participants. According to Jordan (2015), qualitative research is an in-depth research using a range of techniques which aims to understand why people think, feel, react and behave in the way that they do. This becomes the best approach which can be used by the researcher in relation to studying or interrogating the Johanne Marange Apostolic Church believer's experiences. Rahman (2016: 123) says "qualitative research is interested in analysing subjective meaning or the social production of issues, events, or practices by collecting non-standardised data and analysing texts and images rather than numbers and statistics". The advantage to the researcher is that they focus on the societal issues affecting the Johanne Marange Apostolic Church.

The research design of this study was the phenomenological design. Lester (1999) claims that the purpose of the phenomenological approach is to illuminate the specific and to identify phenomena through how they are perceived by the actors in a situation. In the human sphere, this normally translates into gathering deep information and perceptions through inductive qualitative methods such as interviews, focus group discussions and participant observation, and representing it from the perspective of the research participant. Phenomenology is concerned with the study of experience from the perspective of the individual, bracketing taken-for-granted assumptions and usual ways of perceiving. Creswell (2017) alludes that phenomenological study explores what people experienced and focuses on their experience of the phenomena. Phenomenology is an approach to qualitative research that focuses on the commonality of a lived experience within a particular group. For Neubauer (2019) phenomenology is a form of qualitative research that focuses on the study of an individual's lived experiences within the world. The fundamental goal of the approach is to arrive at a description of the nature of the particular phenomenon (Creswell, 2017). With the advantages postulated in the above context, it is important to reiterate that the phenomenology research design was the ideal research design to be used in this study. Neubauer (2019) further notes that the phenomenological approach brings out that since each researcher is one-sided with previously revealed preferences and suppositions about the challenge that he or she is taking into consideration, this predisposition can rather be put aside, and find unknown experiences that are faced on a daily basis. A population is a collection of objects, events or individuals having some common characteristics that the researcher is interested in studying. The target population for this research were the members of the Johanne Marange Apostolic Church and they were asked on the effects of COVID-19 vaccination rollout on the church. The study was conducted in Mberengwa under Chief Maziofa at the Johanne Marange Apostolic Church stationed there. The researcher made use of convenience sampling. Crossman (2019) defines convenience sampling as non-probability sample in which the researcher uses the subjects that are nearest and available to participate in the research study. It can be postulated that one of the main disadvantages of convenience sampling is that it is not inclusive of many participants but it gives precedence to those who are in the proximity and vicinity of the research while ignoring other significant contributors to the research. Crossman (2019) views a sample size as part of or a subset of the target population from which data can be collected to estimate phenomena about the whole population. The research used ten participants in the study who contributed immensely to the effects on COVID-19 vaccination rollout in the Johanne Marange Apostolic Church. Research implemented the use of the semi-structured interviews. In-depth interviews bring out the probability to make investigations and act in response further to each of the participants' reactions with an end objective to advance the quality of information put together from these personal encounters. Cohen et al. (2011) reiterate that interviews are the best because they create an opportunity where interviewees can air their perceptions and views outside of the generally asked questions by the researcher. The interview guide also consisted of the demographical data of participants. The data was collected from the Johanne Marange Apostolic Church.

The research ethics which are fundamental to the implementation of the interview guide were of a virtue rather than vice. According to McLeod (2014) interview schedules have a standardised format which means the same questions are asked to each interviewee in the same order. This was important in the research as it made sure that consistency and methods free from bias were used. This was the procedure which was instigated by the research so as to avoid all the genres of bias which can be cultural, methodological and item bias.

Findings

This section of the chapter has brought into consideration the information and responses of the Johanne Marange Apostolic Church members from Mberengwa. Ten families were interviewed through the use of focus groups discussions to relay the impact of COVID-19 on the Johanne Marange Apostolic Church. The key aspects of the research were guided by the three research questions which guided the study and these were: How was the Johanne Marange Apostolic Church doctrine affected by the prevalence of COVID-19? What challenges were predominant in the church due the vaccination program? What was the overall impact or possible mitigation for

COVID-19 challenges on the Johanne Marange church in Mberengwa District under Chief Maziofa?

One female member highlighted that:

> The problem associated with COVID-19 in our church was that the pandemic came with the strict requirement of people to be vaccinated for churches to be attended physically and it is our church belief that God through his angel Raphael heals us, hence no need for injections and medication.

A different view was given by Lovemore Mativenga, one of the church members who said:

> COVID-19 affected our churches because the morale of the church members was greatly affected by the deaths which were being paraded daily in the mainstream media outlets and phone devices and this had a dent on the level of spirituality of the congregants. For the holy trinity to be amongst us there is the need for the congregants to sing and the prophets will go into ecstasy, thus being spiritual but when the morale was low due to the unprecedented pandemic this really affected the level of spirituality of the church.

The Mabuwa family pointed out thus:

> Theologically, our prophets within the church were not able to give a spiritually detailed account of COVID-19 and its implications and many church members lost faith in the process towards the church as confusion was now amongst them because external influences on vaccination were having an edge over them and that was a challenge to the church.

Another different perception and perspective to the saga was brought out by Mr Danmore Mandinyenya who asserted that:

> We do not believe in COVID-19, it's a common infection like influenza and never affected us because we continued with our church services normally, our church hierarchy which consists of Elder of the church, Youth leaders, Prophet of the church, Healers of the church, Nyamukuta of the church and owner of the church (regionally) all agreed that there is nothing as COVID-19. It is just an influenza and it never affects our church activities.

Abraham Hove from the Hove family asserted that:

> The COVID-19 pandemic had no impact on the church because we always conducted our church services without fear and on the issue of vaccination, even the government is aware of the fact that our church members do not visit the medical institutions because it is within the church doctrine to be

healed by the Holy Spirit, hence I do not think that COVID-19 had an impact on the church activities in any manner.

Zhou Shemunyoro, an elder brother to Zhou Munodawafa, articulated that:

> We cannot really say that the church activities were affected by COVID-19 not even despite the government stipulation that all church activities are banned were continued as normal because at the shrine that's where we are delivered, unless COVID-19 affected individuals within the church that yes I agree because we had our church members whose relatives were infected with COVID-19 and they passed away and this was one of the main impacts in the church because it affected the level of spirituality of the church members, in that manner and perspective yes I agree the church was affected by COVID-19.

Saliwe Sithole, a prominent Johanne Marange church member, also alluded that:

> Individuals within the church were affected by the pandemic and that is so true, but to state that the church was impacted by COVID-19 is just a fallacy, because the Holy Spirit continued to guide us and this *denda* (pandemic) was prophesied hence nothing affected us as we had been advised by the church leadership about the nature of the infection and how we can protect ourselves, so this was not something which was new to us, hence the effects and impact which is being spoken about not in the church but as components of the church yes.

In the same argument, Tendiso Chinhanga, another member of the church residing within the Mberengwa District, said:

> We are located in the rural areas where we have restricted movements and our houses are not haphazardly located like the ones in the urban centres and with the COVID-19 regulations stating that we should socially distance, our church daily practiced that, and we would attend our church gathering without any intimidation from the law authorities.

Another member, Tarubvira also postulated that:

> Economically, our church does not really survive on church offerings as it is prohibited to pay large amounts of money to the church because we neither have any rentals to pay and most of our church leaders are employed by different organisations and have their own businesses so, economically the church was not affected at all because our shrine is an open space we do not have any electricity bills or water bills or pay rentals to the rural district council or fund for an opulent life for our church elders, thus economically we were never affected.

However, the Mapiravana was of the different view and said:

> Inasmuch as most of the church's procedures of doing things were not
> heavily altered, since the induction of COVID-19 most people were now
> reluctant on sharing their things because of the fear of being given the infec-
> tious disease and this antagonised the collectivistic approach to life which
> is mainly spearheaded by the church and this can be attributed to be one of
> the main impacts which the church realised with regards to the emergency
> of COVID-19 within the world and the country as most church members
> now shunned the idea of sharing their valuables for fear of contracting the
> infectious diseases and this was the impact.

The policy towards responding to COVID-19 which was stated by the government antagonised the beliefs held by members of the Johanne Marange
Apostolic Church and this had an effect on their beliefs and health as well.
From the responses which were given by all of the participants, all of the
participants in the research agreed that they have never visited any hospital
since childhood and their church shrine through the intervention of the Holy
Spirit has healed them uncountable times, therefore, the forced hospitalisation of the church members who would have been forcefully diagnosed with
COVID-19 and shunning the shrine for help affected the congregants and
church elders as most of those who were forced to be hospitalised eventually
died, therefore one of the major effects of COVID-19 towards the Johanne
Marange Apostolic Church. They would interpret this type of death as a bad
omen, not the will of God.

The utterances and responses of the congregants highlight that indeed the
closure of churches due to the prevalence of COVID-19 affected the Johanne
Marange Apostolic Church members because many of the participants were
of the view that their church is the only place in which they could be delivered,
hence the closure of the church during a pandemic was not ideal. Others
also castigated the decision by the government to open churches to the fully
vaccinated, asserting that it is tantamount to the banishment of the Johanne
Marange Apostolic Church because most government dignitaries including
the president of Zimbabwe are aware of the fact that they do not visit hospitals
and they must respect their beliefs, hence forced hospitalisation and vaccination is affecting the church deeply.

The responses given by the Johanne Marange church members highlight
that the church as an entity was not affected because despite the emergency
of the pandemic they narrated that their church activities should continue as
normal. The reason why their services continued as normal can be attributed
to the fact that they worship in the bush very far away from the village and
shops such that the law enforcement agent would hardly reach for them or
the law enforcement agents chose not to arrest them for reasons best known
to them. Twelve participants responded to the questions which the researcher
were asking and the majority of the participants highlighted that indeed while

church members as individuals were affected by the effects of the pandemic which culminated in the form of deaths, the church activities were rarely affected by COVID-19.

The analysis and observations made by the researcher were that many of the participants in the study were less informed about what coronavirus is and the only stipulation and obligation which they obeyed was the wearing of masks and this was done because on any given instance and circumstance it was contravening the church doctrine unlike the vaccination programme which is being initiated by the government. This shows that the members of Johanne Marange respect their Church doctrine and their leaders more than the government and law enforcement agents. They said that they are protected by prayer (The Zimbabwe Mail, 2021) rather than those COVID-19 containment measures.

The government has asked religious groups to endorse the COVID-19 vaccine. The Catholic Church, evangelical and adventist groups have done so. But with a tradition of not seeking or trusting medical help, some of the "white garment" Churches such as Johanne Marange Apostolic churches are refusing to encourage congregations to get vaccinated.

With millions of followers across southern Africa, Johanne Marange Church's stance to refuse vaccines undermined Zimbabwe's attempts to vaccinate 60% of the population by December 2021. "We believe in God, and science is entirely subject to God's will." These are some of the sayings that were uttered by Johanne Marange members. "I grew up on my parents' prayers and I am passing it down to my children. My family will not take the vaccine because we are protected by prayers", some would be heard saying.

The Apostolic position threatens the success of vaccination programmes in southern Africa, according to research published in the *Journal of Religion and Health* in 2017, which linked it directly to the rise of measles outbreaks in 2009 to 2010. More than 85% of Zimbabweans identify as Christian, and 37% belong to the Apostolic church. Sentiments include "I believe we should not be forced to get vaccinated. For us who grew up without medicine, vaccinations are an insult to our faith and religion. Surely the authorities can achieve whatever they want to do without involving us." These are some of the general utterances that were witnessed during the research.

A majority of the members of Johanne Marange Apostolic Church believe they do not need a vaccine. "Our preacher gave us a clear instruction that if we use these little stones and holy water, he prayed for, nothing will happen to our families. Since COVID-19 began last March, our family and I have never suffered from this disease, we are as strong as ever", says one of the female congregants. She further alludes to the fact that, "My children are strong, so I have no cause to fear. I have always believed in prayers and this is how I choose to go through this pandemic." While the government mandates only the vaccinated can attend religious services, it is tough to enforce in the Apostolic churches, who meet outdoors on hilltops and in fields.

Prosper Chonzi, Harare's health services director, said the authorities are running campaigns on the benefits of vaccination to increase uptake. Despite the efforts to continue engaging the church many people are still sceptical about the vaccine.

There are fears that once vaccinated, one will not be fertile anymore. This misinformation is scaring many Johanne Marange men since they are polygamous and believe that marriage is for procreation. They said that on vaccination the government should leave an individual to make a personal decision and not be cajoled into taking the vaccination. "Telling people to stay away from church if they are not vaccinated is the same as forcing the vaccination, which is not right", one Johanne Marange follower insisted.

Discussion

The responses alluded to by the church members of the Johanne Marange stipulate that the church as an institution was not affected by the emergency of the pandemic. This observation, which was communicated by members of the church, is different from what the scholars have concluded. According to Pillay (2020) most churches were used to the physical presence of the congregants and this would eventually boost the economic standpoint of the church. From the above stipulated, it can be argued that the differences in effects of COVID-19 is based on the notion that church members of the Johanne Marange did not stop going to church and like most African initiated churches it does not have any infrastructural developments which require the payment of electrical and water bills and since they do not pay it can be understood why they alluded that the church economically was not affected by the emergency of the COVID-19 pandemic.

Nyangoni (2021) noted that some churches did not close and were not affected because they had the political shield of those who are in the top echelons of power. The same sentiments were echoed by some of the participants in the study who highlighted that despite the government ban on churches, the members of the Johanne Marange Apostolic Church continued with their church gatherings. This shows the reluctance of the national laws on the African initiated churches unlike the mainstream churches which are operating in the government. This can be further ascertained by the sentiments and utterances of the church members that the government is conscious and aware of the fact that the Johanne Marange congregants do not get vaccinated because the Holy Spirit is responsible for curing them in the emergency of a pandemic. The government had directed that all church members can only attend after they have been fully vaccinated but members of the Johanne Marange Apostolic Church continued to go to church without being vaccinated and this highlights the notion why many participants in the church stated that the church was not affected by the presence of COVID-19.

The majority of the participants who participated in the study noted that the emergence of the pandemic affected most of their church rules and doctrines which are sacred and should be followed accordingly. The participants stated that their church doctrine stipulates that in moments of gatherings they share everything, since this gives an insight into the themes which were uttered by Jesus Christ himself which among others is inclusive of sharing but the regulations which included social distancing and avoiding handshakes and holy kiss meant that the church's doctrine, with its emphasis on collectivism, was undermined. In response to the call by government to avoid meeting in numbers, the Johanne Marange Apostolic Church members continued to attend their church gatherings despite the ban by the government and subsequently the unvaccinated continued to attend.

The findings also reflected that the Johanne Marange Apostolic Church was not affected by mandatory vaccination programme as the church members stated that the government was aware of the fact that the Holy Spirit guides and protects them from pandemics, thus all the government's calls regarding the pandemic were unaccepted in the Johanne Marange church.

Economically, most of the reviewed literature effectively reflected that most churches' financial standpoints were affected by the emergency of COVID-19. Musoni and Chitando (2022) argue that most local churches in Zimbabwe were affected by the emergency of the unprecedented COVID-19 because when the churches were closed, they could no longer collect tithes and this meant that most churches' financial stability was affected. However, the responses generated by the participants who happen to be members of the Johanne Marange church stated that the economic position of the church was not affected because the church unlike most of the contemporary churches does not have any buildings which require electricity and water bills but they occupy spaces which are not paid for.

The results generated also noted that it is not the obligation and mandate of the church members to take care of the church's leaders as they are all employed and they provide for themselves. Thus, economically, the pandemic had no impact on the church as evidenced by the answers and responses echoed by the church members. The majority of the participants agreed to the fact that the presence of psychological challenges to the church members was inevitable and this affected the morale of the church. The participants mentioned that due to the prevalence of psychological challenges such as anxiety and panic disorder the morale and level of spirituality in the church decreased.

Conclusion

The results collected and information gathered from the participants clearly highlighted that the Johanne Marange Apostolic Church based in Mberengwa did not experience the magnitude and effects of COVID-19. As for government directives the church was on the safe side, hence stipulations such as the closure of churches, vaccination programmes did not affect the church as it was business as usual. What did not go well with the church members was the idea of forced vaccination which they did not adhere to despite the government's call. They even said that they told the vaccination team to go and call the president of the republic of Zimbabwe whom they claim knows that they do not go to hospital.

Recommendations

The study makes the following recommendations:

- Members of the Johanne Marange church are recommended to follow the stipulations as asserted by the government because this will make sure that their church members are protected by the laws of the country as no one is above the law.
- Members of Johanne Marange should be made to know that vaccination is not just for the government to reach 60% herd immunity but is a measure to safeguard people's lives including theirs too.
- The government of Zimbabwe should take a radical stance against the Johanne Marange church and make sure that like all the other churches it follows the rules and regulations of the country so that in times of a pandemic all the citizens abide by government pronouncements.

References

Primary Sources

Ms X, Munene Hospital (12/10/2021)
Lovemore Mativenga, Danga (13/10/2021)
The Mabuwa Family, Mpandashango Primary School (21/10/2021)
Mr Danmore Mandinyenya, Vutika School (17/10/2021)
Abraham Hove, Rengwe Shopping Centre (29/10/2021) from the Hove Family
Zhou Shemunyoro, Danga (29/10/2021)
Saliwe Sithole, Rusvinge Village (26/10/2021)
Tendiso Chinhanga, Mpandashango Primary School (22/10/2021)
Mr Takesure Tarubvira, Mwembe Village (17/10/2021)
Mrs Chipo Mapiravana, Vutika School (07/10/2021)

Secondary Sources

Cohen, L., Manion, L., and Morrison, K. 2011. *Research Methods in Education*. 6th edition. London: Routledge.
Creswell, J.W. 2017. *Qualitative Inquiry and Research Design: Choosing among Five Traditions*. London and Thousand Oaks, CA: Sage.
Crossman, A. 2019. *Convenience Samples for Research*, https://thoughtco.com/convenience-sampling-3026726
Dewey, J. 1993. *How We Think: A Restatement of the Relation of Reflective Thinking to the Educative Process*. Boston, MA: D.C. Heath & Co Publishers.
Fitzgerald, L., Heston, M., and Tidwell, D. 2009. *Research Methods for Self-Study of Practice*. New York: Springer.

Freeby, R. 2015. *A Phenomenological Observation of Two Theatrical Learning Environments.* Adult Education Research Conference. https://newprairiepress.org/aerc/2015/papers/24

Jordan, B. 2015. Importance of qualitative research and the problem of mass data gathering, Accessed on: https://Linkedin.com/pulse/importance-qualitative-research-problem-mass.data-gathering-talbot

Lester, S. 1999. An introduction to phenomenological research. Taunton UK, Stan Lester Developments. Retrieved from wwwsld.demon.co.uk/resmethy.pdf

Masondo, S.T. 2014. The African indigenous churches spiritual resources for democracy and social cohesion. *Verbum et Ecclesia*, 35(3), 1–8. DOI: https://doi.org/10.4102/ve.v35i3.1341

Mcleod, K. 2014. Orientating to assembling: Qualitative inquiry for more-than-human-world, Accessed at https://doi.org/10.1177/160940691401300120

Musoni, P. and Chitando, E. 2022. Spiritualisation of the causes of illness: An analysis of the Zimbabwe–born white garment churches' theological position on the origin and treatment of COVID-19. *Exchange Journal*, 51(4), 361–376.

Muyambo, T. 2022. Social distancing in the context of COVID-19 in Zimbabwe: Perspectives from Ndau religious indigenous knowledge systems. In F. Sibanda, T. Muyambo, and E. Chitando (Eds), *Religion and the COVID-19 Pandemic in Southern Africa*. London and New York: Routledge, pp. 37–51.

Neubauer, B.E. et. al. 2019. *How Phenomenology Can Help Us Learn from the Experiences of Others*, pubmed.ncb.nlm.n.h.gov/30953335/

Nyangoni, K. 2021. Zimbabwe Police 'shield' Marange Sect. *The Standard*, 18 July. Accessed at: http://allafrica.com/stories/202107190655.html

Ohlamann, P., Frost, M., and Grab, W. 2016. African Initiated Churches' potential as development actors. *HTS Theological Studies*, 72(4), 1–12. Accessed at: https://hts.org.za/index.php/hts/article/view/3825

Pillay, J. 2017. The Church as a transformation and change agent. *HTS Theological Studies*, 73(3). Pretoria. http://dx.doi.org/10.4102/hts.v73i3.4352

Pillay, J. 2020. COVID-19 shows the need to make church more flexible. *Transformation: An International Journal of Holistic Mission Studies,* 37(4), 266–275. https://journals.sagepub.com/doi/epub/10.1177/0265378820963156

Rahman, S.M. 2016. The advantages and disadvantages of using qualitative and quantitative approaches and methods in languages. Testing and assessment research: A literature review. *Journal of Education and Learning*, 6(1), 102 Accesed at: https://Doi:10.5539/,el.v6n1p102

Spitzeck, H. 2018. *African Instituted Churches: Close to God and the People, Organisation of African Instituted Churches*. Accessed at: https://oaic.org/African-instituted-churches-close-to-god-and-the people/

Taylor, S., et.al. 2020. A proactive approach for managing COVID-19: The importance of understanding the motivational roots of vaccination hesitancy for SARS-CoV2. *Sec. Health Psychology*, 11. https://doi.org/10.3389/fpsyg.2020.575950

Triandis, H.C. 2012. The self and social behaviour in differing cultural contexts. *Psychological Review*, 96, 506–520.

Welby, J. 2020. *A Message from Archbishop Justin Welby on Responding to Coronavirus.* Available at: www.archbishopofcanterbury.org/speaking-writing/articles/message-archbishop-justin-welby-responding-coronavirus (accessed 16 June 2023).

World Health Organization. 2020a. *Coronavirus Disease (COVID-19) Pandemic. Press Conference.* www.who.int/emergencies/diseases/novel-coronavirus-2019

World Health Organization. 2020b. Updates on COVID–19. Accessed at: www.who.
int>covid-19>information

Xinhua Net (12 August). 2021. *Zimbabwe allows Vaccinated People to Resume Church
Services*, www.xinhuanet.comzenglish.2021-08

The Zimbabwe Mail (8 November). 2021. "We are protected by Prayers": *Sects
Hampering Vaccine Rollout*: www.thezimbabwemail.com/religion/we-are-protected-
by-prayers-sects-hampering-vaccine-roll-out/

11 'Disconcerting Vaccination Voices'

Experiences of Diasporic Zimbabweans in the United Kingdom

Nomatter Sande and Silas Nyadzo

Introduction

The COVID-19 pandemic began to attract media attention when China executed a military-type lockdown of the city of Wuhan. Like in other European countries, the British media reported that the pandemic seemed a distant outbreak in which their interest focused on the civil liberties of the citizens of Wuhan. When the World Health Organization declared it a world pandemic on 11 March 2020, it triggered diverse reactions. For instance, there were many predictions, theories and mitigatory solutions. By and large, 'confusing voices' characterised the effort to identify the emergence of COVID-19. The increase in deaths caused diverse actors and institutions to step forward and contribute towards addressing the challenge. Media reports indicated that although Asians and Africans constitute a tiny minority of the British population, deaths from COVID-19 were proportionally very high among them. It is critical to understand the interface of religion, politics, and responses to COVID-19 vaccination in the context of religious diasporic Zimbabweans in the United Kingdom.

Methodology

The study employs a qualitative approach to evaluate grey literature. The increase in deaths caused diverse actors and institutions to step forward and contribute to the challenge. Since COVID-19 was emerging, methodologically we decided to employ a phenomenological observation qualitative research. Phenomenological observation is a process of observing events, people, processes, and objects while avoiding attachment and inputting the observer's prior prejudices, opinions, or dogmas (Freeby, 2015). The researchers are part of the African Pentecostal church in the diaspora. The researchers did not only observe but participated in pastoral ministry with and to believers. The main question of this study was focused on understanding how COVID-19 could have triggered diverse 'disconcerting voices' from politics, economics, medicine, religion, and responses to COVID-19 vaccinations.

DOI: 10.4324/9781003388630-11

Furthermore, how do these disconcerting voices in diasporic contexts out-line lessons learnt for the future in terms of the interface of epidemics, religion, politics, and responses to vaccinations? We analysed the data gathered for responses to vaccines through three thematic issues, namely, the religious voices; political voices; and scientific/medical voices. Our reflections were based on "assumption interrogation". Fitzgerald, Heston and Tidwell (2009) argue that "assumption interrogation" allows the researcher to cross-examine data through a reflective process to come up with new information that may emerge. This study moves from descriptions into the proactive engagement of these 'disconcerting vaccination voices'. The process of reflection is "active, persistent and careful consideration of any belief or supposed form of know-ledge in the light of the grounds that support it and the further conclusions to which it tends" (Dewey, 1993: 9). Our reflective process was skewed towards the enhancement of knowledge for social justice in responses to COVID-19 vaccinations.

Disconcerting COVID-19 Vaccination Voices

Many conspiracy theories and uncertainties about the origins of COVID-19 brought fear to many people. In the case of the diasporic Zimbabweans in the United Kingdom, COVID-19 created disconcerting voices about vaccinations. The voices included the religious, political, and medical realms. The United Kingdom is a multicultural context where there is connectivity amongst the religious, political, and scientific/medical worldviews toning down the drive of competition for supremacy. Therefore, paying attention to diverse disconcerting vaccination voices and how they impact the religious Zimbabweans in the United Kingdom is critical. We found out that diasporic Zimbabweans who adhere to both African Traditional Religions and Christianity predominately believe that nothing simply happens – there are forces which affect the health and well-being of people. For instance, from the African traditional religions perspective aggrieved or alien spirits cause illness and consulting traditional healers and herbal treatment solves the maladies (Chavunduka, 1978). While most Zimbabwean Christians do not necessarily deny that spirits cause diseases, however, the disagreement with the African Traditional Religions is about the source of the power of healing. Some Zimbabwean Christians, especially African Pentecostals in general understand the source of healing in African Traditional Religions as demonic (Sande, 2019). Resultingly, the advent of COVID-19 was understood from such diverse perspectives and intrinsically this has an impact on diasporic Zimbabwean vaccine acceptance and/or hesitancy.

Religious Voices

The study revealed that religion played a pivotal role for the religious Zimbabweans in the United Kingdom to either accept or deny COVID-19 vaccinations. Religious Zimbabweans remember that the missionary David Livingstone came from these shores and were not afraid to exercise their faith. The African immigrant Christians were vocal against vaccinations and galvanised its church membership, the wider community, respective national communities back in Africa and the UK government into fervent prayer. While it is known that there is a decline of mainline Christianity in the United Kingdom, Sande and Samushonga (2020) argue that the African Pentecostals are altering their experiences due to the demand of the changing socio-cultural context. There was a time when special prayers were organised to pray for the then Prime Minister Boris Johnson, who spent more than a two-week stint at Number 10 Downing Street, and St Thomas Hospital, before moving to Chequers with COVID-19 infection. Prime Minister Johnson must have been informed of the prayers of the Christians for his survival from COVID-19 (Roberts et al., 2020). As part of the African community, the overall feeling was that Christian Zimbabweans in the United Kingdom quickly resorted to prayers as a way of asking God to provide solutions which came in the form of vaccines. When the vaccines were introduced, the African Pentecostals viewed prayer as the premium.

The present study showed that even the monarchy was no longer keen on Christianity. Although the late Queen gave a speech about COVID-19 vaccinations, she completely avoided the mention of 'God' in her address as the Head of both the Church of England and the Government. This was contrary to diasporic Zimbabweans' views who felt that God had answered their prayers through the provision of vaccines. Similarly, some African politicians publicly highlighted the role of God in the context of COVID-19, especially in finding vaccines. For instance, John Magufuli, the late Tanzanian President, declared that COVID-19 is a "devil's tool" formed to disturb people from worshipping God in a time of crisis. He declared that "These Holy places are where God is [...] Coronavirus cannot survive in the body of Christ; it will burn" (Taylor et al., 2020). One of the issues that emerged from these findings was an appeal to religion by leaders in times of crisis. For most African Pentecostals the answer was not, therefore, in vaccines but in fervent prayer to God to save his people.

Commenting on the speech by Archbishop Welby is critical to this study. He made a speech on 13 March 2020. His message called on the British citizens to comply with government guidance and regulations; nurture the gifts of hope, faith, and courage through personal prayer; keep contact with others; help the neighbour while keeping social distancing; pray for the National Health Service (NHS) frontline staff; and lastly meditate on Psalm 46, "God is our refuge and strength, an ever-present help in trouble" (Welby, 2020). It is not fair, however, to be too harsh on Archbishop Welby since he followed the precedent which was set during the Spanish influenza pandemic of 1918 (Greg, 2020).

In the USA, where the Administration is closely linked with the Evangelical Alliance, several pastors defied their State Governors' orders to close their churches (Allen, 2020). A few of those who did sadly died from COVID-19

(Boorstein, 2020). There are no reports of British Evangelical or Pentecostal preachers taking the cue from their American colleagues. The COVID-19 pandemic forced Christian doctors and other medical staff to practice their faith openly. The *Church Times* reported, "Christian doctors and nurses have described how their faith has helped them through the fear, anxiety, and physical toil of working on the NHS frontline during the COVID-19 crisis. Many have prayed, and asked for prayers, for patients' healing and for staff to cope with the challenges" (Fry, 2020). With social distancing keeping most chaplains away from hospital beds, such Christian medical staff filled in the gap to provide spiritual support to themselves and any patients who needed them. This was very important in the UK where public space is highly secularised. Maybe the developed nations tend to neglect religions because they have other alternatives to deal with diseases. In 2009–10 media reports dominated the news of a Devon nurse who was moved from the ward to a desk job for refusing to remove her crucifix, with the Employment Tribunal endorsing that decision (Woodward, 2020). A British Airways employee, who was sacked for also wearing a crucifix in 2013, ended up winning her case in the European Court of Human Rights (Ralph, 2020). Even as recently as 2017, an NHS nurse was fired for offering to pray for a cancer patient who was going into surgery (Chibundu, 2020). So to hear that some staff at Northwick Park Hospital started their shift with a prayer to be able to cope with the overwhelming work becomes quite significant since it is not the norm. While these examples illustrate the centrality of prayer in health scares, experiences of African Pentecostals in the United Kingdom indicate that prayer comes first before vaccines. For them, the most important thing is not the end (vaccines) but the means (prayer). Diasporic Zimbabweans in the United Kingdom did not easily embrace COVID-19 vaccinations as was the case in Zimbabwe as shown by other chapters in this volume.

The *Birmingham News* made news in 1918 when they offered to print sermons, service outlines, and announcements for various clergy in Birmingham (Greg, 2020). This time around, in this COVID-19 pandemic, the term 'virtual church' has been coined for the various media platforms through which the clergy interact with their congregants without gathering in one place. The University of Birmingham wrote a brief titled, 'Rapid Adaptation: Telemediated Worship, COVID-19, and Virtual Services' to discuss the several initiatives by the various churches to remain connected with their congregants (Bryson and Davies, 2020). The study revealed that due to easy accessibility of online religion equipment in the UK, African Pentecostals did not see vaccinations as a prerequisite to church services as was the case back home in Zimbabwe.

Most smaller church leaders established their 'do it yourself' television channels which were linked to mainly YouTube and Facebook, with most funerals conducted through online 'Zoom', an interactive platform. The development of such channels affected the content of most sermons as preachers had to cater to the international audience instead of their local church audience. Online church services had mixed participation, popular preachers had a heavy subscription while others may struggle to be watched by even 50 subscribers. The audience is no longer limited to national boundaries. After COVID-19, it is not clear what church membership is going to be like since members have now been exposed to other external preachers of their preference. Due to this scenario gatherings were no longer possible and people saw no need to take vaccines. They would attend church in the comfort of their homes.

During this COVID-19 pandemic, Psalm 91 has been adopted by most Pentecostal/Charismatic and Evangelical churches throughout the world, including the Zimbabwean diasporians in the UK to encourage the faith of the faithful. Using anecdotal evidence from our experience as Pentecostal pastors, church members have established prayer networks across denominations to pray against COVID-19, and for those infected by it. Some ministers encouraged their members to participate in vaccinations. We have encountered several stories of survivors of COVID-19 who were subject to these fervent prayers. Using the Apostolic Faith Mission International Ministries UK (AFMIM UK) where we belong as an example, we have lost less than five members out of a membership of over 3000. Our view is that God has protected our membership in answer to prayer. However, further empirical research post-COVID-19 is required to make definite findings with regard to the role and effectiveness of prayer during COVID-19. From what is happening at the time of this writing, it can be argued that while the mainline British society has pushed 'science' to the centre through COVID-19 vaccinations, the African, particularly Zimbabwean diaspora has found the opportunity to force God to the centre in the public space in dealing with this existential threat. In the same line of thought, it is probably fair to argue that while the British do not explicitly express their faith publicly, the Africans in the diaspora exhibit a public spirituality in the context of a crisis, the COVID-19 crisis.

The nation's sense of panic even tolerated Christian prayers in public places, but mainstream media appeared to ignore such news. The Government's mantra that they are to be led by science was just a political game to push away blame when convenient. As discussed above, there were divergent voices which did not 'sing' from the same hymn sheet. The Zimbabwean Christians in the diaspora believe that the United Kingdom should go back to God and bring back God in the public space rather than merely relying on COVID-19 vaccinations. They contended that once God is back in schools and government, the nation would be better equipped holistically to deal with all the social, medical, and economic challenges.

Christian voices were very loud but it did not mean that the Zimbabweans who adhere to African Traditional Religions were not doing anything. The problem is that the solutions from African Traditional Religions are secretive. It is believed that if people know about one's herbs then the herbs lose their power. While the world was advocating for scientific vaccinations, Zimbabweans also latched their hopes on Zumbani (*lappia javanica*) tea. In the United Kingdom, 100g of Zumbani was sold for £9.99 (Mwanaka Fresh Farm Foods, 2021). Mwanaka Farm Fresh Foods is owned by a Zimbabwean who sells all products from Zimbabwe. According to Thebe (2022: 313) "home remedies (the most fashionable being steaming and *Zumbani* tea) are used simultaneously with Western medicines".

In general, all faith organisations, particularly other religions like Buddhism, Islam, and Hinduism invariably encouraged compliance with government directives and guidance to handle COVID-19 and vaccinations (The Interfaith Network, 2020). These faith organisations' primary focus appears to have been on how to navigate liturgical concerns for their congregants during essential festivals. All other faiths did not fare any better in terms of providing a religious prophetic voice to the government and the public. The implication of this is the possibility that religion is losing grip in the British but still firmly holding to diasporic Africans.

It clear that the religious voice made diasporic Zimbabweans in the UK hesitant to accept vaccines because of the continued prayers and herbal treatment of Zumbani and steam heating which emanated most from an African Traditional Religion perspective. However, it is worth noting that many diasporic Zimbabweans, including Pentecostals and African Tradition Religions traditionalists accepted the scientific jab as a result of the social desirability bias, not because they saw agency in vaccines.

Political Voices

The UK response to the outbreak of COVID-19 has generally been described as cynical, lacklustre, and not severe enough. The outbreak of COVID-19 in Wuhan was initially treated as a political game between China and the West. The UK appeared to agree with most Western countries that the emergency measures China had taken in Wuhan were draconian and infringed on human rights (Smith, 2020). The outbreak of COVID-19 in the United Kingdom wrought panic in the public which manifested mainly in panic buying of foodstuff and curiously toilet paper. To calm the nation, the Prime Minister, who was still revelling in his electoral victory and Brexit accomplishment, lulled the nation into complacency. Perhaps Boris Johnson, the then UK prime minister, was taking the cue from his 'special relationship' partner, Donald Trump. In one of his trademark tweets, the former US President Donald Trump wrote, "So last year 37,000 Americans died from the common Flu. It averages between 27,000 and 70,000 per year. Nothing is shut down; life and the economy go on. At this moment there are 546 confirmed cases of COVID-19 with 22 deaths. Think about that!" (Brooks, 2020). Politically, the emergence of COVID-19 has caused many labels at the expense of dealing with the pandemic. Other common labels include 'Wuhan virus', and yet others used the phrase 'Kung flu'. Besides the way the virus was affecting the Western countries, some African politicians argued that the pandemic was a way in which God was punishing the USA and the West for imposing economic sanctions on them. It follows, therefore, that while political actors' primary focus was to deal with COVID-19, they were blinded by their political differences thereby sending a wrong signal to the people. The vaccine hesitancy that followed the political bickering was indicative of the disconcerting voices.

It seems the UK was not taking COVID-19 seriously, WHO warned (Sinclair and Read, 2020). The European Union made block plans for procuring personal protective equipment (PPE) in bulk, but the UK opted out of that arrangement (European Commission, 2020). Probably, the UK could not join supposedly in the spirit of Brexit. It is debatable whether cooperation with the EU would have helped the UK in its fight against COVID-19 because while the EU set up the machinery to coordinate national responses to COVID-19 with the boast, 'This is European solidarity at its best', Italy was already suffering alone. On 12 March 2020, Boris Johnson announced a state of emergency and the opposition parties concurred with this decision. However, the Government emphasised that they would be guided by scientific and medical advice. It can thus be suggested that in developed nations, science takes the leading role as far as medical issues are concerned. The British Prime Minister admitted in the House of Commons on 27 May 2020 that the UK was unprepared for COVID-19 concluding with, "We didn't learn the lesson on SARS and MERS".

The British Monarch also gave a speech on COVID-19 from Windsor Castle. Queen Elizabeth II recalled the time she gave another speech from the same room during the Second World War. Echoes from those years conjure up the idea of the nation under siege, the cohesive effort to fight the attack, and the resolve and tenacity in the face of danger. She singled out the NHS for a special thank you while also thanking all citizens for their cooperation with Government guidance. It is significant to notice that the Queen might have been appealing to the British virtues of fortitude, bravery, determination, and resilience which saw Britain survive and weather the blitzkrieg. It shows that it is important in times of crisis to turn back and check lessons from history.

Economically, Her Majesty's Treasury through the UK Government provided arguably the most robust programme to support the economy by undertaking a furlough scheme (Sunak, 2020). The economy is a significant part of the body politic of any nation. The furlough scheme is basically an arrangement where the Government undertook to pay private workers 80 per cent of their wages. "We will support jobs, we will support incomes, we will support businesses, and we will help you protect your loved ones. We will do whatever it takes." boomed the Chancellor of the Exchequer in his 17 March 2020 statement in response to COVID-19. It is interesting to note that in the UK, through the lockdown, the government supported the vulnerable, and saved people's livelihoods.

The Bank of England also gave a statement to commit to underwriting the financial obligations of the Government during the COVID-19 lockdown and its aftermath (www.bankofengland.co.uk). Despite all such good intentions, the real test was in the implementation process. By 10 April 2020 media reports were suggesting that as many as 3 million Britons were going hungry because of the lockdown (https://foodfoundation.org.uk). The number of those going hungry shot up to a fifth of UK homes with children, according to *The*

Guardian of 5 May 2020. Some businesses and the public have volunteered to donate foodstuffs at the doorsteps of the most vulnerable people. The question can be, What lessons can this approach proffer to COVID-19, frontline health personnel, and health facilities in 'less developed' countries? A strange phenomenon of 'Rainbow' flags and banners on house windows and hospitals and some streets have etched firmly in the British collective memory during this COVID-19 lockdown. Perhaps the rainbow is symbolic of the diversity of various voices, which have represented the different sections of British society, as they speak about the COVID-19 pandemic. Considering the sorry state of economies and health facilities in many African countries, the evidence is awash that if COVID-19 is (and in fact has) to hit Africa as hard as it did in China, Europe, and the USA, the results would have been even more devastating. A curious sideshow about the 'rainbow flags', though, was the complaint by the Lesbians, Gays, Bisexual, and Transgender community that the six-striped flag had been 'stolen' by the NHS (Wareham, 2020). The political voices in most ways have made diasporic Zimbabweans to be hesitant to accept scientific jabs.

Scientific/Medical Voices

The pandemic started to get world attention as a 'pneumonia of unknown cause', when reported to the WHO on 31 December 2019. By 13 January 2020, the disease was now being referred to as the 'novel coronavirus' before the name changed to '2019-nCov' as January 2020 ended. The WHO Director-General announced on 11 February 2020 that finally the name of the disease would be called 'COVID-19'[1].

British scientists appeared to be silent on the developments of research on COVID-19 in the early stages. We noticed some activity by 5 February 2020 when a UK scientist joined global efforts to find a vaccine against COVID-19. Professor Robin Shattuck reported that in 14 days, Imperial London College had managed to develop a vaccine ready to be tested on animals. All they needed was further funding for the vaccine to be ready for human use by the summer of 2020.[2] By 17 April 2020 scientists from Cambridge University also published a paper suggesting that COVID-19 may have started as early as September 2019 and not in Wuhan, but in a southern province (Best, 2020). The objective of that research seemed to identify the origin of the disease to prevent future outbreaks. The UK Government's commitment to scientific research can be measured by its contribution of "£20m to CEPI, the Coalition for Epidemic Preparedness Innovations, an international agency set up in 2017 to deal with health crises exactly like this one" (Joshi, 2020). Professor Adrian Hill of Oxford University also joined in the race to produce a vaccine to treat COVID-19. By 20 May 2020, the UK Government announced a further £84m for research at both Imperial London College and Oxford University. The Oxford experiments which started in January 2020 have advanced to human testing as of April 2020. No definitive findings have been discovered from the sample of 510 volunteers as results were expected by mid-June 2020 (Gartner et al., 2020).

It is worth noting that scientists are working on re-purposing drugs which are approved to treat other diseases like Ebola, Malaria, and HIV to boost immunity against COVID-19 (Gartner et al., 2020). While the UK Government pitched the scientific voice to be the 'loudest' in determining its policy, procedures, and practices, the devolved administrations have been able to make different autonomous decisions. On 12 March 2020, the Prime Minister stated, "At all stages, we have been guided by the science, and we will do the right thing at the right time" (Johnson, 2020). The above position has made it possible for the Government to shift the blame to the scientists for anything that went wrong with the containment procedures. Scientists have been providing the UK Government advice through an agency called the Scientific Advisory Group for Emergencies (SAGE). When a government minister suggested that the COVID-19 death toll was too high due to 'wrong' scientific advice (McGuinness, 2020), SAGE was quick to defend itself by asking the Government to publish the advice in question (Siddique, 2020). The conflict highlighted above, therefore, makes it difficult for the public to believe the policies and instructions given by the Government in efforts to contain the spread of COVID-19 and save lives.

Further confusion was brought about by the formation of another, independent 'SAGE', this time the Independent Scientific Advisory Group for Emergencies led by a former Scientific Chief Adviser, David King (Vaughan, 2020). The latter appears to act as an independent peer review mechanism to the official advice given to the Government by SAGE. There appeared to be no such confusion in Scotland, Wales, and Northern Ireland. When the UK Government changed from 'Stay at Home, Protect the NHS, and Save Lives' based on scientific evidence, the devolved administrations remained with that policy. Nicola Sturgeon is reported to say that scientists provide advice, but it was up to the government leaders to make decisions. Only England, therefore, moved to 'Stay Alert, Protect the NHS, and Save Lives'. The meddling of politicians in the scientific project can never beat suggestions from President Trump of the USA who, so it appears, never ceased to grab onto anything that would make headlines in the media about COVID-19. Arguably the most dramatic and bizarre idea he suggested on 24 April 2020 was that COVID-19 patients might benefit from having injections of disinfectants. The Medical Doctor who accompanied President Trump to his daily COVID-19 briefings could only stare at the floor when Trump waxed lyrical, "Right, and then I see the disinfectant, it knocks it out in a minute, one minute and is there a way we can do something like that by injection inside or almost a cleaning, 'cause you see it gets on the lungs, and it does a tremendous number on the lungs" (Sky News, 2020).

On 30 January 2020, the WHO declared the 2019-nCov (as it was then) outbreak a Public Health Emergency of international concern thereby allowing for the Emergency Committee to convene. The key medical recommendation agreed "that early detection, isolating and treating cases, contact tracing and social distancing measures – in line with the level of risk – can all work to interrupt virus spread". The UK's Government's performance is measured against the major pillars cited above, namely, early detection, isolating and treating cases, social distancing measures, and contact tracing (WHO, 2020).

In line with their stance of being led by scientific evidence, the UK Government thrust the National Health Service (NHS) into the centre of the frontline to combat the ravages of COVID-19. The NHS became the last bastion against the onslaught of COVID-19, but there were other preventive measures which were adopted to contain the spread of the infection. In a laissez-faire attitude, accompanied by a show of bravado, Boris Johnson announced hygienic measures on the one hand while flouting the same on his escapades throughout the country. Containment and control measures were brought into effect as a knee-jerk reaction, perhaps in response to high-profile people, Prince Charles and Prime Minister Johnson included, who had contracted COVID-19. The ill-equipped NHS was thrust into the forefront and ended up suffering many casualties. The medical and scientific voices made many Zimbabweans accept the vaccine jab. Some diasporic Zimbabweans accepted that they were coerced because it was mandatory for those who were working in hospitals and nursing care homes to be jabbed. The majority of Zimbabweans do medical-related jobs (Mbiba et al., 2020).

Conclusion

The study showed that within the United Kingdom, there were disconcerting voices towards dealing with the COVID-19 pandemic including vaccinations. The medical voice worked alongside the scientific one, with the political one at the centre coordinating the fight against COVID-19. The political voice has faithfully stuck to the secular script to the hilt. Most of the political voices in this study showed that politics plays a role in the issue of public health by encouraging vaccinations. While religions have a special role within the UK, in the context of COVID-19 religious institutions rallied behind fervent prayer that led science to develop vaccinations. Therefore, the relationship between science and religion should be seen as one influencing the other. Religions in the United Kingdom were accorded virtual space and discouraged physical meetings and encouraged the use of vaccinations. There is less competition between science and religion for proffering solutions to the pandemic. Thus religious Zimbabweans in the United Kingdom received many disconcerting voices that influenced them to either be hesitant or to accept COVID-19 vaccinations.

Notes

1 @DrTedros #COVID19 pic.twitter.com.
2 www.imperial.ac.uk

References

Allen, N. 2020. US evangelical megachurches to open for Easter Sunday so 'Satan doesn't win'. Retrieved 31 May 2020 from www.telegraph.co.uk/news/2020/04/10/us-evangelical-megachurches-open-easter-sunday-satan-doesnt/

Best, S. 2020. UK scientists believe coronavirus outbreak may have actually started in September. Retrieved 27 May 2020 from www.mirror.co.uk/science/coronavirus-outbreak-started-september-british-21882200

Boorstein, M. 2020. Prominent Virginia pastor who said 'God is larger than this dreaded virus' dies of COVID-19. Retrieved 26 May 2020 from www.washingtonpost.com/religion/2020/04/13/virginia-pastor-church-dies-coronavirus/

Brooks, B. 2020. Like the flu? Trump's coronavirus messaging confuses public, pandemic researchers say. Retrieved 29 May 2020 from www.reuters.com/article/us-health-coronavirus-mixed-messages/like-the-flu-trumps-coronavirus-messaging-confuses-public-pandemic-researchers-say-idUSKBN2102GY

Bryson, J. and Davies, A. 2020. Rapid adaptation: Telemediated worship, COVID-19 and virtual services. Retrieved 30 May 2020 from www.birmingham.ac.uk/news/the birminghambrief/items/2020/04/rapid-adaptation-telemediated-worship-covid-19-and-virtual-services.aspx

Chavhunduka, G. 1978. *Traditional Herbal Medicine and Healing in Zimbabwe.* Gweru: Mambo Press.

Chibundu, O. 2020. Why is it wrong for a nurse to offer prayers? Retrieved 30 May 2020 from www.theguardian.com/commentisfree/2016/dec/12/nurse-prayers-sarah-kuteh-christian-faith-patients

European Commission. 2020. Coronavirus response. Retrieved 22 May 2020 from https://ec.europa.eu/info/live-work-travel-eu/health/coronavirus-response_en

Fry, M. 2020. More people praying during lockdown, survey suggests. Retrieved 31 May 2020 from www.churchtimes.co.uk/articles/2020/1-may/news/uk/more-people-praying-during-lockdown-survey-suggests

Gartner, A., Roberts, L., and Hope, C. 2020. How close are we to a coronavirus vaccine? Latest news on UK and US trials. Retrieved 28 May 2020 from www.telegraph.co.uk/global-health/science-and-disease/covid-19-vaccine-update-news-clinical-trials-coronavirus/

Greg, G. 2020. What clergy said when influenza closed churches in 1918. Retrieved 30 May 2020 from www.al.com/coronavirus/2020/04/what-clergy-said-when-influenza-closed-churches-in-1918.html

The Interfaith Network. 2020. Retrieved 2 June 2020 from www.interfaith.org.uk/news/faith-communities-and-coronavirus

Johnson B. 2020. PM statement on Coronavirus: 12 March 2020. Retrieved 26 May 2020 from www.gov.uk/government/speeches/pm-statement-on-coronavirus-12-march-2020

Joshi, A. 2020. Coronavirus: 'Significant breakthrough' in race for vaccine made by UK scientists. Retrieved 27 May 2020 from https://news.sky.com/story/coronavirus-significant-breakthrough-in-race-for-vaccine-made-by-uk-scientists-11926469

Mbiba, B., Chireka, B., Kunonga, E., Gezi, K., Matsvai, P., and Manatse, Z. 2020. At the deep end: COVID-19 experiences of Zimbabwean health and care workers in the United Kingdom. *Journal of Migration and Health*, 1–2, 100024. https://doi.org/10.1016/j.jmh.2020.100024

McGuinness, A. 2020. Coronavirus: Minister says 'wrong' advice at start of COVID-19 outbreak could have led to mistakes. Retrieved 28 May 2020 from https://news.sky.com/story/coronavirus-minister-says-wrong-advice-at-start-of-covid-19-outbreak-could-have-led-to-mistakes-11990896

Mwanaka Fresh Farm Foods and Butchery. 2021. Mwanaka Organic Zumbani Herbal Green Tea. Retrieved 7 April 2023 from www.mwanakafarmshop.com/product/orga nic-zumbani-herbal-green-tea/

Qulity-Harper, C. and Liverpool, L. 2020. Covid-19 news: People in the UK are sleeping less well under lockdown. Retrieved 28 May 2020 from www.newscientist.com/arti cle/2237475-covid-19-news-people-in-the-uk-are-sleeping-less-well-under-lockdown/ #ixzz6OQlmTGzP

Ralph, T. 2020. Nadia Eweida, Christian British Airways employee, wins discrimination case. Retrieved 30 May 2020 from www.pri.org/stories/2013-01-15/nadia-ewe ida-christian-british-airways-employee-wins-discrimination-case

Roberts, L., Fawehinmi, Y., Davies, G., Gartner, A., and Global Health Security Team. 2020. www.telegraph.co.uk/global-health/science-and-disease/coronavirus-news-lat est-uk-cases-covid-19-boris-johnson-updates/

Sande, N. 2019. Greening faith and herbology in Pentecostalism in Zimbabwe. *Journal of Religion in Africa*, 49, 59–72.

Sande, N. and Samushonga H.M. 2020. African Pentecostal ecclesiastical practices and cultural adaptation in a changing world. *Journal of the European Pentecostal Theological Association*, 40(1), 17–31.

Siddique, H., 2020. UK scientists must not be blamed for giving advice, says Royal Society head. Retrieved 28 May 2020 from www.theguardian.com/world/2020/may/ 20/uk-scientists-must-not-be-blamed-coronavirus-advice-says-royal-society-head

Sinclair, I. and Read, R. 2020. 'A national scandal': A timeline of the UK government's woeful response to coronavirus crisis. Retrieved 27 May 2020 from https://bylineti mes.com/2020/04/11/a-national-scandal-a-timeline-of-the-uk-governments-woeful-response-to-the-coronavirus-crisis/

Sky News. 2020. *Coronavirus: Trump Under Fire for Suggesting Disinfectant as COVID-19 Treatment*. Retrieved 30 May 2020 from https://news.sky.com/story/coronavirus-trump-under-fire-for-suggesting-disinfectant-as-covid-19-treatment-11977958

Smith, N. 2020. Coronavirus: Fears rise of Chinese cover-up as 56 million in lockdown and hospitals overwhelmed. Retrieved 14 May 2020 from www.telegraph.co.uk/news/ 2020/01/24/coronavirus-fears-rise-chinese-cover-up-40-million-lockdown/

Statement on the Second Meeting of the International Health Regulations. 2005. *Emergency Committee Regarding the Outbreak of Novel Coronavirus* (2019-nCoV). Retrieved 28 May 2020 from www.who.int/news-room/detail/30-01-2020-statement-on-the-second-meeting-of-the-international-health-regulations-(2005)-emergency-committee-regarding-the-outbreak-of-novel-coronavirus-(2019-ncov)

Sunak, R. 2020. HM Treasury and Chancellor of the Exchequer, Rishi Sunak on COVID-19 response. Retrieved 19 May 2020 from www.gov.uk/government/speec hes/chancellor-of-the-exchequer-rishi-sunak-on-covid19-response

Thebe, P. 2022. Home remedies as agency in the face of COVID-19 in Zimbabwe. *The Oriental Anthropologist*, 22(2), 313–335.

Vaughan, A. 2020. Independent scientists criticise UK government's COVID-19 approach. Retrieved 28 May 2020 from www.newscientist.com/article/2243236-inde pendent-scientists-criticise-uk-governments-covid-19-approach/

Wareham, J. 2020. *Why Some LGBT+ People Feel Uneasy At The Sight Of NHS Rainbow Flags*. Retrieved 31 May 2020 from www.forbes.com/sites/jamiewareham/ 2020/05/06/should-the-lgbt-community-call-out-nhs-appropriation-of-rainbow-flag/ #34fc3f3cd544

Woodward, J. 2020. Nurse who refused to hide crucifix loses case. Retrieved 29 May 2020 from www.independent.co.uk/news/uk/home-news/nurse-who-refused-to-hide-crucifix-loses-case-1937269.html

12 Vaccination Uptake and Power Dynamics

Insights from African Initiated Churches and Traditional Healers in Masvingo Province, Zimbabwe

Excellent Chireshe and Mavis Thokozile Macheka

Introduction

In 2021, the World Health Organization (WHO) reported that more than three million fatalities and 1.55 billion cases had been recorded globally (WHO, 2021a). Realising the threat and global impact of the COVID-19 pandemic, scientists made efforts to introduce vaccination against the novel coronavirus as one of the most effective strategies for fighting the disease. It was argued that more than 100 vaccines had gone beyond the pre-clinical development phase with more than half of these reaching the clinical development phase (WHO, 2021b). Scholars further explained that herd immunity for SARS-CoV-19 could be reached by vaccinating about 60–72% of the population (Anderson et al., 2020). Therefore, the rate at which people uptook the vaccines was critical in containing the virus. As for Africa, for instance, it was documented that the region was lagging behind in COVID-19 vaccination rollout, with only 10.2% of its population fully vaccinated, compared to 55.5% globally (WHO, 2022). The WHO further reported that between January and August 2021, the low vaccination coverage was due to insufficient availability of vaccines but since August 2021, vaccine supply in the African region increased significantly as a result of the introduced COVAX facility, which donated 69% of all vaccines received in the African region.

Apart from the supply challenges highlighted, the vaccine rollout and uptake were a contested terrain characterised by both willingness to get vaccinated and vaccine hesitancy in the wake of misinformation and disinformation propagated mostly through social media. Vaccination uptake is voluntary but due to COVID-19 vaccination resistance and hesitancy and the need to reach herd immunity for SARS-CoV-19, governments in power have to implement various strategies to encourage their population to accept vaccination. The Government of Zimbabwe was no exception as it embarked on a vaccine rollout programme. Against this background, this chapter seeks to examine the different lived realities of some members of African Initiated Churches (AICs) and traditional healers in terms of their vaccine uptake and attitudes towards

DOI: 10.4324/9781003388630-12

the same. As existing COVID-19 vaccine studies have barely concentrated on religious factors influencing vaccine uptake, this chapter seeks to address the following research questions: What were the perceptions and attitudes of AICs and traditional healers towards COVID-19 vaccination? What intervention strategies were employed by the different sectors of society to encourage vaccine uptake? What factors influenced COVID-19 vaccine acceptance and hesitancy among members of the AICs and traditional healers? It is these questions that the study will need to address to establish the influence of power dynamics in the ultimate decision and action towards vaccination.

Contextual Background

The outbreak of the COVID-19 pandemic caused by the SARS-CoV-2 and its devastating consequences challenged governments the world over to institute control measures. The responses included, among others, aggressive implementation of suppression strategies, such as case identification, quarantine and isolation, contact tracing, and social distancing (Yamey et al., 2020). As the WHO warned the world of possible immediate outbreaks (Mahfound et al., 2020), the development of COVID-19 vaccines was perceived as the lasting solution (Yamey et al., 2020). Despite the existence of scientific evidence that the development of vaccines usually takes up to a decade, the available new manufacturing platforms, structure-based antigen design, computational biology, protein engineering, and gene synthesis have provided the tools to now make vaccines with speed and precision (Graham, 2020). It is because of this that the COVID-19 vaccines were developed in record time. Though it was hoped that the acceptance and uptake of the vaccines could bring the COVID-19 pandemic under control, the vaccines were received with mixed feelings by the public. There was vaccine hesitancy globally.

The issue of vaccine hesitancy is not unprecedented. As Galagali et al. (2022) argue, vaccine hesitancy is a complicated and multi-faceted phenomenon that dates back to the first vaccinations performed by Dr Zabdiel Boylston (1721) and Edward Jenner (1796–1798). They add that, in 2019, the WHO named vaccine hesitancy as one of the top ten threats to global health. Vaccine hesitancy, so goes the argument, limits vaccine uptake and ability to achieve collective immunity and possible solutions. A study of vaccine hesitancy and refusal by Dube et al. (2015) revealed that even though scientists recognise vaccination as one of the most successful public health measures, there were anti-vaccination movements that were blamed for lowering vaccine acceptance rates and the increase in vaccine-preventable disease outbreaks and epidemics. For instance, in the 1990s, there were anti-vaccination movements against the hepatitis B vaccine and multiple sclerosis in France that resulted in the suspension of the universal vaccination programme (Francois et al., 2005). Similarly, at the end of the nineteenth century, anti-vaccination activists in North America campaigned against smallpox vaccines (Betsch et al., 2010).

Vaccination has always been associated with resistance since time immemorial due to varied anti-vaccine conspiracy theories and beliefs. An investigation into the influence of such conspiracy allegations on vaccination intentions has been carried out in a British community. Anti-vaccine conspiracy beliefs result in a negative attitude towards vaccines and misinterpretation of vaccination intention and are mostly caused by the perceived dangers of vaccines, and feelings of powerlessness, disillusionment and mistrust in authorities (Jolley and Douglas, 2014). This issue of vaccine hesitancy was not only for pandemics. In more recent studies on the vaccination of children against some chronic conditions, vaccine hesitancy is also popular. In Italy, for instance, despite a majority of parents acknowledging that children with chronic diseases are at greater risk of complications from vaccine-preventable diseases and that these diseases are dangerous for their children, some parents were still doubtful about vaccination (Napolitano et al., 2022). Napolitano and colleagues argue that reasons for hesitancy range from a concern about the potential side effects of the vaccines, the belief that vaccination administration was not useful, to accessing the information on recommended vaccination from the Internet, social and mass media. In Amasya, parents refused to vaccinate their children because of suspicion that there are harmful substances in the vaccine, that the vaccine would harm the child and lack of confidence emanating from the fact that all childhood vaccines come from abroad (Sonkaya and Ozturk, 2022).

With regard to COVID-19 vaccine hesitancy and acceptance, it has been documented that vaccine acceptance was higher in developing countries than in developed countries. The scientifically proven efficiency of vaccines in curbing the spread of COVID-19 did not automatically lead to a decrease in global vaccine hesitancy (Gerussi et al., 2021; Paul et al., 2021). A comparative study of at least ten low-middle income countries, Russia (upper-middle income) and the USA (high-income country) revealed a significantly higher willingness to take a COVID-19 vaccine in low-middle income countries, compared with the USA and Russia (Solis et al., 2021). Again, despite the surge of the deadly Delta variant among the US populations, there was a suboptimal vaccine acceptance rate (Agley et al., 2021; Liu et al., 2021; Baack et al., 2021). Similarly, another study of vaccine hesitancy in the USA demonstrates that vaccine hesitancy is a challenge for the success and optimal implementation of COVID-19 immunisation programs in the USA (Wang and Liu, 2022). They argue that it is mainly due to vaccine-related conspiracy/misinformation from social media. Some factors influencing vaccine acceptance and hesitancy in the USA were noted by several scholars as minority race, gender, low socioeconomic status, religious considerations, community norms, media information and healthcare resources (Mercadante and Law, 2021; Daly and Robinson, 2021; Szilagyi et al., 2021; Ruiz and Bell, 2021). Another systematic review of vaccine acceptance and hesitancy established that the highest COVID-19 hesitancy rate was found in Arabian countries compared with other parts of the world (Cascini et al., 2021). The results of that review point to reasons for having a negative perception of vaccine efficacy, safety, convenience and price and it was mainly among the marginalised groups.

In Africa, it is argued that the existing negative experiences with the healthcare system and general distrust towards the government fuelled distrust and suspicion towards COVID-19 vaccines (Ackah et al., 2021). Further, the region which historically struggles with adequate supplies and equitable access to healthcare also faces a new hurdle—insufficient vaccine uptake. Several factors contributed to either accepting or rejecting the COVID-19 vaccines across Africa. In Nigeria, for instance, reasons for vaccine hesitancy included distrust, inadequate information, fear of long-term effects and infertility-related rumours (Iliyasu et al., 2021a), marital status, respondents' age and Christian denominational affiliation (Uzochukwu et al., 2021), doubts about the existence of COVID-19, mistrust of authorities, and popular credence to rumours and conspiracy theories (Iliyasu et al., 2021b) and concerns and worries about the 'speed' with which the vaccines were being produced, the possibility of future adverse effects from vaccination, misinformation, and level of preparedness in the health system to implement the vaccine campaign (Chokwuocha et al., 2022).

On the other hand, scholars also identified factors that led to vaccine acceptance. A study in Bangladesh, India, Myanmar, Kenya, the Democratic Republic of the Congo (DRC) and Tanzania revealed that perceived social norms, perceived positive and negative consequences, perceived risk, perceived severity, trust, perceived safety, and expected access to COVID-19 vaccines, perceived self-efficacy, trust in COVID-19 information provided by leaders, perceived divine will and perceived action efficacy of the COVID-19 vaccines led to COVID-19-vaccine acceptance (Davis et al., 2022). A survey of six Sub-Saharan African populations, namely, Burkina Faso, Ethiopia, Malawi, Mali, Nigeria and Uganda also established that information, sensitisation and engagement campaigns raised acceptance for a COVID-19 vaccine in the richer and more educated households (Kanyanda et al., 2021). Health personnel across the continent were also not a challenge when it comes to accepting vaccination (Nzaji et al., 2020; Wiysonge et al., 2021).

Through these works, we have a fair understanding of vaccine hesitancy and acceptance across the globe. There is, however, a limitation on data related to the influence of religious beliefs on either acceptance or hesitancy towards vaccination. Again, the data for reviewed works are more generalised where scholars were assessing the community in general. We acknowledge that African spiritualities and values are anchoring for most Africans regardless of religious denomination and thus we need to explore how African spiritualities shape and inform the community's responses to COVID-19 vaccination. In particular, we will draw our readers to experiences of AICs and traditional healers in Masvingo province, Zimbabwe, on vaccine acceptance and hesitancy. We will further establish the influence of power dynamics in their decisions and actions towards vaccination.

Materials and Methods

Data discussed in this chapter were drawn from a qualitative study through key informant interviews and focus group discussions with participants from Masvingo and Bikita districts. The study adopted a sociological approach where we examined how religion influences societal decisions on vaccination acceptancy and hesitancy. This qualitative study commenced with an examination of secondary sources in order to acquaint the researchers with the available literature on vaccine hesitancy and acceptance. Data from literature review were complemented with key informant interviews and focus group discussions. Twenty-eight purposively sampled key informant interviews were conducted with traditional leadership, religious leaders, traditional healers, faith-based organisations (FBOs) and Ministry of Health and Child Care officials. A total of nine focus group discussions with church members and traditional healers were conducted.

The participants were engaged to understand the emergent dynamic ushered when African spiritualities intersect with uncertainties, risks and insecurities that are associated with COVID-19 vaccination. We engaged traditional leaders such as chiefs and councillors to understand their experiences of encouraging people from different religious backgrounds to uptake COVID-19 vaccination. Religious leaders and faith-based organisations from both Christianity and African traditional religion (traditional healers) were engaged to understand their perceptions and attitude towards COVID-19 vaccination and the strategies they employed to encourage or discourage their members to accept vaccination. Environmental Health Technicians from the Ministry of Health and Child Care were also part of this study because they were mandated by an Act of Parliament to be responsible for encouraging and vaccinating the community. They were included because they had experienced everyday challenges and successes in vaccinating the community and reasons thereof. Church members and community were engaged to understand their perceptions towards vaccination and to explore factors that influenced their decisions towards vaccination/non-vaccination.

Data were subjected to thematic analysis and detailed descriptions, narrative vignettes and direct quotes from interviews and focus group discussions were presented following the themes. Further, ethical considerations such as debriefing, informed consent, voluntary participation, confidentiality and respect of culture were mainstreamed.

Results and Interpretation

This section presents and analyses findings obtained from the empirical study. Interviews and focus group discussions with key informants revealed different perceptions and attitudes towards the COVID-19 vaccine. The presentation is centred on vaccine uptake and the attitudes related to such. The following issues namely: (1) perceptions and attitudes towards COVID-19 vaccination, (2) strategies to encourage vaccination uptake, (3) factors influencing vaccine uptake, and (4) factors influencing vaccine hesitancy, were the major recurrent themes identified during data analysis. The study established diverse responses to the COVID-19 vaccination programme. The responses were partly influenced by the conceptualisation of the pandemic.

Perceptions and Attitudes Towards COVID-19 Vaccination

Perceptions and attitudes towards COVID-19 vaccination were varied. They were a function of a number of factors. As some scholars noted earlier, vaccination received mixed reactions from people (Dube et al., 2015). There was both acceptance and negation of the vaccine. In Masvingo and Bikita districts, leaders were a critical feature in the formation of attitudes towards the vaccine. Whereas some religious leaders showed support for government programmes by accepting the vaccine, other religious leaders were not supportive. They repelled vaccination and, in the process, discouraged their members from getting vaccinated. Many political leaders exerted force on the people by using threats to get them vaccinated. On the other hand, religious leaders were persuasive. Apart from religious leaders, media, especially social media, was very critical in information dissemination. Social media was associated with misinforming people through conspiracy theories. From the study, it can be noted that at first most people were resistant to vaccination. They were suspicious due to the bombardment of misinformation that was being circulated through social media. People were confused because what the government was commanding them to do and what social media circulated, were at variance. Attitudes towards COVID-19 vaccination were reflected through vaccine acceptance and hesitancy, as well as associated justifications. Findings from village workers show that churches that appreciated the dangers of COVID-19 were supportive of the government-initiated vaccination programme and allowed their members to get vaccinated.

Vaccine Acceptance

Various strategies were used by those in authority (political figures, religious leaders in AICs, traditional healers, and other community leaders, as well as healthcare workers) to get people vaccinated. The strategies were both coercive and non-coercive. Religious leaders set examples for their followers to follow. Those leaders who got vaccinated encouraged their followers to do the same. They encouraged their followers by setting examples. Because religious leaders wield influence upon their members, what they say and do is likely to have great influence on the conduct and beliefs of their members. This applies to vaccination. The following sub-sections discuss in detail experiences of communities under study.

Encouragement by Influential People, Through Words

It came out that church and traditional leaders, traditional healers and healthcare workers encouraged people to get vaccinated. They encouraged people to follow the WHO guidelines as mandated by the government. Some leaders from AICs encouraged their members to follow government regulations on COVID-19 management. In connection with this, one pastor, a focus group member, said:

> We encouraged our members to get vaccinated just as the government encouraged everyone to get vaccinated. We followed government rules on COVID-19 management. As such, we encouraged those who were willing to get vaccinated to do so, without using force.[1]

In a similar vein, a focus group member from a Zionist Church said that their bishop advised them to follow what they were told by village healthcare workers. When the vaccine came, their bishop encouraged them to get vaccinated. It also emerged that the government tried to persuade people to get vaccinated by telling them that vaccination was going to render the masks unnecessary as it was a panacea to the pandemic. Given that many people were not comfortable with putting on face masks, this was an incentive for vaccination. As a result of the encouragement, several people got vaccinated.

Some religious leaders encouraged their followers to get vaccinated by assuring them that the COVID-19 vaccine was safe as it was just like child vaccination against child killer diseases such as measles and polio. Since it is a norm for most people, apart from members of the Johanne Marange Church, to have their children vaccinated, the analogy resulted in people shedding suspicion on vaccination against COVID-19. Challenging conspiracy theories that the vaccinated were going to die or suffer negative health consequences, some religious leaders indicated that no government would want to kill its people and, therefore, the members were to rest assured that the vaccine was safe.

Encouragement by Influential People, Through Setting an Example

The study revealed that traditional healers and most church leaders supported vaccination as a solution to the COVID-19 pandemic. They encouraged their clients/followers to get vaccinated and led by example. Leaders from Pentecostal churches that participated in the study indicated that they were vaccinated because they were both loyal to the government and convinced that the vaccine was an effective remedy to COVID-19. Another reason was to set an example for their followers to follow. Concerning this, one leader said:

> We got vaccinated so that those who follow us can do the same. It is not possible to encourage someone to do something that you have not done. We

encouraged them to get vaccinated to protect themselves and their families. We explained to them the benefits of vaccination as we had learnt from healthcare officials.[2]

This led to a significant number of followers accepting COVID-19 vaccination.

Responses from focus groups lend support to responses from key informant interviews. In terms of strategies employed to encourage COVID-19 vaccination, one focus group member belonging to a Zionist church said:

> Our Bishop was the first one to get vaccinated. He showed us his vaccination card and encouraged us to go and get vaccinated.[3]

The bishop is further reported as having presented his COVID-19 vaccination card to his congregants as evidence that he was vaccinated. The bishop was further quoted as saying:

> It is a lie that those who are vaccinated are going to die. I was vaccinated, but I'm still alive. Go and get vaccinated. As a church we allow vaccination.[4]

Another focus group member from the Zionist Church added:

> Because of the example of our bishop, we all went for vaccination. What encouraged us to get vaccinated was the support that we got from our church leaders. They encouraged us to support the COVID-19 vaccination programme that was initiated by the government.[5]

One church leader reiterated what the church members said in terms of setting examples for others to follow. He said:

> When the vaccine came, we leaders were vaccinated. This gave us the energy to encourage our members to get vaccinated.[6]

Responses from councillors indicate that they worked collaboratively with village health workers. To encourage people to get vaccinated, they explained to them the benefits of the vaccine and that they had been vaccinated and did not experience any negative side effects. This strategy was helpful because it saw several people joining the vaccination queues. Traditional healers also encouraged their clients to get vaccinated. They displayed their vaccination cards in their surgeries for clients to see that they walk the talk when it comes to vaccination. They also assured their clients that they would not die because of vaccination and so they should not hesitate to get vaccinated. Traditional healers taught that the use of traditional medicine alongside vaccination was helpful in the face of COVID-19. This contributed to vaccine acceptance; a finding that corresponds with findings from earlier studies conducted in some Sub-Saharan African countries, namely, Burkina Faso, Malawi, Uganda, Mali, Ethiopia and

Nigeria, as reported by Kanyanda et al. (2021). The studies established that information and sensitisation raised acceptance for a COVID-19 vaccine.

Since leaders, especially religious ones, command respect among their followers, their influence on the followers is significant, hence the acceptance of vaccines, following the example of their leaders. This finding corresponds with the view of scholars such as Davis et al. (2022) that trust in COVID-19 information provided by leaders led to vaccine acceptance.

Coercion Through Threats and Policies

Politicians encouraged people to get vaccinated, through both persuasion and the use of threats. The use of threats by the government forced some people to accept vaccination. While on the one hand, the government said no one was going to be forced to get vaccinated, threats of the unvaccinated not being able to access social services forced some people to get vaccinated. The following verbal quote from a ward councillor highlights the government's coercive tendencies:

> When the government realised that the vaccination uptake was low it resorted to threats. It instilled fear in the people by telling them that they were not forced to get vaccinated but there shall come a time when the unvaccinated would not be allowed to board the Zupco buses, to attend church services, or to join social gatherings.[7]

This left people with little choice but to get vaccinated so that they would be able to go to church, to board the Zupco buses and to join gatherings.

Later, the government moved from threat to action. It gave the directive that only the vaccinated should be allowed to attend church services and that the number of participants was supposed to be controlled. Church leaders were tasked to ensure that all those who attended their services were vaccinated. They were supposed to check vaccination status upon entrance and take a record of those who had attended the church service. In addition, they were supposed to prevent the unvaccinated from attending church services. Many people's love for church attendance resulted in some of them getting vaccinated. However, some leaders from AICs did not observe the guideline on church attendance by only those who were vaccinated. Many religious leaders felt that it was not their responsibility to ensure that only the vaccinated attended church. Furthermore, most religious leaders felt that it was morally wrong to send away someone who would have come to church to fellowship with others on the grounds that they had not been vaccinated.

While religious leaders felt that they could not prevent church members from attending church services because they were not vaccinated, there were threats by political leaders. The threats were intended to force church leaders and their congregants to get vaccinated. One ward councillor had this to say:

> To enforce compliance we were making threats. We said we're going to send the police force to all churches. The police officers would demand

vaccination certificates from church participants. We were giving them examples of places that police officers visited and demanded vaccination certificates from participants. Those church members who were found to be without certificates were arrested along with their leaders. This resulted in many people getting vaccinated whether they liked it or not.[8]

Thus, what drove some people to get vaccinated was that they wanted to attend church services and it was emphasised that churches were supposed to open their doors to the vaccinated only. It can thus be noted that vaccination was both voluntary and non-voluntary. Based on the foregoing, it can be noted that the COVID-19 vaccination programme had mixed fortunes, that is, both acceptance and non-acceptance.

Witnessing COVID-19 Related Sickness and Death of Close Relatives and Associates

Different categories of participants, including chiefs, councillors, traditional healers, healthcare workers, church leaders and laypeople indicated that a rise in COVID-19 related sickness and death challenged people, who initially were hesitant, to get vaccinated. Some participants from a Zionist focus group discussion indicated that although at first some of them were hesitant to get vaccinated, they later changed their minds upon witnessing COVID-19 related sickness and death in their communities. They indicated that COVID-19 was a reality that required real, practical solutions, including vaccination, as they had been convinced by village health workers, their religious leaders and environmental health technicians. A religious leader from a Zionist church said that the number of COVID-19 related deaths instilled fear in the people from various religious backgrounds and made them want to be vaccinated. This was also highlighted by traditional leaders.

Initial resistance to COVID-19 vaccination among Christians from AICs was also attested by traditional leaders, ward councillors and healthcare workers who indicated that, initially, when COVID-19 had not yet presented itself as a significant health threat, people did not have much fear of it. The preaching was that God was the protector and that those who died, would die according to God's plan. As such, they did not take seriously government-decreed COVID-19 management measures, including vaccination. The preaching during the early days of COVID-19 was that when God decides to take a person, He will do so at His time. Based on this, it was held that death happens according to God's plan. However, later, when the pandemic became more pronounced, there was an appreciation of the deadliness of the disease. This resulted in people taking COVID-19 control measures more seriously, so much so that when the COVID-19 vaccine came, several people were willing to get vaccinated and prevent themselves from dying of COVID-19. The following verbal quote from a councillor illustrates this:

Some people witnessed COVID-19 related deaths in their areas and this challenged them to get vaccinated.[9]

This includes some healthcare workers and some Christians from AICs who normally do not want to go to hospitals for medication because of their belief in the strength of spiritual healing.

Taking advantage of the spate of COVID-19 deaths, a ward councillor encouraged members in her ward to get vaccinated to prevent themselves from getting sick or dying of COVID-19. She stated that she told members of her ward that dying was now a choice (*"kufa kuda"*) because there was prevention in the form of COVID-19 vaccination. The ward councillor indicated that she was working in collaboration with the village health workers and village heads to mobilise people, especially those from AICs that tended to spiritualise the pandemic and so downplayed the role of vaccination. This resulted in long queues at vaccination centres. In getting people to vaccinate, the message propagated was that people must be vaccinated to live because COVID-19 kills. However, members of the Johanne Marange Apostolic Church remained adamant because of the church doctrine.

A ward councillor indicated that some members from an Apostolic Church were willing to get vaccinated but they did not want to be vaccinated during daytime in public places, so they requested to be vaccinated privately. The ward councillor granted their request and so invited them to her place. She requested healthcare workers to come and vaccinate them at night. She realised that although only a few had talked to her, the number that gathered at her place was much bigger. All those who came were vaccinated. What seems to be clear is that the pandemic had reached such an alarming level that even those Christians whose churches did not encourage vaccination felt that they needed vaccination to survive the pandemic. It can be inferred that private vaccination was meant to hide from other church members because perhaps the act seemed to be at variance with public church teachings concerning COVID-19.

Fear of Losing Jobs

A ward councillor indicated that some people were vaccinated to maintain their jobs. There was a time when some employers demanded vaccination certificates from their employees. The demand was non-discriminatory. Whether one was a Christian or not, one was supposed to present the vaccination certificate to maintain their job. This led many people, including members of AICs, to get vaccinated.

Compatibility of African Indigenous Healthcare Systems and Modern Healthcare Systems

According to traditional healers, African indigenous healthcare systems and modern medical healthcare systems are complementary. There is no friction. They asserted that African people consult modern healthcare systems, prophets and traditional healers. There are times when Western medication is the most appropriate therapy, whereas in some cases, it is traditional therapy that is more appropriate. For this reason, they supported COVID-19 vaccination. They indicated that they were vaccinated and encouraged their clients to get vaccinated. They said they drew their clients from among Christians and non-Christians alike. Some Christians who professed a negative attitude towards traditional healers during the day were reported to be going to traditional healers during the night for assistance on various health-related matters. It is to such Christians that traditional healers gave the advice to get vaccinated. In view of this, it can be noted that some Christians from an African initiated Christian background consulted traditional healers and during the process were advised to seek vaccination. Most of these, according to the traditional healers, were vaccinated. In this regard, what motivated vaccine acceptance among some members of AICs was not the advice of their church leaders but that of traditional healers.

Traditional healers indicated that it is necessary to obey civil authorities, whether what they would be doing was satisfactory or not.

> As members of the Zimbabwe Traditional Healers Association (ZINATHA), we are obliged to obey government regulations including those related to the COVID-19 pandemic. Therefore, we accept and encourage vaccination as one of the COVID-19 control measures.[10]

Vaccine Hesitancy

The study revealed that vaccine hesitancy is a function of diverse and interlocking factors. This concurs with Galagali et al.'s (2022) argument that vaccine hesitancy is a complicated and multi-faceted phenomenon. Factors influencing vaccine hesitancy include conspiracy theories involving misinformation circulating, especially through social media, and other social communication channels, denial of the existence of the pandemic, church doctrine which negates modern healthcare systems, which prohibits church members from seeking medical care from clinics, hospitals and other modern healthcare systems, belief that people are protected by God against COVID-19, and the belief that COVID-19 is a spiritual problem that requires spiritual solutions, forcing people to get vaccinated, and inconsistent conduct by politicians, which left people confused.

Misinformation and Suspicion

Misinformation and rumours, circulating mainly through social media, emerged as one of the most significant factors that led to vaccine hesitancy. This finding confirms Jolley and Douglas' (2014) argument that anti-vaccine conspiracy beliefs result in a negative attitude towards vaccines and misinterpretation of vaccine intention. Furthermore, the role of social media as a transmitter of misinformation and conspiracy theories has been noted in the literature (for example, Mercadante and Law, 2021; Ruiz and Bell, 2021; Wang and Liu, 2021).

When the government first rolled out the COVID-19 vaccination programme many people were not prepared to get vaccinated because of conspiracy theories that were circulating, especially through social media. Social media was doing a disservice to those who were teaching people about COVID-19 and encouraging them to be vaccinated. All participants in the study revealed that social media was detrimental to the successful implementation of the COVID-19 vaccination programme because it circulated information that made people fear being vaccinated. From the Evangelical Fellowship of Zimbabwe focus group discussion, it emerged that efforts by church leaders to conscientise people about COVID-19 and to encourage them to get vaccinated were compromised by wrong information circulating through social media. Misinformation about COVID-19 vaccination was moving fast. In connection with this, one member of the focus group discussion said:

> As preachers, we do not have a monopoly over our audience. Those who listen to you also listen to other voices. So as soon as we are through with them, having taught them what we were taught by healthcare officials, someone else is going to speak to them through social media. Some are circulating wrong information to the effect that those who are vaccinated are going to die within two years.[11]

What was even more disturbing, according to some participants, is that some healthcare workers, including nurses and doctors, were transmitting wrong information to scare people away. One Pentecostal church leader said that he had heard a nurse telling the youth that they should not get vaccinated as vaccination causes sterility. Infertility-related rumours are one of the reasons for vaccine hesitancy (Iliyasu et al., 2021a). Some doctors were also implicated in transmitting conflicting information on the effects of the COVID-19 vaccine. Under such circumstances, it became difficult for church leaders to convince their congregants to get vaccinated. Misinformation about COVID-19, resulting in people rejecting the vaccine, is well documented (for example, Chokwuocha et al., 2022; Daly and Robison, 2021; Iliyasu et al., 2021b; Ruiz and Bell, 2021; Uzochukwu et al., 2021).

Vaccine hesitancy was also due to suspicion that since the vaccines came from abroad, they were potentially dangerous to Africans as they could be used as weapons to wipe away Africans (see Chapter 9, this volume). The suspicion was grounded in colonial history wherein Africans were ill-treated by whites, making it difficult for some Africans to believe that anything good for Africans could come from the West. As one chief said:

> The relationship between blacks and whites since colonial times has been one of friction. The suspicion that the white people cannot produce medicines for Africans to live has made some people, both Christian and non-Christian, to repel COVID-19 vaccination.[12]

In this regard, COVID-19 vaccines were considered harmful to health. The suspicion that vaccines from abroad could be harmful confirms the findings of a study conducted by Sonkaya and Ozturk (2022) in Amasya which indicate that vaccine hesitancy is caused by the suspicion that vaccines coming from abroad could be harmful.

Denial of the Existence of the Pandemic

Some religious groupings among AICs believed that there was no COVID-19. Village healthcare workers revealed that some Christians from AICs believed that COVID-19 was not real; it was a 'newspaper disease', as one participant put it. This effectively implies that people who hold such beliefs would not take steps to prevent COVID-19 or to seek treatment if they have contracted the virus that causes the disease. Village healthcare workers and ward councillors stated that many members of the Johanne Marange Apostolic Church did not believe that there was COVID-19. Apart from the Johanne Marange Apostolic Church members, there were also other AIC members who denied the existence of COVID-19 and instead attributed COVID-19 related sicknesses to witch-craft. This was revealed by the ZINATHA focus group members who indicated that some Christians from AICs clandestinely visited them for help, believing that they had been bewitched. Doubts about the existence of COVID-19 are documented in the literature as a reason for vaccine hesitancy (for example, Iliyasu et al., 2021b).

Church Doctrines which Negate Modern Healthcare Systems

Most participants indicated that the Johanne Marange Apostolic Church teaches against seeking help from modern healthcare systems. There is an emphasis on faith healing. Village healthcare workers indicated that of all churches, the Johanne Marange Church was the most difficult to work with when it comes to COVID-19 vaccination. Members of the Church did not receive vaccination because of their beliefs, even if one tried to move door to door trying to convince them to get vaccinated. They maintained that they did not consume medicines and they did not want medicines in their bodies. A ward councillor quoted a member of the Johanne Marange Apostolic Church as saying:

> Our church does not allow us to get vaccinated or to take medicines. We pray and believe that when a child gets sick, he/she is taken to the shrine to be prayed for. If he/she dies, we believe it is God's will.[13]

Some AIC members were reported by village healthcare workers as saying that the pandemic was prophesied long back, and it is written in the Bible that incurable diseases shall come during the last days. The perception was that COVID-19 was a mark of the last days. The Christians concerned repelled COVID-19 vaccination arguing that there was no need to get vaccinated against an incurable disease. That vaccine acceptance and hesitancy are also influenced by religious considerations has been noted by Mercadente and Law (2021), Daly and Robinson (2021), Szilagyi et al. (2021) and Ruiz and Bell (2021), among others.

Spiritualisation of COVID-19

The study found that some Christians from AICs and traditional healers tended to conceptualise the pandemic in spiritual terms, in terms of origin and treatment. Some believed since they were prayerful, they were protected by God against COVID-19. Some church leaders who participated in the study revealed that there are biblical texts such as Psalm 91 which show that God is a refuge, a protector, even against COVID-19. Village healthcare workers revealed that such Christians had confidence that since they have Jesus who is alive, they would not contract COVID-19. Given this, they did not see the relevance of COVID-19 vaccination, hence their refusal to get vaccinated. Related to the belief that God is the protector against COVID-19, is the belief that COVID-19 is a spiritual problem that requires a solution. Some Christians claimed that they were immunised against COVID-19 by the founders of their churches, for example, Paul Mwazha and Johanne Marange. Others belonging to Johanne Masowe Apostolic churches claimed that they had been immunised spiritually at their religious shrines and so there was no need to get vaccinated. It also came out that some AIC Christians believed that death comes at God's appointed time, and no one can prevent it, thus effectively rendering COVID-19 vaccination unnecessary. One councillor reported that some Christians said:

> When God decides to take a person [through death], He takes him/her at His time.[14]

From an Apostolic focus group discussion, it came out that at first, some Christians were not willing to get vaccinated because they associated the vaccine with Satanism. Concerning this, one focus group participant said:

> When the vaccine came, at first people were not willing to get vaccinated. They believed it was a means of making them join Satanism.[15]

Participants said that later on, with more education from health care workers and encouragement from church leaders and politicians, many people got vaccinated.

Forcing People to Get Vaccinated

One reason why some people were suspicious of vaccination was that it was forced. Results from the Pentecostal grouping focus group discussion revealed that people were not willing to be vaccinated because politicians were forcing it upon them, using threats. As one participant from the focus group said:

Some of our members began to question why COVID-19 vaccination was forced if it was helpful to them. Why did the president say "No one is forced to get vaccinated but there shall come a time when you will not be able to attend church or board the ZUPCO buses if you are not vaccinated?" If vaccination was a noble exercise, then words that instil fear in the people were not supposed to come out. As ministers of religion, we try our best to educate people about COVID-19 and encourage them to get vaccinated but when politicians put fear in them to force them to get vaccinated, they get confused and come back to us asking "but why?"[16]

This is an expression of suspicion and distrust of the government, leading to vaccine hesitancy. As Ackah et al. (2021) point out, distrust towards the government fuels suspicion towards COVID-19 vaccines.

Inconsistent Conduct by Politicians

It emerged that the behaviour of politicians was confusing to the people. It was reported that some politicians believed that COVID-19 chooses whom to kill (*inotora vainoda*) which suggests that to them COVID-19 vaccination was unnecessary. Some participants accused politicians of acting as if they were immune to the virus and of politicising COVID-19 vaccination when they discriminated against some churches when it came to COVID-19 vaccination surveillance, that is, some churches were considered more prone to the virus than others, hence police officers were sent there to demand vaccination cards. This raised a red flag and discouraged some congregants from getting vaccinated.

The foregoing discussion on vaccine hesitancy suggests that many factors militated against people's acceptance of COVID-19 vaccination. This lends support to Napolitano et al.'s (2022) argument that reasons for hesitancy range from a concern about potential side effects of the vaccines to the belief that vaccination administration was not useful. The study has revealed that vaccine hesitancy is an impediment to the successful implementation of the vaccination programme in Zimbabwe, as elsewhere, for example, in the USA (Wang and Liu, 2022). As noted earlier, according to the WHO, vaccine hesitancy is one of the top ten threats to global health.

Conclusion

The study has revealed that attitudes towards COVID-19 vaccine rollout by the government and uptake of the vaccine, manifesting in vaccine acceptance, hesitancy or rejection, were a function of diverse factors, chief of which was African spirituality. The conceptualisation of, and relationship to, spiritual beings had a bearing on the conceptualisation of COVID-19 and the attendant acceptance or rejection of the COVID-19 vaccine. Those who saw COVID-19 as a spiritual phenomenon in terms of origin and treatment tended to have negative attitudes towards vaccination against the disease. Those who viewed the pandemic in both biomedical and spiritual terms tended to support the vaccine rollout programme and got themselves vaccinated. It should be noted that both AICs and traditional healers shared an understanding that COVID-19 had some spiritual dimension. However, while all traditional healers supported the vaccination programme and encouraged their clients to do the same, some branches of AICs did not support the programme, partly because of their spirituality and partly because of misinformation that was circulating mainly through social media. Although strategies such as awareness campaigns and threats were used to make people accept the vaccine, others remained adamant. Given this, government officials had to work closely with church leaders that repelled COVID-19 vaccination to achieve herd immunity and as such control the spread of the pandemic. Given that the study revealed that traditional healers were side-lined by the Government when it comes to COVID-19 management, it is recommended that in the future government engages them so that pandemics are more effectively dealt with. A multisectoral approach to dealing with the pandemic is likely to result in better support for government initiatives, including vaccination programmes. Since the use of threats to compel people to get vaccinated led to resistance among some, it is recommended that government officials use persuasive language to make people voluntarily present themselves for vaccination. Spirituality has emerged as both a resource and an impediment to the management of COVID-19. In view of this, it is recommended that government engages religious communities to secure their support when pursuing health-related and other initiatives.

Notes

1 Focus group discussion, Masvingo District.
2 Interview with a church leader, Bikita District.
3 Focus group discussion, Bikita District.
4 Interview with church leader, Bikita District.
5 Focus group discussion, Bikita District.
6 Interview with church leader, Masvingo District.
7 Interview with Councilor, Masvingo District.
8 Interview with Councilor, Masvingo District.
9 Interview with Councillor, Bikita District.
10 Interview with traditional healer, Masvingo District.
11 Focus group discussion, Masvingo District.
12 Interview with traditional leader, Masvingo District.
13 Interview with Councilor, Bikita District.
14 Interview with councilor, Masvingo District.
15 Focus group Discussion, Masvingo District
16 Focus group discussion, Masvingo District.

References

Ackah, B.B.B., Woo, M., Stallwood, L., et al. 2021. COVID-19 vaccine hesitancy in Africa: A scoping review, *Global Health Research and Policy*, 7(21), 1–20.

Agley, J., Xiao, Y., Thompson, E.E., et al. 2021. Factors associated with reported likelihood to get vaccinated for COVID-19 in a nationally representative US survey. *Public Health*, 196, 91–94.

Anderson, R.M., Vegvari, C., Truscott, J., and Collyer, B.S. 2020. Challenges in creating herd immunity to SARS-CoV-2 infection by mass vaccination. *Lancet*, 396, 1614–1616.

Baack, B.N., Abad, N., Yankey, D., et al. 2021. COVID-19 vaccination coverage and intent among adults aged 18–39 Years–United States, March–May 2021. *Morbidity and Mortality Weekly Report*, 70(25), 928–933.

Betsch, C., Renkewitz, F., Betsch, T. et al. 2010. The influence of vaccine-critical websites on perceiving vaccination risks. *Journal of Health Psychology*, 15(3), 446–555.

Cascini, F., Pantovic, A., Al-Ajlouni, Y., et al. 2021. Attitudes, acceptance and hesitancy among the general population worldwide to receive the COVID-19 vaccines and their contributing factors: A systematic review. *EClinicalMedicine*, 40, 101113.

Chukwuocha, U.M., Emerole, C.O., Iwuoha, G.N., et al. 2022. Stakeholders' hopes and concerns about the COVID-19 vaccines in Southeastern Nigeria: A qualitative study, *BMC Public Health*, 22(1), 330.

Daly, M., and Robinson, E. 2021. Willingness to vaccinate against COVID-19 in the US: Representative longitudinal evidence from April to October 2020. *American Journal of Preventive Medicine*, 60(6), 766–773.

Davis, T.P., Yimam, A.K., Kalam, M.A., et al. 2022. Behavioural determinants of COVID-19 vaccine acceptance in rural areas of six lower–and middle-income countries. *Vaccines*, 10, 214.

Dubé, E., Vivion, M., and MacDonald, N.E. 2015. Vaccine hesitancy, vaccine refusal and the anti-vaccine movement: Influence, impact and implications. *Expert Review of Vaccines*, 14(1), 99–117.

Francois, G., Duclos, P., Margolis, H., et al. 2005. Vaccine safety controversies and the future of vaccination programs. *Pediatric Infectious Disease Journal*, 24(11), 953–961.

Galagali, P.M., Kinikar, A.A., Kumar, V.S. 2022. Vaccine hesitancy: Obstacles and Challenges. *Current Pediatrics Reports*, 10, 241–248.

Gerussi, V., Peghin, M., Palese, A., et al. 2021. Vaccine hesitancy among Italian patients recovered from COVID-19 infection towards influenza and Sars-Cov-2 vaccination. *Vaccines*, 9(2), 172.

Graham, B.S. 2020. Rapid COVID-19 vaccine development. *Science*, 368(6494), 945–946.

Iliyasu, Z., Garba, M.R., Gajida, A.U., et al. 2021a. "Why should I take the COVID-19 vaccine after recovering from the disease?" A mixed-methods study of correlates of COVID-19 vaccine acceptability among health workers in Northern Nigeria. *Pathogens and Global Health*, 116(4), 254–262.

Iliyasu, Z., Umar, A.A., Abdullahi, H.M., et al. 2021b. "They have produced a vaccine, but we doubt if COVID-19 exists": Correlates of COVID-19 vaccine acceptability among adults in Kano, Nigeria. *Human Vaccines & Immunotherapeutics*, 17(11), 4057–4064.

Jolley, D. and Douglas, K.M. 2014. The effects of anti-vaccine conspiracy theories on vaccination intentions. *PLoS ONE*, 9(2), 1–9.

Kanyanda, S., Markhof, Y, Wollburg, P., et al. 2021. Acceptance of COVID-19 vaccines in Sub-Saharan Africa: Evidence from six national phone surveys. *BMJ Open*, 11, e055159.

Liu, T., He, Z., Huang, J., et al. 2021. A comparison of vaccine hesitancy of COVID-19 vaccination in China and the United States. *Vaccines (Basel)*, 9(6), 649.

Mahfoud, F., Azizi, M., Ewen, S., et al. 2020. Proceedings from the 3rd European Clinical Consensus Conference for clinical trials in device-based hypertension therapies. *European Heart Journal*, 41(16), 1588–1599.

Mercadante, A.R. and Law, A.V. 2021. Will they, or won't they? Examining patients' vaccine intention for flu and COVID-19 using the Health Belief Model. *Research in Social and Administrative Pharmacy*, 17(9), 1596–1605.

Napolitano, F., Miraglia del Giudice, G., Angelillo, S., et al. 2022. Hesitancy towards childhood vaccinations among parents of children with underlying chronic medical conditions in Italy. *Vaccines*, 10, 1254.

Nzaji, M.K., Ngombe, L., Mwamba, G.N., et al. 2020. Acceptability of vaccination against COVID-19 among healthcare workers in the Democratic Republic of the Congo. *Pragmatic and Observational Research*, 11, 103–109.

Paul, E., Steptoe, A., and Fancourt, D. 2021. Attitudes towards vaccines and intention to vaccinate against COVID-19: Implications for public health communications. *Lancet Regional Health-Europe*, 1, 100012. DOI:10.1016/j.lanepe.2020.100012. PMID:33954296; PMCID:PMC7834475.

Ruiz, J.B. and Bell, R.A. 2021. Predictors of intention to vaccinate against COVID-19: Results of a nationwide survey. *Vaccine*, 39(7), 1080–1086.

Solís Arce, J.S., Warren, S.S., Meriggi, N.F, et al. 2021. COVID-19 vaccine acceptance and hesitancy in low–and middle-income countries. *Nature Medicine*, 27(8), 1385–1394.

Sonkaya, I.Z. and Ozturk A. 2022. Vaccine hesitancy and refusal: A case study of Amasya. *Turkish Journal of Pediatric Disease*. Available at https://dergipark.org.tr/en/download/article-file/2645968

Szilagyi, P.G., Thomas, K., Shah, M.D., et al. 2021. National trends in the US public's likelihood of getting a COVID-19 vaccine—1 April to 8 December 2020. *JAMA*, 325, 396–398.

Uzochukwu, I.C., Eleje, G.U., Nwankwo, C.H., et al. 2021. COVID-19 vaccine hesitancy among staff and students in a Nigerian tertiary educational institution. *Therapeutic Advances in Infectious Disease*, 8, https://doi.org/10.1177/20499361211054923

Wang, Y. and Liu, Y. 2022. Multilevel determinants of COVID-19 vaccination hesitancy in the United States: A rapid systematic review. *Preventive Medicine Reports*, 25, 101673. DOI:10.1016/j.pmedr.2021.101673. PMID:34934611; PMCID:PMC8675390.

WHO. 2021a. WHO Coronavirus (COVID-19) Dashboard. Accessed 10 January 2023. https://covid19.who.int/

WHO 2021b. *Draft Landscape of COVID-19 Candidate Vaccines*. Geneva; www.who.int/ publications/m/item/draft-landscape-of-Covid-19-candidate-vaccines

WHO 2022. *Covid-19 Vaccination in the WHO African Region*, Monthly Bulletin, February 2022.

Wiysonge, C.S., Ndwandwe, D, Ryan, J., et al. 2021. Vaccine hesitancy in the era of COVID-19: Could lessons from the past help in divining the future? *Human Vaccines & Immunotherapeutics*, *18*, 1–3.

Yamey, G., Schäferhoff, M., Hatchett, R., Pate, M., Zhao, F., McDade, K.K. 2020. Ensuring global access to COVID-19 vaccines. *Lancet*, 395(10234), 1405–1406.

13 The Bible and COVID-19 Vaccination in Zimbabwe

Critical Reflections on the Influence of the Bible on both Vaccine Acceptance and Hesitancy

Makomborero Allen Bowa

Introduction

The COVID-19 pandemic is a serious health crisis that has been highly disruptive to everyday life since its outbreak. Indeed, the pandemic quickly became the world's most pressing emergency which swept across the globe causing death, untold suffering and unprecedented disruption across the broad spectrum of society (Sibanda et al., 2022: 1; Muyambo, 2022: 37; Bowa, 2022: 186; Sipeyiye, 2022: 52). This development prompted the scientific community to develop several COVID-19 vaccines with the sole intention of containing the spread of this deadly virus. However, massive controversy has surrounded these COVID-19 vaccines due to the proliferation of numerous conspiracy theories. As Fuchs (2021: 147) rightly points out, the emergence of COVID-19 gave momentum to the anti-vaccination movement that created and spread new conspiracy theories about the disease and COVID-19 vaccines. Interestingly, some of these conspiracy theories have emerged precisely from the interpretation of the COVID-19 pandemic in the light of the biblical apocalyptic traditions relating to the end of the world. Indeed, the Bible has played a significant role in not only shaping the politics around COVID-19 but also in influencing how people have experienced and responded to COVID-19 even in the Zimbabwe context. This puts into perspective Sibanda et al.'s (2022: 13) observation that the other form of politics that emerged from the religious engagement with COVID-19 relates to biblical interpretation. It is thus clear that multiple interpretations of the Bible exist in the wake of COVID-19 (Sibanda et al., 2022: 13), which interpretations have a direct bearing on both vaccine acceptance and hesitancy in society.

Ultimately, biblical fundamentalists and some mega-church leaders have associated the COVID-19 pandemic with signs of the end times and, more significantly, the COVID-19 vaccines with the 'mark of the beast' described in the apocalyptic Book of Revelations. As Bodner et al. (2021: 148) put it, the authoritative piece of literature on end times for Christians is the Book of Revelation. It is in this context that biblical interpretation has contributed to the prevalence

DOI: 10.4324/9781003388630-13

of vaccine hesitancy, which in essence embodies the unwillingness to receive vaccines by some Christians in spite of the existence of sound scientific evidence supporting the safety and efficacy of these vaccines. McAbee et.al (2021: 2) define vaccine hesitancy as the delay in acceptance or refusal of vaccination despite the availability of vaccination services. In this respect, several vaccines have been developed but many among Christians remain sceptical about these vaccines as a result of the influence of the Bible. Consequently, vaccine hesitancy remains one of the greatest threats to all efforts to combat the COVID-19 pandemic as it contributes to the failure to achieve or sustain herd immunity, thus unnecessarily perpetuating the pandemic and causing untold suffering and deaths. Consequently, all efforts to reduce the burden of the COVID-19 pandemic through vaccination have been further compounded by the emerging threat of vaccine hesitancy (McAbee et al., 2021: 2). Indeed, vaccine hesitancy emerges as a serious global health threat despite the fact that vaccines have proven to be one of the most effective public health strategies to protect against infectious diseases, such as COVID-19 (McAbee et al., 2021: 1). This is the situation existing in the Zimbabwean context as the vaccination process has been associated with confusing information such that the initial response was characterised by complacency in embracing the vaccination drive (Humbe, 2022: 77). More significant to note is the idea that the factors contributing to vaccine hesitancy in Zimbabwe are multifaceted and thus require equally complex strategies to be addressed (Dzanamarira, 2021: 7). Certainly, the manner in which the Bible has been interpreted by some Church leaders has played a substantial role in fomenting vaccine hesitancy in the Zimbabwean context.

Conversely, some religious authorities have engaged the Bible to support the use of vaccines as safe and effective, essential for curtailing the COVID-19 pandemic. A substantial number of Church leaders have sought to provide a religious backing on the use of vaccines through the use of the Bible with the view of fostering vaccine acceptance in the broader Zimbabwean context. As such, biblical interpretation has been used to defuse some of the conspiracy beliefs that have been fuelling vaccine hesitancy. Generally, as McAbee et al. (2021: 2) observe, socio-cultural and religious beliefs also play a significant role in COVID-19 vaccine acceptance in Africa, as the majority of the population is religious. Indeed, McAbee's observation is consistent with developments in the Zimbabwean context, especially with regard to the use of the Bible in promoting vaccine acceptance and uptake. Against this backdrop, this chapter examines how the Bible has played an ambivalent role in fostering both vaccine acceptance and hesitancy in the wake of the COVID-19 pandemic, particularly in the Zimbabwean context. Using Festinger's theory of cognitive dissonance, the chapter critically examines how the Bible has informed people's behaviours and attitudes towards COVID-19 vaccines. Fundamentally, the chapter demonstrates how it is challenging to counter some of the retrogressive effects of conspiracy theories and misinformation relating to COVID-19 vaccines without a comprehensive understanding of how the Bible has been used to both support and resist vaccination initiatives. The findings of the research have important implications for the development of tailored and targeted strategies to address the challenge of vaccine hesitancy which threatens efforts to address the COVID-19 pandemic in Zimbabwe.

Theoretical Framework and Methodology

This chapter draws insights from Festinger's theory of cognitive dissonance. This has been one of the most influential theories in social psychology, from which much has been learned about the determinants of attitudes and beliefs, the internalisation of values, the consequences of decisions and other important psychological processes (Harmon-Jones and Mills, 2019: 3), especially those associated with catastrophic developments in society. Basically, cognitive dissonance takes place when a certain development causes a serious discrepancy between two of an individual's cognitions or beliefs (Cooper, 2007: 2, 6; Harmon-Jones and Mills, 2019: 3). Cooper (2007: 5) further states that the premise of the cognitive dissonance theory is that people do not tolerate inconsistency very well. As such, the very basic observation of this theory is that human beings do not like inconsistency because it creates psychological discomfort. Thus, the evidence that dissonance occurs is found in observable manifestations of attempts to reduce dissonance (Jenkins, 2013: 9). Essentially, people experience stress or discomfort as a result of conflicting cognitions and they attempt to alter their attitudes and beliefs as a way of not only reducing the discomfort but also restoring consistency. The greater the magnitude of the dissonance, the greater is the pressure to reduce dissonance (Harmon-Jones and Mills, 2019: 3). As such, the existence of dissonance, being psychologically uncomfortable, motivates the person to reduce the dissonance and leads to avoidance of information likely to increase the dissonance (Cooper, 2007: 7; Harmon-Jones and Mills, 2019: 3). Basically, Festinger indicated that there are three ways to cope with cognitive dissonance: (a) changing one or several involved elements in the dissonance relationship, for example moving an opinion to fit behaviour; (b) adding new elements to reduce the inconsistency, for example adopting opinions which fit behaviour; and (c) reducing the importance of the involved elements. (Cooper, 2007: 2–3, 9; Harmon-Jones and Mills, 2019: 4). Thus, it is in the attempt to restore consistency that human beings come up with narratives that account for the inconsistency between their individual expectations and reality. This is the context in which conspiracy theories must also be appreciated. Fundamentally, as Prooijen and Douglas (2017: 324) argue, crisis situations often elicit sense-making narratives which take the form of conspiracy theories among citizens in their attempt to understand and explain why certain events occurred, particularly in the case of negative or unexpected events.

Adopting the theory of cognitive dissonance in this chapter helps to illustrate the psychological impact of the COVID-19 pandemic, particularly in the lives of Christians. It is beyond any doubt that the pandemic created cognitive dissonance among many Christian believers in the world. Some of the core beliefs of devoted followers of the Bible were disconfirmed by the devastating pandemic. The belief that God would protect Christians from the pandemic was thwarted by the reality of many Christian believers succumbing to the pandemic. Certainly, this created discomfort among many believers. Against this backdrop, insights from the cognitive dissonance theory provide a deeper understanding of the psychological processes that have been triggered by all catastrophic developments associated with the COVID-19 pandemic. The theory provides a lens through which Christian responses to the COVID-19 pandemic in Zimbabwe can be examined, particularly focusing on how the Bible has been used to deal with the incomprehensible situation caused by the pandemic. Furthermore, the theory provides invaluable insights that help in appreciating the psychological process underpinning the development of various COVID-19 conspiracy theories, including those conspiracies emerging from biblical interpretation.

In terms of methodology, this highly qualitative chapter employs a multi-method approach to data collection which includes desk review, observations and video analysis in order to facilitate the triangulation of results. Desk review is used to gather all important information relating to the devastating impact of the COVID-19 pandemic across the broad spectrum of society in Zimbabwe and beyond. More importantly, given that most Church leaders held virtual services as a result of social distancing and lockdown protocols, video analysis invaluably helps in collecting data that demonstrates how Church leaders have made sense of the COVID-19 pandemic in the light of biblical traditions. In essence, video analysis helps in understanding the influence of biblical interpretation in fostering both vaccine acceptance and hesitancy in the Zimbabwean context.

The COVID-19 Crisis and the Emergence of Conspiracy Theories: History in Perpetuity

Contrary to common assumptions, belief in conspiracy theories has been prevalent throughout human history as people continuously experience substantial uncertainty and fear due to societal crisis situations (Prooijen and Douglas, 2017: 323). Indeed, there is a consensus among experts that crisis situations breed and spread conspiracy theories. Evidence drawn from past developments demonstrates that the tendency to believe in conspiracy theories is part of human nature and that people have been susceptible to such beliefs throughout history as a way of coping with the uncertainty caused by crisis situations (Prooijen and Douglas, 2017: 325). From a cognitive dissonance perspective, conspiracy theories are not only part of people's attempts to deal with the psychological discomfort associated with a crisis but also coping mechanisms that help in restoring consistency in the wake of a crisis. Generally, as Bodner et al. (2021: 325, 246) argue, conspiracy theories create order from events that sometimes have no coherent explanation and offer a sense of control and a way of understanding change and causality. Accordingly, Prooijen and Douglas (2017: 327) contend that conspiracy theories provide people with simplified answers, specifically to questions of how a certain crisis situation emerged. Fundamentally, these answers play a significant role in helping people to cope with any devastating crisis situation. Thus, the relationship between uncertainty and conspiracy beliefs has substantial implications for understanding how people psychologically cope with adversity in their everyday life (Prooijen and Douglas, 2017: 328). Accordingly, this relationship has implications for understanding how people cope with devastating existential crises such as the coronavirus crisis.

Since the outbreak of the COVID-19 pandemic various conspiracy theories have emerged and circulated, particularly through social media into public consciousness, thereby negatively affecting the way people saw the pandemic and the vaccination programme. Social media is indeed the most important and sustaining mode of communication in the contemporary world which has acted as a double-edged sword of communication, facilitating smooth connectivity on one hand, while on the other hand, providing pathways for spreading very crude, unreliable and false information which has been as a source of emotional disturbances and unnecessary panic (Ponde-Mutsvedu and Chirongoma, 2022: 108). Indeed, the rapid emergence of COVID-19 gave rise to several conspiracy theories which have enjoyed considerable coverage on various social media platforms. The emergence of conspiracy theories is not unique to the COVID-19 crisis but rather one that has also characterised other preceding crises, hence the fundamental argument that this is indeed history in perpetuity. Undoubtedly, the COVID-19 pandemic created uncertainties throughout the world, a development that has triggered the proliferation of conspiracy theories as people attempt to make sense of the crisis. Consequently, the public space in Africa and beyond has been awash with multiple interpretations of the origin of the pandemic, its signification and routes of resolution (Sibanda et al., 2022: 11). Interestingly, most of the conspiracies relating to the COVID-19 pandemic have emerged precisely from the religious fraternity. It is in this context that the Bible has played a role in influencing how people have made sense of the COVID-19 pandemic and the vaccination initiatives. Indeed, the Bible has been the source that has provided the impetus for the emergence and proliferation of COVID-19 conspiracies.

To illustrate the above point, Bodner et al. (2021: 150) argue that to understand the layout of conspiracy theories spreading in Christian communities, we also need to understand the biblical context and characters involved. Prevalent almost in all Christian communities worldwide is the association of the COVID-19 pandemic with signs of end times. Consequently, as Bodner et al. (2021: 143) highlight, some of the conspiracy theories circling COVID-19 pertain to a New World Order and extra-biblical approaches to end times, making a connection between vaccination, contact tracing and 'the Mark of the Beast' described in the Book of Revelations. This is quite representative of interpretations in the broader African context and more particularly the Zimbabwean context. This puts into perspective Sibanda et al.'s (2022: 12) observation that, with COVID-19 paralysing in-person religious gatherings, some African Pentecostal leaders sought to reclaim authority by making pronouncements on the pandemic. Biblical interpretation has primarily informed some of the pronouncements on the origins of the pandemic, its signification and routes of resolution by these Church leaders. Thus, the devastating impact of COVID-19 pandemic, particularly in Southern Africa, has seen the retrieval and use of images of apocalypticism (Sibanda et al., 2022: 11), predominantly drawn from the Bible. Notably, some of these conspiracy theories are a serious public health threat since they undermine all efforts to combat the spread of the pandemic. Indeed, as Bodner et al., 2021: 246) generally observe, the social, economic and health crises brought on by COVID-19 have been exacerbated by conspiracy theories, exploitation, amplification, astroturfing and proselytising from believers. Accordingly, writing in the context of Southern Africa, Sibanda et al. (2022: 6) indicate that some religious leaders have generated and circulated messianic and apocalyptic messages, which have essentially downplayed the value of official public health guidance, and offering religious panaceas that have been detrimental to good public health practice.

The Role of Biblical Interpretation in Fostering COVID-19 Vaccine Hesitancy in Zimbabwe

It is undisputedly known that the Bible has sometimes played a retrogressive role in fostering vaccine hesitancy in the Zimbabwean context. Several biblically grounded conspiracy theories have emerged, especially from charismatic and African Pentecostal Church leaders who have sought to make sense of the pandemic and the rolling out of vaccines in the light of biblical traditions (Sibanda et al., 2022: 11). With regard to COVID-19 vaccination in Zimbabwe, some outspoken religious leaders with huge followings have spoken against COVID-19 vaccines, associating them with the devil's intention to destroy mankind (Masiyiwa et al., 2021). Indeed, the issue of vaccines has been a highly contentious issue, with some Pentecostal leaders fomenting resistance to the vaccines (Sibanda et al., 2022: 12). For instance, Kwaramba (2021) indicates that initially, at the outbreak of the pandemic, a prominent African Pentecostal leader such as Emmanuel Makandiwa in Zimbabwe reassured his followers that they would be spared from the virus through prayer and divine protection. The basis for such an approach to the COVID-19 pandemic was grounded in texts such as Psalm 121: 5–8 which reads;

> The LORD watches over you. The LORD is your shade at your right hand; the sun will not harm you by day, nor the moon by night. The LORD will keep you from all harm – he will watch over your life; the LORD will watch over your coming and going both now and forevermore.

and Psalm 91:10–11 which also reads:

> no harm will overtake you, no disaster will come near your tent. For he will command his angels concerning you to guard you in all your ways.

In essence, prominent African Pentecostal leaders, including Makandiwa, sought to explain the origins of the pandemic and to reassure their followers of divine protection (Sibanda et al., 2022: 12), using the Bible as their primary source of this knowledge.

Another perspective advanced in Makandiwa's engagement with the Bible in the wake of the COVID-19 pandemic was the association of COVID-19 vaccines with the 'Mark of the Beast' described in Revelations 13: 16–18 which reads:

> Also it causes all, both small and great, both rich and poor, both free and slave, to be marked on the right hand or the forehead, so that no one can buy or sell unless he has the mark, that is, the name of the beast or the number of its name. This calls for wisdom: let him who has understanding reckon the number of the beast, for it is a human number, its number is six hundred and sixty-six.

Indeed, Makandiwa's interpretation insinuated that COVID-19 vaccines were the 'mark of the beast', especially considering that only those who presented vaccination cards were allowed to enjoy certain freedoms that the unvaccinated could not enjoy. In his reflections, the whole idea of COVID-19 vaccines and vaccination cards fit perfectly well in what is described in Revelations. Consequently, Makandiwa was accused of perpetuating conspiracy theories through making allusions to the 'mark of the beast' (Kwaramba, 2021).

Generally, as Sibanda et al. (2022: 12) observe, there were insinuations that some devilish plan was underway to exterminate Africans, or that the vaccines were designed to alter the DNA of those who would be injected, thereby tampering with God's plan and form regarding humans. Undoubtedly, such insinuations characterised Makandiwa's understanding of COVID-19 vaccines in the context of biblical traditions. Indeed, Makandiwa courted controversy when he said that his followers were protected from coronavirus and that the vaccines distorted people's DNA because they contained microchip implants (Shumba, 2021; Kwaramba, 2021, Humbe, 2022: 77–78). Makandiwa's sentiments on COVID-19 vaccine were heavily criticised, especially by those who embrace science as a proven and authentic response to the pandemic (Humbe, 2022: 77–78). In essence, being as charismatic as he is, Makandiwa's utterances and sentiments in the wake of the pandemic contributed to vaccine hesitancy and reluctance among his followers (Shumba, 2021), on essentially two levels. First, Makandiwa's assurance of divine protection influenced some among his followers to disregard all public health measures to combat the spread of pandemic including vaccines. For them only God would provide the best protection that no other human initiative could do. Second, Makandiwa's association of the COVID-19 vaccine with the 'mark of the beast' essentially deterred some among his many followers from taking up the vaccines. Consequently, given the numbers that follow him, a significant share of the population was sceptical and opposed vaccinations. Important to note here is the fact that while Makandiwa later on retracted his utterances on COVID-19 vaccines (Humbe, 2022: 77–78), his initial unproven utterances had already caused much damage, especially with regard to fostering vaccine hesitancy in Zimbabwean society.

In one of the videos posted on his YouTube channel, Makandiwa urged people to intercede and pray over the issue of COVID-19 vaccines.[1] A critical analysis of his message in this video reveals quite a number of conspiracies which have fuelled vaccine hesitancy in Zimbabwe. First, Makandiwa insinuates that COVID-19 vaccines are not a genuine initiative to curb the spread of the pandemic but rather such vaccines are part of a grand scheme by the rich and powerful to inflict diseases in people. Second, Makandiwa insinuated that the real pandemic would start after the vaccination process. In essence, Makandiwa suggested that the vaccines were not to be trusted because they were flawed. In the video, Makandiwa remarked that:

> if there was something wrong with the test kits, there will definitely be something wrong with the vaccine … people don't understand the destruction that is man-made. I am trying to deliver people from the snare of the devil … There is a trap … So if we are to seek for God's intervention against the vaccine, we have to be successful … We want that level of anointing to work in God's people where we see the fulfilment of a declaration by Jesus over his disciples that you will tread upon scorpions and serpents. When that day arrives and they put poison in your body … You will survive the attack … the power of God will heal us … Start praying … I am calling out for the intercessors to pray for the healing of the nations that the people with money are going to inflict pain and diseases on people in the context of prevention … The actual outbreak will start after the vaccine, let us be ready now. We can't trust these people, let us trust God. They will stop at nothing for as long as they see money, you are not safe. Let us trust God. Only God can deliver us from this affliction and I know that the anointing that we have will work for our own good. Everything works out for good for those that love the Lord.

Evidently, the above extract illustrates that the preacher's utterances were drawn from and informed by biblical traditions from the New Testament. In his deliberations, Makandiwa made reference to biblical ideas captured in texts such as Luke 10:19 which reads "Behold, I have given you authority to tread upon serpents and scorpions, and over all the power of the enemy; and nothing shall hurt you", and Romans 8:28 which reads "We know that in everything God works for good with those who love him, who are called according to his purpose". Indeed, the prominent Pentecostal leader used ideas drawn from such texts to assure his followers that God would protect them, not only from the pandemic, but also from the devastating effects of the pandemic. Undoubtedly, the preacher's utterances fuelled scepticism towards COVID-19 vaccines and contributed to the challenge of vaccine hesitancy.

Another prime example that demonstrates how the Bible has been used to foster vaccine hesitancy is seen in Apostle Chiwenga's sermon on YouTube entitled "The Pestilence: Understanding COVID-19".[2] In this sermon, Apostle Chiwenga engaged several biblical texts in his attempt to make sense of the COVID-19 pandemic. What is clear from the sermon is the association of the COVID-19 pandemic with divine punishment for disobedience. To accentuate this idea, the Apostle made reference to texts such as Deuteronomy 28: 15–22, which reads

> But if you will not obey the LORD your God by diligently observing all his commandments and decrees, which I am commanding you today, then all these curses shall come upon you and overtake you. Cursed shall you be in the city, and cursed shall you be in the field. Cursed shall be your basket and your kneading bowl. Cursed shall be the fruit of your womb, the fruit of your ground, the increase of your cattle and the issue of your flock. Cursed shall you be when you come in, and cursed shall you be when you go out. The LORD will send upon you disaster, panic, and frustration in everything you attempt to do, until you are destroyed and perish quickly, on account of the evil of your deeds, because you have forsaken me. The LORD will make the pestilence cling to you until it has consumed you off the land that you are entering to possess. The LORD will afflict you with consumption, fever, inflammation, with fiery heat and drought, and with blight and mildew; they shall pursue you until you perish.

In the video, Chiwenga also made reference to Leviticus 26:25 which reads:

> I will bring the sword against you, executing vengeance for the covenant; and if you withdraw within your cities, I will send pestilence among you, and you shall be delivered into enemy hands.

Indeed, at various intervals in the video the preacher referred to Matthew 24:7–8, Luke 21 and 2 Samuel 24:15ff, which texts project the idea that God sometimes sends pestilences as punishment. In his interactions with various biblical texts, Chiwenga insinuated that the COVID-19 pandemic was punishment from God. Indeed, with such interpretations prevailing, one wonders therefore: Is the COVID-19 pandemic a curse from God? If it is, will vaccines be effective in curtailing its devastating effect? Undoubtedly, many people struggled to find answers to these questions. These are indeed serious questions whose answers provide important insights relating to the role of the Bible in fostering vaccine hesitancy in the Zimbabwean context. Clearly, Chiwenga's interpretation of the COVID-19 pandemic in the light of biblical traditions was quite problematic in that it explicitly fostered the idea that the pandemic was punishment for humanity's wickedness and as such, there could be no human intervention, even in the form of vaccines, that could halt this God-ordained pandemic until a point where God decided to stop it. This kind of interpretation left many in a state of cognitive dissonance where they were uncertain of what they were supposed to do in the wake of the devastating pandemic.

For Chiwenga, the pandemic was a God-ordained pestilence that was designed to bring people to repentance. It is clear in the video that the preacher is convinced that no human intervention will be effective in stopping the pandemic. In his sermon, Chiwenga vehemently indicates that:

> You can't defeat a pestilence by observing hygienic practices … A pestilence is a God-ordained plague, it will kill the people it was designed to kill and when God is satisfied with the number of people, God will stop the pestilence.

Undoubtedly, the very idea that the pandemic would only end when God desired it to, fuelled complacency to take up vaccination among his followers. The preacher's utterances had serious implications on vaccine acceptance as his interpretation of COVID-19 in the light of the biblical narratives suggested that vaccines were ineffective. Consequently, many among his followers were reluctant to take up vaccines. Given that conspiracy theories have the unfortunate side effect of isolating people, as Bodner et al. (2021: 36) point out, the argument advanced here is that many people were isolated from the COVID-19 vaccination initiative on the basis of conspiracy theories that emerged from speculations related to end time events and misinterpretations drawn from the Bible. Indeed, Church leaders like Chiwenga were responsible for not only forming but also perpetuating some of these conspiracies.

Backing up his sentiments on the COVID-19 pandemic, Chiwenga made further reference to texts such as 2 Chronicles 7:12–16 which reads:

> Then the LORD appeared to Solomon in the night and said to him: "I have heard your prayer, and have chosen this place for myself as a house of sacrifice. When I shut up the heavens so that there is no rain, or command the locust to devour the land, or send pestilence among my people, if my people who are called by my name humble themselves, pray, seek my face, and turn from their wicked ways, then I will hear from heaven, and will forgive their sin and heal their land. Now my eyes will be open and my ears attentive to the prayer that is made in this place. For now I have chosen and consecrated this house so that my name may be there forever; my eyes and my heart will be there for all time."

and Luke 13:3 which reads:

I tell you, No; but unless you repent you will all likewise perish.

The preacher's reading of such texts clearly suggested that the COVID-19 pandemic will only come to an end when humanity has fully repented. By implication, the Apostle advanced the idea that no other initiative besides repentance will curtail the spread of the pandemic. To put it somewhat differently, the Apostle insinuated that the pandemic would stop causing untold suffering and deaths only when people have repented in a manner that makes God revoke the so-called COVID-19 curse. Such utterances have been detrimental to all initiatives to end the scourge of the pandemic since the Apostle's followers take his words to be gospel truth. In essence, such interpretations have fuelled vaccine hesitancy which has undermined public health measures to eradicate the pandemic in Zimbabwe. Generally, vaccine hesitancy can drive outbreaks of vaccine-preventable diseases, lead to slower vaccination rates, and hinder the attainment and sustainability of herd immunity (McAbee et al., 2021: 2). It is against this backdrop that the implications of certain interpretations of the Bible, especially by African Pentecostal leaders on vaccine hesitancy, must be appreciated. It is quite unfortunate that a number of congregants succumbed to the novel pandemic, on account of some wrong biblical interpretations (Shumba, 2021). Evidently, these facts point to the reality that it is indeed challenging to counter some of the retrogressive effects of conspiracy theories and misinformation relating to COVID-19 vaccines without a comprehensive understanding of how the Bible has been used by those who have been resisting vaccination initiatives.

The Bible and COVID-19 Vaccine Acceptance in Zimbabwe

While the interpretation of the COVID-19 pandemic in the light of some biblical traditions has fomented vaccine hesitancy as demonstrated above, the same Bible has been engaged by some Church leaders in their endeavour to promote COVID-19 vaccinations. Since the beginning of the pandemic there have been calls for Church leaders to collaborate with government and non-governmental entities as well as health experts in the fight against the pandemic, particularly in promoting vaccine acceptance (Masiyiwa et al., 2021). As Maiden (2021: 2) puts it, faith leaders are critical partners in addressing many known barriers to the uptake of health and other essential services, including vaccines. Commenting on developments in the Zimbabwean context, Dzanamarira (2021: 7) indicates that the national COVID-19 vaccination programmes of Zimbabwe could benefit from champions such as artists, politicians and religious leaders providing the correct information to raise community awareness and ensure vaccine acceptance.

Indeed, some religious leaders headed the call to collaborate with government in encouraging people to get vaccinated. Definitely, as experts indicated, the collaboration between Church leaders and health experts could invaluably help in shifting negative perceptions about the COVID-19 vaccines that had been attributed to widespread misinformation emanating precisely from reflections of the COVID-19 pandemic in the light of some biblical traditions. In fact, as Maiden (2021: 2) observes, some religious leaders noted with concern that the spread of too much unfiltered information and misinformation undermined people's trust in the COVID-19 vaccines. As such, some Church leaders sought to dispel some of the conspiracies associated with the COVID-19 pandemic using the Bible. In Zimbabwe, Church leaders, from the Zimbabwe Council of Churches (ZCC), the Evangelical Fellowship of Zimbabwe (EFZ), the Zimbabwe Catholic Bishops Conference (ZCBC) and the Zimbabwe Indigenous Inter-Denominational Council of Churches (ZIIDCC) led by Bishop Nehemiah Mutendi were invited by government to take part in the vaccination programme (Kwaramba and Madzimure, 2021).

Accordingly, some of the Church leaders who openly complemented the government in the fight against COVID-19 by urging their members to embrace vaccines, adhere to COVID-19 guideline measures include Bishop Nehemiah Mutendi of the Zion Christian Church, and Apostle Andrew Wutawunashe of the Family of God Church (Zinyuke, 2021). By accepting the vaccines, these Church leaders inspired confidence in their followers so that they would equally accept the COVID-19 vaccines. Some of these leaders even sought to foster vaccine acceptance using biblical narratives. For instance, Apostle Andrew Wutawunashe is quoted to have said:

> people should not be misled by falsehoods being peddled on social media since the word of God did not prohibit the use of vaccines, hence there was no excuse for Christians not to take it. This is to inspire others to be vaccinated, especially those who are being misguided by falsehoods that it is 'unchristian' and against the word of God to be vaccinated ... I keep saying the first vaccination was in Exodus 15:26 when Moses was given a tree to vaccinate the water.
>
> (Zinyuke, 2021)

Similarly, the Zimbabwe Episcopal Area Bishop of the United Methodist Church, Eben K. Nhiwatiwa, encouraged people to receive vaccinations after having received his second dose. In his remarks, the Bishop encouraged people to get vaccinated as a sign of showing love to another. He stated that:

> The message for all Zimbabweans ... is showing love for one another ... If you get a vaccine, you are loving your neighbour. You are protecting your neighbour and loved ones.
>
> (Chikwanah and Londe, 2021)

Evidently, the Bishop's utterances were drawn from New Testament texts such as Matthew 22:37–39 and Mark 12:30–31 which emphasise the idea of loving one's neighbour as oneself. By implication therefore, this fostered vaccine acceptance by associating the idea of getting vaccinated with God's commandment of always considering others in the same way that one would want to be considered. As such, the Bishop used the Bible to emphasise the idea that getting vaccinated was an initiative that would protect everyone. Undoubtedly, many among his followers must have heeded the call to be vaccinated, especially considering that the Bishop's message was grounded in the scripture that many consider to be authoritative in their lives.

Furthermore, some Church leaders supported the COVID-19 vaccination programme in Zimbabwe by demonstrating that there was no biblical basis for not taking vaccines. For instance, Bishop Peter Mukwena from the Family of God Church remarked that:

> The good news is that we have received thousands of vaccines so I encourage all Christians to take it … There is nothing wrong in taking a vaccine because it is a preventative measure against the disease just like washing your hands, eating good food and wearing masks that we have already been doing. There is nothing wrong biblically or scientifically with getting the vaccine.
>
> (Zinyuke, 2021)

Indeed, since the outbreak, some Church leaders have effectively engaged the Bible in their drive to foster compliance with WHO and government recommendations and guidelines on vaccination. A prime example is Rev Alan Masimba Gurupira from the United Methodist Church, who supports the vaccination exercise by making reference to the parable of the wedding banquet in Matthew 22:11ff, in which he argued that Jesus emphasised compliance (Chingwe, 2021). It is on the basis of his understanding of this text that he encouraged all to comply to WHO and government advice and be vaccinated. Accordingly, Rev Gurupira made reference to Luke 5:14 in which the lepers were required to show themselves to the priest, a certificate of cleansing. By implication therefore, he advanced the idea that vaccines are a way of cleansing people from the COVID-19 plague. More importantly, this kind of engagement with the text fostered the idea that people were only safe if they vaccinated. It is thus in this respect that biblical interpretation played a critical role is demystifying certain conspiracies surrounding COVID-19, thereby fostering vaccine acceptance in the broader Zimbabwean societal landscape. Fundamentally, the Bible was effectively used by other religious leaders in an effort to overcome opposition to the coronavirus vaccine with the sole view of fostering vaccine acceptance.

Conclusion

This contribution has examined the interface between the Bible and COVID-19 vaccination in the Zimbabwean context. Building on the insights from the cognitive dissonance theory, the chapter examined the psychological processes that characterised Christian responses to COVID-19, particularly focusing on how the Bible was used to deal with the incomprehensible situation caused by the pandemic. The chapter also reflected on the relationship between societal crisis situations and the emergence of conspiracy theories and argued that the emergency of several conspiracy theories in the wake of COVID-19 is essentially history in perpetuity. The core argument advanced in the chapter is that the Bible has played an ambivalent role in fostering both vaccine acceptance and hesitancy in the context of Zimbabwe. The reality on the ground was that religious opinions on the pandemic emanating from the Bible had far-reaching implications on both vaccine hesitancy and acceptance in the country. Citing examples from selected African Pentecostal leaders, the chapter demonstrated how the Bible has been interpreted in a manner that ultimately fostered vaccine hesitancy. Through these examples, the chapter demonstrated how some of the COVID-19 related conspiracies which are prevalent almost worldwide have emerged from some forms of biblical interpretation. This contribution also highlighted the threats associated with vaccine hesitancy in the wake of the pandemic and argued that a comprehensive understanding of how the COVID-19 pandemic has been interpreted in the light of biblical traditions is imperative in the endeavour to counter some of the retrogressive effects of conspiracy theories in as far as curbing the spread of the pandemic is concerned. More importantly, the chapter demonstrated by way of examples, how some Church leaders have engaged the Bible in raising community awareness and ensuring vaccine acceptance in the Zimbabwean context. Indeed, some Church leaders have played a critical role in demystifying certain conspiracies surrounding COVID-19 through biblical interpretation, clearly demonstrating that there is no biblical basis for rejecting vaccines. Through such initiatives, these Church leaders have contributed immensely in the fight against COVID-19 through fostering vaccine acceptance.

Notes

1. A Call To Intercede: Important Announcement From Emmanuel Makandiwa, Streamed live on 25/05/20, Accessible at: www.youtube.com/watch?v=IX-_vtF1-LY&t=379s
2. The Pestilence: Understanding Covid 19, Apostle T Chiwenga, Mid-Week Service streamed live on 25/03/20, Accessible at: www.youtube.com/watch?v=lhyAcjv5MGk

References

Bodner, J., Welch, W., Brodie, I., Muldoon, A., Leech, D., & Marshal, A. 2022. *COVID-19 Conspiracy Theories QAnon, 5G, the New World Order and Other Viral Ideas.* Jefferson, NC: McFarland.

Bowa, M.A. 2022. The coronavirus pandemic and persons with disabilities: Towards a liberating reading of the Bible for Churches in Southern Africa. In F. Sibanda, T. Muyambo, & E. Chitando (Eds), *Religion and the COVID-19 Pandemic in Southern Africa.* London: Routledge, 186–201.

Chikwanah, E., & Londe, C.T. 2021. Church promotes COVID-19 vaccines in Africa, *UM News*. Accessible at: www.umnews.org/en/news/church-promotes-covid-19-vaccines-in-africa

Chingwe, K. 2021. Zimbabwe churches reopen to vaccinated, unvaccinated, *UM News*. Accessible at: www.umnews.org/en/news/zimbabwe-churches-reopen-to-vaccinated-unvaccinated

Cooper, J.M. 2007. *Cognitive Dissonance: 50 Years of a Classic Theory*. New York: Sage Publications.

Dzinamarira, T., Nachipo, B., Phiri, B., & Musuka, G. 2021. COVID-19 vaccine roll-out in South Africa and Zimbabwe: Urgent need to address community preparedness, fears and hesitancy. *Vaccines*, 9(250), 1–10.

Fuchs, C. 2021. *Communicating COVID-19: Everyday Life, Digital Capitalism, and Conspiracy Theories in Pandemic Times*. Emerald Publishing Limited.

Harmon-Jones, E. 2019. *Cognitive Dissonance Re-examining a Pivotal Theory in Psychology*. Washington DC: American Psychological Association.

Humbe, B.P. 2022. Living with COVID-19 in Zimbabwe: A religious and scientific healing response. In F. Sibanda, T. Muyambo, & E. Chitando (Eds), *Religion and the COVID-19 Pandemic in Southern Africa*. London: Routledge, 72–88.

Jenkins, T. 2013. *Of Flying Saucers and Social Scientists: A Re-reading of When Prophecy Fails and of Cognitive Dissonance*. London: Palgrave Macmillan.

Kwaramba, F. 2021. COVID-19 vaccination: Experts red-flag sceptical Church leaders, *The Herald*. Accessible at: www.herald.co.zw/covid-19-vaccination-experts-red-flag-sceptical-church-leaders/

Kwaramba, F., & Madzimure, J. 2021. Parties, churches embrace vaccination call, *The Herald*. Accessible at: www.herald.co.zw/parties-churches-embrace-vaccination-call/

Maiden, J. 2021. Zimbabwe's religious leaders increase efforts to tackle COVID-19 and support vaccines, *UNICEF Zimbabwe*. Accessible at: www.unicef.org/zimbabwe/press-releases/zimbabwes-religious-leaders-increase-efforts-tackle-covid-19-and-support-vaccines

Masiyiwa, G., Chenjerai, E., & Mujuru, L. 2021. Battling the virus when religion and public health collide. *Global Press Journal*: Accessible at https://globalpressjournal.com/africa/zimbabwe/religion-public-health-collide/

McAbee, L., Tapera, O., & Kanyangarara, M. 2021. Factors associated with COVID-19 vaccine intentions in Eastern Zimbabwe: A cross-sectional study. *Vaccines*, 9(1109), 1–10.

Muyambo, T. 2022. Social distancing in the context of COVID-19 in Zimbabwe Perspectives from Ndau religious indigenous knowledge systems. In F. Sibanda, T. Muyambo, & E. Chitando (Eds), *Religion and the COVID-19 Pandemic in Southern Africa*. London: Routledge, 37–51.

Ponde-Mutsvedu, L., & Chirongoma, S. 2022. Tele-evangelism, tele-health and cyberbullying in the wake of the outbreak of COVID-19 in Zimbabwe, In F. Sibanda, T. Muyambo, & E. Chitando (Eds), *Religion and the COVID-19 Pandemic in Southern Africa*. London: Routledge, pp. 103–114.

Prooijen, J., & Douglas, K.M. 2017. Conspiracy theories as part of history: The role of societal crisis situations. *Memory Studies*, 10(3), 323–333.

Shumba, T. 2021. Church must preach gospel of ending the pandemic, *The Herald*. Accessible at: www.herald.co.zw/church-must-preach-gospel-of-ending-the-pandemic/

Sibanda, F., Muyambo, T., & Chitando, E. 2022. Introduction: Religion and public health in the shadow of COVID-19 pandemic in Southern Africa, In F. Sibanda, T.

Muyambo, & E. Chitando (Eds), *Religion and the COVID-19 Pandemic in Southern Africa*. London: Routledge, pp. 1–24.

Sipeyiye, S. 2022. Coping with the coronavirus (COVID-19): Resources from Ndau indigenous religion. In F. Sibanda, T. Muyambo, & E. Chitando (Eds), *Religion and the COVID-19 Pandemic in Southern Africa*. London: Routledge, pp. 52–71.

Zinyuke, R. 2021. COVID-19 More church leaders take vaccine, *The Herald*. Accessible at: www.herald.co.zw/covid-19-more-church-leaders-take-vaccine/

14 Vaccination in African Initiated Churches in Zimbabwe

A Recipe for Church Ideological Bisection

Bernard Pindukai Humbe

Introduction

The country of Zimbabwe is historically, culturally, religiously, socially and linguistically complex. Its Constitutional Amendment Act of 2013 provides for freedom of worship without fear of being discriminated against or persecuted. This makes Zimbabwe not only home to many religious traditions, but assorted indigenous religions as well (Humbe, 2018). Within this religious package, more than 85% of the Zimbabweans identify as Christian, and about 37% of the Christians belong to the Apostolic Church.[1] Based on the above statistical representation, there is no doubt that the Apostolic Churches, commonly known as African Independent Churches (AIC) command large followings in Zimbabwe. Zimbabwean society has been hard hit by the COVID-19 pandemic and this had an impact on the AICs. Since the beginning of the pandemic, the Government demonstrated practically that the scientific route was the only recommended practice to address the situation. Apparently, the national response sidelined religion to manage the pandemic. Yet religion has the capacity to influence the way individuals/groups conduct themselves, interact with others and interpret certain phenomena, in this case COVID-19 (Humbe, 2022; Nyathi, 2021). The Ministry of Health and Child Care (MoHCC) has become the mouthpiece and implementer of World Health Organization (WHO) guidelines and measures on COVID-19 (Humbe, 2022). Strengthening of the national response to COVID-19 was done through deployment of vaccines in line with WHO and African Union guidelines. Using the national vaccine framework, healthcare workers administered the vaccine working together with the Medicine Control Authority of Zimbabwe and local scientists throughout the deployment period and after the deployment.

On 18 February 2021, Retired General Dr Constantino Chiwenga, the Vice President and Minister of Health and Child Care, became the first Zimbabwean person in the country to be inoculated with Sinopharm vaccine from China (Humbe, 2022). Against this backdrop, the chapter focuses on the confluence between the AICs and COVID-19 vaccination. Vaccination is considered to be one of the greatest public health achievements of the twentieth century, which has helped to build a society free of vaccine preventable diseases and saved

DOI: 10.4324/9781003388630-14

lives of millions across the globe. While vaccines are viewed as the greatest achievement of public health recommended to be the panacea to harness the coronavirus, Zimbabwe witnessed an era of vaccination refusal. The response to the vaccination drive in Zimbabwe has been associated with resistance, complacency and hesitancy especially in the context of AICs. Relatively, no studies have explored the vaccination drive as a recipe for church ideological bisection in AICs. This chapter begins by considering 'strictness' as an ideological concept which aids in understanding the nature of AICs' response to the COVID-19 vaccination exercise in Zimbabwe. The notion of strictness is substantiated with information coaxed through interviews, observations and documentary analysis. In this vein, the study advances the premise that AICs can be understood as institutions that shape their followers' behaviour traits. The churches in their various outfits supply their adherents with variable behavioural incentives for participation in religious activity, which in turn have systematic implications for participation in the vaccination drive. The AICs have been known to stick to certain proscribed injunctions which gave scholars in religious studies the impetus to group them in the same cluster of African Christianity. They are well known for conflating traditional African beliefs with a Christian doctrine, defiance in use of modern medicine and demand followers seek healing or protection against disease through spiritual means like prayer and the use of holy water. With the 'strict' church framework, the chapter unpacks why a COVID-19 medical procedure is shunned by some believers, especially in the African churches.

On the other hand, the chapter sheds light on factors which triggered AIC followers to shift from their dominant healthcare system of faith healing to modern medical services such as embracing COVID-19 vaccination. Thus the analysis divides AICs into various branches which depict conservatism and liberal/semi conservatism in ideology. This ideological bisection is basically division in opinion among members of different AIC sects (used here in a non-evaluation way to simply mean 'diverse groups') as well between members of the same sects (Chingono, 2021). Those who are pro-vaccination are described in this chapter as liberal and the anti-vaccination supporters are understood as conservatives. The liberals emphasise an accommodating stance towards modernity characterised by modern health delivery systems, a proactive view on issues of social justice and pluralism in their tolerance of varied individual beliefs. This is in contrast to the conservatism whereby the adherents believe in maintaining the strict church doctrines, choices about vaccination being driven by church teachings of defiance against modern medicine, adhere to church and government directives against one's responsible use of liberty. Further, the chapter interrogates whether different religious beliefs are, in themselves, real exception for vaccination (Gordana et al., 2016). In this vein the study further notes that there are some in AICs who readily accepted vaccines on the basis of some extra-religious reasons. At the end, the chapter concludes that the response of AICs to COVID-19 vaccination in Zimbabwe was characterised by ambivalence which has fanned church ideological bisection.

The 'Strict' Churches Ideological Framework

This study employed an advanced compelling theory regarding the institutional features of AICs to be what is known as 'strict' churches (Campbell, 2004). Strictness refers to the existence of particular expectations, and enforcement of such expectations, for churches' members or active congregants (Flynn, 2010: 4). Flynn (2010) admits that leading thinkers such as Dean Kelley perceive strictness as a characteristic of many conservative churches, though conservatism should not be viewed as the same thing as strictness. This chapter maintains the idea that strictness embellished in conservatism is relevantly applicable in AICs. Justification of this understanding is made on the understanding that AICs as strict churches demand congregants to make sacrifices, such as worship in open spaces, wearing a prescribed dress code, keeping of beads, abstaining from conventional public health programmes and consumption of a prescribed diet. As the sacrifices are implemented, it resonates with the idea that strict churches are those having high tension with their surroundings (Campbell, 2004). More often than not members of these churches usually receive criticism from various commentators, whether Christians or not, with regard to their strict ideology.

To concretise the notion of strictness, adopting three distinct, but related, traits of AICs was found to be imperative: absolutism, conformity and fanaticism (Flynn, 2010: 4). Absolutism refers to a rejection of all beliefs or explanations of life except for the church's or the denomination's (Flynn, 2010: 4). When churches are being described as absolutist, it implies that in praxis they have a closed system of beliefs and meaning, believing that they are the only ones who know the real truth about God. In absolutism, the general trend has been that members of such churches attach themselves to the churches' value sets without critically evaluating them (Flynn, 2010: 4). An application of absolutism in this study is made by examining a strong sense of purpose and regarding teachings, deeds, doctrines and traditions as foundational sources of AICs' response to COVID-19 vaccination programme. These churches are older than COVID-19, their absolutist tendency could not be tempered with by demands of a secular approach to manage the pandemic. Strictly related to absolutism is fanaticism. Fanatics have a strong missionary zeal, feeling that they must share their knowledge of God with others, and are unwilling to hear others' views regarding God (Flynn, 2010: 4). Fanatics may isolate themselves from the views of the outside world, or they may drown out other views with a flood of messages proclaiming their own versions of the 'Good News' of how one might receive salvation from eternal damnation. They force their views upon others without believing that other people's views have value (Flynn, 2010: 4). It explains why they regard people who do not subscribe to their religious disposition as lost. In line with this concept of fanaticism, this chapter explores how AICs understood the nature of COVID-19 vaccination based on their belief systems. In some instances, AICs claim to have received prophecies about the pandemic before it had emerged on the scene and how it should be managed.

If some of these AICs were aware of the pandemic, the chapter further examines whether they have the zeal to participate in propagating the secular approach in managing the COVID-19 pandemic. Another important word in this chapter is conformity. A church that values conformity does not tolerate deviance or dissent among its members, shunning those who dare go against the church's teachings. As a result, members of a church may display some traits that set them apart from the rest of the population (Flynn, 2010: 4). Shunning vaccination is one good example of how an AIC sect distinguishes itself from other Christian groupings. At the same time the chapter understands believers' acceptance of vaccination as a way of conformity to the church's teaching, especially if it is a call made by the church leader as a response to a new pandemic situation. Paradoxically, conformity may be realised as the result of personal conviction and influence of state policy.

The last term to be employed in this chapter is free-riding. A term borrowed from political science and economics, free-riding refers to the tendency of individuals who are part of a group to enjoy the benefits of the group without making significant contributions to its demands. In the context of this study, free-riding means being affiliated with AICs without making a meaningful contribution to preserve the strictness of the church from influences of the outside world, whether it is secular world or some other religious traditions. Since they are free-riders they have seen nothing weird about vaccination since it is meant to save lives of the people from the deadly COVID-19 pandemic. Certain factors other than religious are preeminent in their desire to get vaccination.

Based on the meaning of the above terms, people who belong to strict churches share a deep-seated faith in the correctness of their church's tenets, leading to a sense of moral certainty (Flynn, 2010). Strict churches enforce compliance with the tenets of the faith by pulling their members into a tight social network composed of fellow believers. When there is a health pandemic, it is this social network which dictates the expected response to the situation, in some instances instigating a spirit of detaching themselves from the world which they might believe is the cause of the problem. However, there is an intriguing insight in the theory's application. This is because while strict churches are able to overcome collective action dilemmas like those associated with mandatory vaccination, the strictness costs of membership has also bred free-riders who have embraced COVID-19 vaccination.

Strictness as an Ideology

In Zimbabwe, strict churches easily collaborate with the ZANU-PF ruling government, viewed by many as a totalitarian regime, for they share with them the same ideology of anti–Western regime change agenda. Marriage between AICs and ZANU-PF started during the colonial era in a bid to dislodge Western imperialism and the relationship continued to flourish in postcolonial

Zimbabwe. Several AIC leaders are on record saying the country's ZANU-PF leaders are God ordained and should not be removed. So anyone wishing to have them voted out is against God's wish. The ideology of strictness functions in the realm of theology in the same way as they do everywhere else: they stereotype the truth; make it more comprehensible and translatable into social and health action (Hovorun, 2016). This comes at the expense of various aberrations in the perception of truth about vaccination. It is this amalgamated AICs–ZANU-PF ideological quandary that vaccination was resisted or accepted, based on a believer's inclination either to the civil rule, church teaching or both. To this end, ideologies polarise religious groups. They make the church "divided between traditionalists and progressives, conservatives and liberals, those accentuating identity and those stressing dialogue ... and so on" (Hovorun, 2016). There are situations where the church and its followers provide a framework where ideologies would not harm: "The terrible paradox is that ideology penetrates into Christianity and is not recognised as opposite to it" (Hovorun, 2016). Ideologies thus should be recognised in the church, and the church should accept that it is dangerous to be identified with them (Hovorun, 2016). Thus, many observers suggest that AICS in Zimbabwe serve to mobilise their members to follow the politics of the ruling ZANU-PF party, yet the same churches encourage members to withdraw from the ZANU-PF government's health policies. The tight social networks formed through their rigorous spirituality can at times facilitate rapid and intense mobilisation against vaccination.

The Spirit of AICs and Health Matters Confronted by COVID-19

Right from the outset, the chapter outlines some institutional characteristic features of AICs which pertain to their participation and non-participation in national health programmes. The acronym AIC has proved to be multivalent in its use. Among other applications, it is understood as African Indigenous Churches, African Initiated Churches and/or African Independent Churches. In the context of this study, an appealing definition of an African Independent Church is proffered by Appiah-Kubi (1977: 117) when he says that "these are churches founded by Africans for Africans in our special African situations. They have all African membership as well as all African leadership." Movements of these churches include Zionist, Apostolic and Ethiopian Churches as well as Pentecostal-Charismatic Churches. They usually regard themselves as Spirit-type churches (Muguranyanga, 2011) or *chechi dzeMweya*, and consequently base their religious beliefs and practices primarily on *Mweya* (Spirit) or *Izwi* (Voice of God). They receive advice and/or guidance from the Holy Spirit or Voice of God through the mediation of prophets or church leaders. However, the special African situations in which these churches are thriving make them heterogeneous. Thus, the AICs in Zimbabwe have been characterised by con-tinuous intensification and expansion, with smaller units emerging from mother bodies. So there is a need to exercise caution when making generalisations about their total belief systems and practices (Humbe, 2018).

In recent times differences between AICs have become more apparent in their response to COVID-19 vaccination exercises. Because of the peculiarities, this chapter uses the term 'sects' to describe them. Some of the AIC movements believe that COVID-19 emerged because of the bad works of the secular world. Therefore COVID-19 is tantamount to an evil spirit. The sects believe that they are aligned to the Holy Spirit or Mweya Mutsvene which is the antithesis of evil spirits like COVID-19, and their duty as Christians is to work hard restoring good health and quality of life of those who are faithful and observe religious tenets, teachings and regulations of the Apostolic churches (Muguranyanga, 2011). Mweya Mutsvene is key in their lives because it is the source of spiritual revelation, prophecy, healing, instruction and protection. Hence, in most cases, Apostolic leaders and faithful "teach faith-healing and regard sickness itself and use of medical services (traditional or modern) as signs of weakness of faith" (Muguranyanga, 2011), and teach that sin can lead to sickness. Thus these sects are epitomised as healing institutes. They emphasise strict adherence to religious teachings and practices, compliance with normative values, and impose penalties on those who violate church regulations and religious teachings (Muguranyanga, 2011).

Church Leaders as Pro-vaccination Agents

When the Zimbabwean government introduced compulsory vaccination, the move generated a perceived value of medical assistance among some AIC members and theology that shapes members' attitudes towards modern medical services. In the proceeding paragraphs the chapter starts by exploring views of AICs who exhibited greater propensity to embrace vaccination. Bishop Nehemiah Mutendi of the Zion Christian Church was among the first AIC leaders to publicly mobilise people for vaccination. Some of his messages trended on social media, confirming the need to be vaccinated. He emphasised the need for vaccination to save lives. His sentiments on vaccination were in support of the government's efforts to reach its target of vaccinating at least 10 million Zimbabweans – or 60% of the population – by the end of 2021.[2] Soon after receiving his first dose of Sinopharm vaccine on 19 March 2021 at Wilkins Hospital in Harare, Bishop Mutendi said: "I urge Zimbabweans to take the vaccine which is offered for free by the government. Prevention is better than cure. We all have to be vaccinated."[3] This understanding of vaccines as preventative remedy to the pandemic by a high-profile faith leader like Mutendi served to entice followers of ZCC and even outsiders to embrace the vaccine.

However, several faith leaders in different AICs questioned the sincerity of Mutendi's call for vaccination. One participant argued that COVID-19 vaccination had put Mutendi's healing powers at bay. Before COVID-19,

Mutendi was well known for addressing health problems to anyone who sought his assistance. While his expressions such as 'prevention is better than cure' were acknowledged by his followers, the beneficial effects of vaccination were sometimes viewed with disappointment, and considered temporary and superficial (Roura et al., 2010) because the vaccine would not offer a definitive cure for COVID-19. A middle-aged female AIC faith healer reiterated that COVID-19 exposed some church leaders like Mutendi to be just ordinary church leaders who have limited powers over diseases. It seems the participants perceived COVID-19 within the framework of Mutendi's *Mapumhangozi* myth. *Mapumhangozi* is a holy rod used by Samuel Mutendi, the founder of ZCC in Zimbabwe. The rod is believed to have mystic powers, especially in warding off anything deemed to be evil. This holy rod was inherited by Samuel Mutendi's son Nehemiah. In this study, the term 'myth' is used in the context of a phenomenological perspective in which myths mean "sacred stories of a community of believers" (Chimininge, 2012). In *mapumhangozi*, the holy staff is used to bless the water by pointing and steering it. The holy water has so many functions in healing and exorcism. Initially followers and even some outsiders had a conviction that Mutendi's *mapumangonzi* had the power to heal the sick and cast out the evil spirit causing this strange sickness. But what became the reality on the ground was that death due to COVID-19 was just equivalent to the vagaries of *ngozi* terminating lives indiscriminately. Thus in their view Mutendi had surrendered his powers to a secular approach in managing COVID-19.

Though Mutendi hailed the vaccination programme, a visit to one of his wellness centres showed that his followers were not feeling totally secured by the vaccine only. Since some people who had been vaccinated were contracting coronavirus, some of his followers were in agreement to think that being vaccinated or not, one should also be protected from the deadly disease by holy waters. They were convinced that vaccination was only done as a sign of adherence to the government's strict national response scientific approach. This follows the close relationship that exists between their church and the ruling ZANU-PF party. At the wellness centre, it was observed that a *Mudzidzisi* (Teacher) had the responsibility of performing body sanitisation using anointed water in a plastic container. What was observed is well captured in a description given by Wepener (2013: 4) in the following words:

> the water is sprinkled over the individual facing the person doing the sprinkling, including the head and feet; after that the person turns around and the same sprinkling is done on the back of his or her body; they turn around again and a bit of water is poured into their hands, which they then use to wash their hands.

The efficacy of anointed water in the indigenous Christian worldview, especially the ZCC Mbungo sect, is centred on the belief that water is closely related to cleansing. Through its sacred powers conferred from God, it protects people from contracting COVID-19, heals the sick and wards off evil which results in people not contracting the virus. Other AICs adherents confirmed that water is very sacral in their spirituality. The followers used it as follows: decoction, concoction, infusion, bathing, steaming and sprinkling homesteads.

Just like Mutendi, another Bishop and founder of the Johane the Fifth of Africa Apostolic Church in the eastern Manicaland province, Andby Makururu, made frantic efforts, encouraging his members to get vaccinated.

> We are transforming the indigenous church to suit global standards. Johane the Fifth of Africa has been on a vaccination drive. In all our preachings, we encourage members to get vaccinations because the Holy Spirit does not cure all these diseases. So I am encouraging the Apostolic sect to go to hospitals and get treatment, I also get treatment and regular check-ups. Sects who deny the benefits of vaccines are out of touch. Those that are still behind are lagging but we are moving with the times.[4]

The above position by Makururu of embracing vaccination in the COVID-19 pandemic is justified on the pretext that modern vaccination has seen the successful treatment, control, and even effective eradication of some of the world's worst diseases.[5] Though his stance among others provided a framework for considering embracing the vaccine to save lives, a close look at his Makururu's views on vaccination shows that these faith leaders have acknowledged the limitedness of faith healing. This created distrust in the Holy Spirit's role in people's social lives. These church leaders have used COVID-19 as an opportunity to showcase the contemporariness of their sects. Modernity in this case is equated to use of science, especially in healing matters. This is a reactionary response to accusations levelled against AIC sects that they were conservatives lagging behind in modern health issues. So what might be derived from Makururu's position is that COVID-19 has created an opportunity for the AICs to be liberal and get realigned with the rest of the modern world. The drive was not influenced by religion but by the desire to be identified with modern global health trends.

This ambiguous and emergent nature of some of the AICs for their lack of authority over diseases is something that some members of the conservative Zion Apostolic Church disputed. The objectors seemed less keen about the goodness of practicing global health standards for this might not be what God wanted for the African Apostles who have a different spirituality from the rest of the world. Adding a voice in the dispute of Apostles receiving vaccination, one fundamentalist, a prophet in the Marange Church, candidly dismissed Makururu's claim that 'the Holy Spirit does not cure all these diseases'. The prophet described Makururu's utterance as blasphemous. He acknowledged the power of the Holy Spirit with its ability to heal diseases like COVID-19 which were regarded as incurable by human beings. So faith healing was a reality depending on the strength of one's faith. This clash of philosophies in AIC circles reflects the essence of their theological standing which shows these sects were started by Africans for specific African situations, and now COVID-19 was one of them.

Are AIC Leaders Leading by Example?

There were some participants who were not comfortable with the position depicted in the preceding paragraphs regarding AIC faith leaders as models in the vaccination exercise. An elderly male participant of the Johane Masowe sect in Masvingo pointed out that it is expected of AIC adherents to follow their leaders in matters to do with faith. He further clarified saying there was a need to exercise extreme caution for the faithful were not expected to uncritically follow the footsteps of their leaders when they side with the secular world. This view demonstrates the conviction of adherents who thought that by receiving vaccination, their leaders had abandoned their most crucial role of defending the church against desecration. So the vaccination driven by the secular world was in violation of AICs' strict religious ideology. It is thought-provoking to note that the leaders who publicly embraced vaccination never equated the coronavirus to evil spirits.

Comparatively, faith leaders who persuaded followers to embrace vaccination were better than those who maintained silence over the matter, as was put across by an AIC evangelist in Mutare. Among other faith leaders, the African Apostolic Church of Paul Mwazha never publicly issued statements on vaccination. Three males and one female Mwazha follower agreed that the muteness of their faith leader created confusion on the part of followers who wanted public confirmation whether they accepted the vaccine or not. As a result followers were subjected into a theological health quandary. Because of lack of clarity and proper guidance believers gave an 'end of times' interpretation to the emergence of COVID-19. Some cited the emergence of diseases and pandemics, the banning of church gatherings as the surest signs of the end of times, thus vaccination was not ideal for them. Accepting the vaccine was tantamount to defiling their bodies which God's temples. The followers became engrossed in the belief that vaccination was *munembo* (Mark of the Beast) which would eventually disqualify people from attaining salvation on the day of judgement. This 'mark' is mentioned in the last book of the Bible and serves as a warning to Christians not to align with the regimes of the world that are antagonistic to God.[6] As long as the directive to administer vaccines to the AICs was not coming from God, it meant the vaccination exercise was not godly. The hesitancy in accepting vaccination makes an impression that Africans have very strong religious beliefs which must be taken into account when health policies are being made as a national response to health pandemics. The proliferation of such an imminent eschatological understanding made them a strict group of the absolute faithful which was staging a fight against Satan and his secular world. In view of the above, AICs viewed themselves as separatists who had nothing to do with the world's troubles. During lockdowns, it was observed that some believers spent most of their times and energy in the forest worshipping. This can be described as 'forest heist'. Believers regarded forests and mountains as hierophanies. Forests and mountains provided the AICs followers with secluded venues for fasting and worshipping, seeking spiritual rejuvenation in the face of a deadly pandemic. This was noted especially when the government implemented a policy of commendatory vaccination which only allowed those who had been vaccinated to gather and attend church services. In their view, frequent visits to their places of worship were a remedy of fighting the coronavirus because they regarded their open places of worship as sacred where they encountered God. At the worship places the following were observed: flouting flags of different colours which range from green, white, red, blue and yellow, artefacts like clay-made bowls (*mbiya*), erected wooden crosses and reeds, among others. At certain worship centres, it was observed that the faith leader used ashes to put a sign of the cross on congregants' forehead, to ensure protection from the perils of coronavirus.

Painful Death but an Indecent Send Off

However, on the other hand, failure to articulate a clear sect's position on the vaccination exercise made some believers take advantage and get jabbed to avoid a 'bad death'. One participant explained that she was fully aware that they would one day die, but dying during the peak of the pandemic was disgraceful because of lack of proper funeral rites for the deceased victim. The participants mentioned the gathering of mourners, singing, dancing and prayers done by the church during funerals as rituals which make the deceased arrive safely into paradise (Nwokoha, 2020: 75). A significant number of believers admitted that they converted to the AICs for the sole purpose of receiving a proper African Christian burial. A male AIC evangelist declared that it was shrewd to get jabbed and live longer so as to be buried properly when the COVID-19 pandemic would have subsided. Based on views from participants, accepting jabbing was determined by a metaphysical disposition of what happens to the deceased when they do not receive proper burial rites. So the obscurity associated with this disease as it causes untimely deaths persuaded the AIC adherents to receive jabbing. An AIC member reiterated that he made a personal choice to be vaccinated due to a disturbing spike in COVID-19 death cases, with Christians also succumbing to the deadly disease. This means Christians were also vulnerable, contrary to claims that they had safe divine protection. In this context, the issue of vaccination was supposed to be viewed side by side with a person's conviction regarding his/her body and personal rights, contrary to the traditional view of the church being in authority over a person's life. This created confusion because AICs do not operate based on individual personal choices but on set principles and guidelines prescribed by the Holy Spirit through intermediaries like prophets and church leaders. Responding to this confusion, a certain faith leader maintained that while his sect believes that the Holy Spirit is the healer of all diseases, COVID-19 included, if a believer's faith was not strong, it was advisable that the person went for vaccination to be protected from the pandemic. Implicitly, those who had strong faith could defy vaccination for it was only for those who had weak faith. In this context, it became a moment to showcase believers' faith and those who defied vaccination were regarded with high esteem.

No to Vaccination

On the contrary, many of the Zion Apostolic Church members were very clear in that they continued following the teachings of their church, that is, of shunning biomedicine. Such members resisted the vaccination drive to such an extent that some even opted to quit their jobs when the government insisted on vaccination. A 22-year-old young man working for a construction company explained that he quitted his job to keep the traditions of the church. He explained that quitting his job was a more glorified move than receiving a COVID-19 jab. He was supported by an old male church elder who said every person shall die regardless of what causes the death, so there was no need to compromise their faith. Such a fundamentalist position was hailed as bold heroism in faith by some of his church members. The elder questioned the contents of injections, reinforcing the widely held myth by AICs that biomedicine is manufactured using suspicious contents. So it was their obligation to keep their bodies clean of Western medication to ensure that they remain pure temples of God. Once believers uphold a myth, it becomes difficult to convince them in dislodging the myth. These claims basically had nothing to do with religious beliefs but reflected some poverty of knowledge on how vaccines are manufactured. This is because they had lack of experience in these jabs since their churches discourage them from using biomedicine. So at the end, they used the church as a scapegoat in shunning vaccination. However, one respondent from a different sect questioned the genuineness of defying vaccination when in actual fact some of these vaccine objectors dubiously acquired fake vaccine cards. This followed a directive by the government that vaccination cards were a prerequisite when travelling. The critic argued that acquiring fake vaccination cards was putting their moral integrity to the test. Responding to this criticism, a female prophet opined that possessing fake cards was done to avoid prosecution.

Some participants in the Zion Apostolic Church believed that once a person was admitted into the church he/she was saved, so no vaccine had salvific values. Looking at this aberration, it seems the believers had just one straightforward purview of a Christian's health life. Yet the COVID-19 situation at stake required practical measures other than just praying to contain the virus from spreading. The response given above was merely referring to the Christian soul's destiny after death. This becomes a challenge in the sense that they perceived the church as providing total salvation to the adherent, yet the vaccine programme harnessed a virus which attacks the physical body. An alternative to vaccination was provided by another respondent in the same sect succinctly in the following words: "Christians should use anointed pebbles for protection from any kind of health threat." This then confirms a pious statement which had already been uttered by her church colleague saying "God, our creator is the absolute vaccine". By using the catchy word 'absolute', the response showed no room for any human-made remedy to harness the problem of COVID-19. Rather efforts to reduce the spreading of COVID-19 had to be sought from God.

Prophecy and COVID-19

A participant from Johane Masowe WeChishanu sect in Buhera questioned why the Zimbabwean government was working within a scientific framework, yet science had failed to predict the coming of this pandemic. He reiterated that his sect had solutions to unanswered questions about the origin of COVID-19. In this line of thinking, the coming of COVID-19 was long back detected by Izwi (God's Voice). Accordingly, what was happening was simply a fulfilment of a 1971 prophecy about a future catastrophe. A certain participant belonging to another Johane Masowe sect in Masvingo concurred saying the following: "The Holy Spirit informed us that in the 2020 season, after experiencing poverty, you will be hard hit by a disease which will be a pandemic, I see open graves, with some men clearing a field without rest." Another voice was added by a congregant in Chivhu who articulated clearly the nature of the disease saying, "a prophecy was given in 2019 saying there shall come a disease which appears like flu resulting in victims having breathing problems as well as losing strength. But the doctors will fail to find a cure to this disease. The disease will kill a lot of people but will eventually come to an end." One sect faith leader emphasised that believers did not have problems in understanding these prophecies because before the coming of Cyclone Idai, the Holy Spirit had already notified the congregants about the impending disaster. However it is important to note that prophecies about the coronavirus only circulated in these AIC sects and were never made public. All respondents cited fear of victimisation by state agents as the sole reason for concealing the information. For them, solutions for the coronavirus were to be provided by God, not through vaccination. Prayer was the remedy. The issue of over relying on science to harness COVID-19 through vaccination was met with serious objections. Thus according to one respondent of the Vadzidzi Apostolic church, "We believe in God, and science is entirely subject to God's will".[7] Because of the strong conviction of living a life full of prayer protection, he declares that together with his family they will not take the vaccine because they were protected by prayers.[8]

The Jabbed Ones Are Regretting

Some AIC adherents regretted having been jabbed. They said they had taken the jab as a sign of loyalty to the state as per teachings of their church. But they now feared that their bodies had been corrupted by the vaccine. A certain faith healer clarified saying she was working on various cases of health problems which included having continuous menstruation, erectile dysfunction and failure to conceive. According to the faith healer and her patients, all these problems developed as a result of vaccination. So what the victims wanted was cleansing of the dirt jab from their bodies for they had received it without proper advice. It explains the religious foundations of the 'Apostolic healthcare system' that emphasises faith-healing, healing rituals, prayer, and Mweya (the Holy Spirit). Healing in the AICs entails the restoration of the imbalances both in an individual and societal sense. Health is defined in terms of the fulfilment of all the roles expected of people in their society. The faith healers play a significant part in the restoration of these imbalances.

Critical Reflections

From the findings, it could be ascertained that as spiritual healing could not be warranted in efforts to harness COVID-19 in Zimbabwe, it implies that God had 'only a part to play' which was complemented by biomedicine fronted by the government. So conformity in the coexistence of spiritual and biomedical approaches to the disease was commonly found in the respondent's responses (Roura et al., 2010). Considering that vaccination was in a very strong sense a compulsory exercise, what seemed acceptable was that spiritual healing was offered more often as a complement than as a substitute for biomedical treatment. It explains why some faith leaders urged their followers to accept vaccination because spiritual healing had limitations which were addressed by the absolute biomedicine. One area which this study found to be complex was that protection from the diseases and or healing of the disease depended on the strength of the faith of those involved. As a result of this uncertainty, the use of both faith healing and biomedicine would generally not be discouraged as it could potentially help in cases where prayer had been unsuccessful. The widely made claim by commentators that white garment churches' doctrinal teachings diminish participation in vaccination programmes diverges from this study. Sects like ZCC Mbungo had their leaders as the first to receive COVID-19 doses.

   The study also established that faith leaders who strongly supported the vaccination drive had some political inclinations to the ZANU-PF ruling party. For example, Mutendi is well known for being a fanatical ally of the ZANU-PF government from the times of then President Robert Mugabe. The ZANU-PF rulers use Mutendi's congregation as a rich minefield of the pro-ZANU-PF electorate. On several occasions he has served as a ZANU-PF mouth piece, ensuring that his followers support the ZANU-PF party programmes. In Masvingo Province, the government's Pfumvudza (agricultural) programme was launched by President Emmerson Mnangagwa at Mutendi's farm. His strong support for ZANU-PF has earned him tremendous benefits from ZANU-PF programmes of indigenisation such as land. Because of that he is on record persuading his followers to support ZANU-PF. Given this scenario, when the issue of vaccination emerged on the scene,

Mutendi as usual was found supporting the programme. The other reason for Mutendi backing vaccination was that his Mbungo Worship Centre is one of Zimbabwe's biggest religious tourist attraction centres. At the site, there is a grand ostentatious church building which was officially commissioned by the then President, Robert Gabriel Mugabe. The tourist centre attracts both locals and foreigners who include ZCC followers and others. It can accommodate up to 20,000 congregants. Based on this understanding, one is persuaded to think that acceptance of the vaccine was meant to show solidarity with the government leader in his efforts to manage COVID-19. He was also setting tourist standards both for his local and international guests who would flock to his shrine. Such superfluous theological motives in health matters were a recipe for ideological bisection.

The government's absolutely strict stance in the vaccination programme made AIC followers buy the idea of receiving jabs. It is part of the church teachings that people should always be allegiant to the ruling government. In some churches like Paul Mwazha's they acknowledge the secular rulers of the country and pray for God's guidance and protection as they execute their duties. So in this case vaccination was an exercise meant to support what the government was implementing since the church commands them to obey state leaders. In situations like this, while the source of division in opinion was based on the strict ideology operating, the difference was whose and what strictness was being appendaged.

The argument here is that while AICs' tight social networks facilitate sporadic mobilisation, the process by which those networks are formed can also serve to deflate their levels of vaccination participation. The study managed to dispel the widely held belief that the Johanne Marange followers abuse the right to health of their children by denying them access to the government's immunisation programmes. In this study it was found that adults detested vaccination citing their faith as a reason for not taking part. This shows consistency in their church's defiance of the modern health delivery system.

Conclusion

The infamous 'vaccination controversy', which has dominated the Zimbabwean religious and health landscape, involved not only an overt political contest since the emergence of COVID-19, but also a more subtle contest over the authority to represent African Christians. The chapter argued that though AICs in Zimbabwe share the same ideology of practising a Christianity grounded on strict indigenous spirituality, divergence of opinion in recent times with regard to health matters, especially COVID-19 vaccination, has appeared to be both theological and non-theological. Vaccine hesitancy was prompted either by strict church ideology or strict state ideology. Based on various responses which opposed vaccination, it can be argued that the potency of AICs in Zimbabwe during pandemics such as COVID-19 is found in their potential for mobilisation, not in their actual mobilisation. This spiritualisation of

COVID-19 influenced AICs followers' attitude and behaviour, primarily driven by their belief that sickness has a spiritual undertone and often requires a religious response. Yet the COVID-19 experiences in Zimbabwe have shown that depending on circumstances, adherents can disarm ideologies.

Notes

1 www.theguardian.com/global-development/2021/nov/01/the-sects-hampering-south ern-africa-covid-vaccine-rollout
2 www.voanews.com/a/zimbabwe-starts-vaccinating-teens-against-covid-19/6297 089.html
3 www.herald.co.zw/covid-19-more-church-leaders-take-vaccine/
4 www.usnews.com/news/world/articles/2021-10-13/its-not-satanism-zimbabwe-chu rch-leaders-preach-vaccines
5 www.abc.net.au//religion/should-christians-be-opposed-to-vaccination/13473770
6 www.abc.net.au//religion/should-christians-be-opposed-to-vaccination/13473770
7 www.theguardian.com/global-development/2021/nov/01/the-sects-hampering-south ern-africa-covid-vaccine-rollout
8 www.theguardian.com/global-development/2021/nov/01/the-sects-hampering-south ern-africa-covid-vaccine-rollout

References

ABC News, www.abc.net.au//religion/should-christians-be-opposed-to-vaccination/ 13473770. Accessed 01/07/2022.
Appiah-Kubi, K. 1977. African theology en route: Papers from the Pan African Conference of Third World Theologians, 17–23 December 1977, Accra, Ghana; https://books.google.com.ng/books/about/African_Theology_en_Route.html
Campbell, D.E. 2004. Acts of faith: Churches and political engagement. *Political Behavior*, 26(2), 155–180.
Chimininge, V. 2012. The ritual of avenging spirit: A case study of the Zion Christian Church of Samuel Mutendi in Zimbabwe. In *Theolgia Viatorum, Journal of Theology and Religion in Africa*, 36(1), 94–124.
Chingono, N. 2021. 'We are protected by prayers': The sects hampering southern Africa's vaccine rollout, www.theguardian.com/global-development/2021/nov/01/ the-sects-hampering-southern-africa-covid-vaccine-rollout.
Flynn, R.A. 2010. Are strict churches really stronger? A study of strictness, congregational activity, and growth in American Protestant churches. *Graduate Theses, Dissertations, and Problem Reports*. 4590. https://researchrepository.wvu.edu/ etd/4590/
Gordana, P., Silvana, K., Galina, L.M., Olga, I.K., Frank, J.L., Michael, C.T., Naoki, M., Suzana, V., and Luka, T. 2016. Religious exception for vaccination or religious excuses for avoiding vaccination. *Croat Med J.*, 57(5), 516–521.
Hovorun, C. 2016. Ideology and religion. *Kyiv-Mohyla Humanities Journal*, *3*, 23–35. National University of Kyiv-Mohyla Academy,
Humbe, B.P. 2018. Indigenous African crusaders of environmental keeping: A phenomenological reflection on the power of AICs' practices in Zimbabwe. In E. Masitera

and F. Sibanda (Eds), *Power in Contemporary Zimbabwe*. New York: Routledge/ Taylor and Francis Group, pp. 85–98.

Humbe, B.P. 2022. Living with COVID-19 in Zimbabwe. A religious and scientific healing response. In F. Sibanda, T. Muyambo, and E. Chitando (Eds), *Religion and the COVID-19 Pandemic in Southern Africa*. London: Routledge, pp. 73–88.

Maguranyanga, B. 2011. *Apostolic Religion, Health and Utilization of Maternal and Child Health Services in Zimbabwe*. Collaborating Center for Operational Research Evaluation, UNICEF, mconsultin group.

Nwokoha, A.2020. Rites and rituals for the dead: Bases for good moral behaviour in Ezzaland, Nigeria. *International Journal of Religion & Human Relations*, 12(1), 67–85.

Nyathi, K. 2021. Religious groups warm up to COVID-19 vaccines in Zimbabwe. (www.unicef.org/zimbabwe/stories/religious-groups-warm-covid-19-vaccines-zimbabwe). UNICEF.

Roura, M., Nsigaye, R., Nhandi, B., Wamoyi, J., Busza, J., Urassa, M., Todd, J., and Zaba, B. 2010. "Driving the devil away": Qualitative insights into miraculous cures for AIDS in a rural Tanzanian ward. *BMC Public Health*, 10, 427.

US News, www.usnews.com/news/world/articles/2021-10-13/its-not-satanism-zimbabwe-church-leaders-preach-vaccines. Accessed 24/06/2022.

Wepener, C. 2013. *Water rituals as a source of (Christian) life in an African Independent Church: To be healed and (re)connected*, CORE, Stellenbosch University SUNScholar Repository.

15 Shona Traditional Religion, Gender and COVID-19 Vaccination in Zimbabwe

The Case of Buhera South, Manicaland Province

Maradze Viriri, Etwin Machibaya and Cuthbert Pisirai

Introduction and Background to the Study

The COVID-19 pandemic virus (coronavirus diseases) has been wreaking havoc on the planet for over two years (Chirisa, 2021). There has been no evidence that the virus' transmission can be totally stopped since it was found in Wuhan, China in December 2019. The major stumbling block is that there seems to be no immediate solution in sight as the virus keeps on mutating.

The negative public perceptions of vaccination was one of the most worrying concerns that occurred when looking at people's response to COVID–19 vaccination programmes rolled out by the government of Zimbabwe (Chirisa, 2021). Hannan et al. (2021) say that this negative attitude towards vaccination was based on the general belief that vaccinations in general include ingredients that are prohibited by certain religious beliefs, making their usage a taboo to their religion. Most religions have no prohibition against vaccination (Chirisa, 2021). However, some have reservations, concerns or restrictions regarding vaccination. The COVID-19 vaccine, like other vaccinations, has the primary goal of protecting the body and building self-defence so that it can be protected from the COVID-19 virus (Chirisa, 2021). The vaccine which was recommended by the government of Zimbabwe to be administered in the country was Sino-pharm BIBP which was first delivered to Zimbabwe in February 2021. This vaccine is meant not only for prevention but also for preventative management while dealing with COVID-19 (Chirisa, 2021). Hannan et al. (2021) say that vaccination serves at least four purposes, namely, reducing COVID-19 related morbidity and mortality; functioning as medical efforts to achieve a level of herd immunity that helps prevent transmission; maintaining or protecting public health as a whole; maintaining productivity and minimising social impacts as a result of COVID-19's spread, including economic, political and educational impacts.

DOI: 10.4324/9781003388630-15

If a person is vaccinated, his or her chance of infection is lower than if he or she has never been vaccinated (Jokwiro, 2020).

The United Nations adopted an international right to freedom of religion more than a half-century ago (Jokwiro, 2020). It also states that this right can be limited when it is necessary to protect the public. This chapter discusses responses to COVID-19 vaccination in Zimbabwe. It focuses on Shona indigenous religion. Just like other religions worldwide, Shona indigenous religion had an influence on the vaccination programme for the COVID-19 virus in Buhera South. Shona religion believes in the existence of God (Tatira, 2016). Mbiti (1975) says that God is at the centre of African religion and dominates all its other beliefs. Bourdillon (1975) says that in the theocentric structuring of African religion, the divinities and certain spirits, usually such as natural phenomena, are described as God's delegates, administrators, servants, vice-regents, and representatives or as intermediaries between God and humans. Among the Shona of Buhera South, the ancestors are very important in their religion because to the Shona ancestors (or ancestral spirits) like divinities and spirits, are often presented as God's representatives or as intermediaries between God and humans. Mbiti (1975) says ancestors are the best group of intermediaries between humans and God. Nabudere (2011) believes that ancestors know the needs of humans, and at the same time, they have full access to the channels of communication with God. Magesa (1997) observed that people and the Shona people, in particular, approach ancestors more often for minor needs of life than they approach God. Machinga (2012: 2) argues that, "The religious beliefs and values play a significant role in the traditional ways of treatment. Rituals, symbolic representatives, dreams, and herbal therapy are some of the methods that have a central place in the traditional healing practice."

Dei (2012) proffers that anthropology is the scientific and humanistic analysis of cultures and society, and by implication it is taken to refer to the way people organise and do different things in their everyday life. COVID-19 called for the ban of social gatherings where most Zimbabwean rural and urban people usually gather for their cultural practices and ancestors' rites. COVID-19 also temporarily stopped the cultural and symbolic death rituals where people usually shake hands with the bereaved (*kubata maoko*) (Kramer, 2021), as a sign of sharing their sorrow. The ancestors had lost their spiritual significance and status because of COVID-19. Its vaccination, medicalised and spreading, had a negative impact on the Shona religion. By implication, COVID-19 severed the Shona social fabric through social distancing, restricting mobility and curtailing social gatherings which have a strong bearing on the Shona religion. Gender dynamics have been seen to be another factor influencing the vaccination in Buhera South. The UN (2020) defines gender as the social or cultural condition of being male or female. It goes on to say that gender refers to male-female differences which are not biological but prescribed by society and culture and as such there are marked differences in male-female gender roles in different societies, cultures and communities.

Theoretical Framework

The chapter is guided by the postcolonial theory which, according to McMillan and Schumacher (2010) falls under the critical research tradition. There was a need for the researchers to be critical of the current situation where a COVID-19 vaccination is presented as one of the study issues in the country. Selected participants were expected to articulate their views and experiences freely as decolonised people on their perspectives on COVID-19 vaccination. The epistemology and methodology of the theory influenced the research processes in this study. Postcolonial theory is concerned with matters of race, ethnicity and gender, with the challenges of formulating a postcolonial national identity. The theory tries to describe how colonised African people's knowledge was used against them in the service of the colonisers' interests and how knowledge about the world is generated under specific relations between the powerful and the powerless. Ndamba (2017) argues that doing research under postcolonial theory is important because it offers some rich and appropriate knowledge that can bring change among the oppressed people and in this case among the Buhera South people. Participants were able to speak for themselves and give solutions and suggestions on COVID-19 vaccination challenges in their area, hoping that their experiences and voices would transform them. Dei (2006) asserts that this theory provides a detailed analysis of colonial and non-colonial issues that are implanted in social and cultural institutes in order to make sense of the current living realities of the colonised.

The theory also encourages the colonised to create strong creative resistance ways and solutions to the coloniser's oppressive ways. According to Subedi and Daza (2008) cited in Ndamba (2017), postcolonialism is used to mean the experiences of those societies which were politically, culturally and linguistically colonised. The culturally colonised were the focus of this study and there were discussions about how colonial culture contributed to the ideology of those who were colonised in Buhera. From this observation, the researchers considered the postcolonial theory an appropriate one for this study which assumes that the people in Buhera South are culturally disadvantaged to accept the COVID-19 vaccination in line with the pandemic requirements. The theory tries to provide a framework that destabilises dominant discourse in the developed world and challenges 'inherent assumptions' and critiques the 'material-discursive legacies of colonialism' (Gavi, 2020).This gave the participants a chance to speak for themselves and give solutions and suggestions on COVID-19 vaccination challenges in their area, hoping that their experiences and voices would transform them. In other words, we can say that the theory liberates and empowers those who were culturally colonised and were no longer believing in their own norms and values.

It must be noted that the theory, according to Ndamba (2017), is an ongoing dialogue by which knowledge is constructed. Nabudere (2011) cited in Ndamba (2017) stated that there is a need for humanity to dialogue with one another as a way of coming up with a meaningful consensus about a new future. This calls for a need to get the views and experiences of the local people in Buhera South on COVID-19 vaccination.

Statement of the Problem

COVID-19 vaccination is being carried out in some countries and in Zimbabwe it has been widely promoted. Specifically, this chapter sought for views from Shona Traditional Religion, gender and women in particular on its application with reference to Buhera South district. There are some traditional beliefs, norms and values that seem to be violated by the mandatory vaccination and there is no research known to us that has been conducted to find out the views and cultural barriers of local people on the vaccination. It is against this background that the chapter investigated the barriers and views of participants in Buhera South in Manicaland province on Shona Traditional Religion (STR), gender and COVID-19 vaccination.

Methodology

This study employed a qualitative research method and descriptive survey method in particular. This design allowed the researchers to gain an understanding of the participants' natural settings (McMillan & Schemacher, 2010). Primary and secondary data were gathered from a variety of sources, including literature such as research papers, information media and statistics data. The postcolonial theory encouraged participants to speak out their views on COVID-19 vaccinations and allows them to come out with possible solutions to their problems.

The study used 20 participants who were purposively selected and data were collected through a qualitative semi-structured interview guide with open-ended questions which were for guidance only. The interviews were flexible and were adapted to the responses, interests and direction indicated by the participants during the interview. The Constant Comparative method by Cohen et al. (2011) was used for analysing data. Using this technique, data were compared and constructed qualitatively. Emerging themes and patterns were noted for analysis (Cohen et al., 2011). All ethical considerations were observed throughout the study and all participants were informed of the intent of the study and their participation was voluntary. The confidentiality of all data collected was ensured. The research results and discussion of findings are presented below.

Results and Discussion

The results were presented qualitatively with two main sub-themes which are *Shona Religion and COVID-19 Vaccination* and *Gender and Vaccination*. These themes are discussed below.

Shona Religion and COVID-19 Vaccination

Results from the research show that certain Shona beliefs of the people of Buhera South hindered the vaccination programme initiated by the government. The people of Buhera South, just like their fellow Africans dotted across Africa, are 'notoriously religious' (Mbiti 1975: 1), and religion is the strongest element in traditional cultures like that of Buhera South under study. Results from this research show that due to some of the beliefs among the Shona of Buhera South, many people resisted the vaccination exercise as they saw it violating some of their beliefs. This stance taken by some of the people of Buhera South concurs with Idowu (1968) who states that the 'Africans in all things are religious'. A close understanding of the religion of the Shona people of Buhera South shows that they are 'incurably religious'. One participant who is a traditional healer **(TH1)** had this to say about the vaccination programme:*"Isu muchitendero chedu chechivanhu tine miti inorapa dzihwamupengo iri zvekuti hatione zviine musoro kuti munhu aende kunobaiwa jekiseni riri kutaurwa nezvaro mazuva ano."* (In our Shona traditional religion we have herbs which can treat this coronavirus and as such we do not see the logic for someone to get vaccinated with this drug which has become so topical these days.)

Such sentiments concur with Mbiti (1975) who says that the moral order of the Shona people is often interpreted as a fruit of religion and as such they are always religious in their day-to-day operations. In sweeping generalisations Mbiti (1975) claims that many African peoples believe that their morals were given to them by God from the very beginning. This is further strengthened by the belief that some of the departed and spirits keep watch over people to make sure that they observe the moral laws and punish them through some misfortunes which include sicknesses when they break them (Tatira 2016). It is from this belief that most of the participants who believed in the Shona traditional religion are of the opinion that their ancestors could safeguard them from the COVID-19 virus hence their resistance to the vaccination programme.

Another traditional healer **(TH2)** who was a participant has this to say, *"Kazhinji pose panouya chirwere kuvanhu vadzimu vedu vanotirotsa miti inoita kuti tirape nayo chirwere saka nekudaro Dzihwamupengo iri tinoguma tikangoriratidzwa muti wekurirapa nawo."* (In most cases whenever there is an outbreak of a diseases our ancestors will show us the herbs to treat it and eventually the ancestors will reveal to us the herb to treat this COVID–19 disease.) Such is the belief in the role of ancestors in their lives that Mbiti (1975) argues that religion has dominated the thinking of African peoples to such an extent that it has shaped their cultures, their social life, their political organisations and economic activities.

Another participant **(M5)** said, *"Hatingambobairwi jekiseni dzihwamupengo chairo, furuwenza yakambouya ikadarika wani midzimu yedu inotidzivirira kubva kuchirwere ichi."* (We cannot get vaccinated against this mere Corona virus, influenza came and went, our ancestors will safeguard against this disease.) Such beliefs from the custodians of Shona tradition led to mixed views regarding the vaccination programme, with a lot of men resisting the programme. One male participant **(M2)** had this to say, *"Hatidi jekiseni iri nekuti rinonzi rakagadzirirwa kuti vose vanenge vabaiwa vasachabereke".* (We do not accept this vaccine because it is meant to render people sterile once they receive it). One male participant, M6, had this to say: *"Iri jekiseni iri harina kunaka zvachose, guhwa rinoti ukaera waribaiwa hauchabereki."* (This drug is not good at all, rumour has it that once you are vaccinated you will not be able to bear children.) This was another myth given by participants. Many participants were very sceptical about the vaccine, though they did not divulge the reasons why they were reluctant to get vaccinated. Another participant **(M1)** said: *"Mushonga uyu unonzi wakagadzirirwa kupedza rudzi rwevanhu vatema vose."* (This drug is meant to wipe out the entire black race) (see Nyatsanza in this volume.) Another participant, **M4**, said: *"Isu pachivanhu chedu nhomba inobayiwa vana vadiki chete kwete vanhu vakuru."* (In our culture we have known that vaccines are meant for infants not elders.) Another male participant **M3** who refused to be vaccinated also said: *"Zvekubaiwa nhomba ndezvevana vadiki kwete, isu tingabaiwa takura kudai nekuti zvambodii?"* (Vaccination is for the infants, old as we are now what is the need for vaccinating us?) Another male participant, **M7**, said: *"Ini ndagara handifariri injection mumuviri wangu kubva ndichiberekwa."* (Personally I hate being injected since birth.) The participant went on to add that they have their own ways of treating diseases in their culture.

The way the participants understand how gender roles, norms and relations and gender inequality influence the access to and the demand for the COVID-19 vaccines in this context is important for this chapter. COVID-19 vaccination planners should incorporate gender-related barriers so that the vaccination exercise reaches everyone, especially those most marginalised (women, those who live with disabilities and children). In the Shona religion, women are the health workers for the family, clan and community at large, and they were most likely to be in patient care roles that expose them to COVID-19. Countries (Zimbabwe included) needed to prioritise essential health workers and rural women as people who receive vaccines at all costs (Campell and Zachary, 2021). Now that the vaccines are for everyone in Zimbabwe, all women should be given the first priority regardless of their location and states because they are at the centre of the family health. The Shona religion expects women to be more submissive to their husbands and the submissiveness includes getting permission from the male figures in their lives for whatever they have to do in life (Tatira, 2016). This is a challenge to most women in Buhera South. Most of the participants stated that they had hard times getting to vaccination centres. They had to ask for permission from men in their families to be vaccinated. One woman, **W6**, who was willing to be vaccinated said: *"Ini zviri kutondinetsa. Varume vangu vanoti ndikabaiwa handizozvari zvekare nokuti kubaiwa uku ndeimwe nzira yevarungu yekutapudza vatema, saka vakatondirambidza."* (As for me, it is so confusing. My husband does not trust the vaccine. He has fears regarding infertility and population control.) By then, most women in Buhera South had heard different visions of the vaccine types and their side effects; most of these were rumours and myths on social media. Some said the vaccines could make women bleed to death; others said vaccines would cause miscarriages, or the women who would take it would not get pregnant again. Another man, **M3**, who refused to allow his wife to get the vaccine said: "*Ini wangu mukadzi haangatombobaiwe nokuti ndichiri kuda vamwe vana*". (My wife cannot get the vaccinated because I still want more children.) In Shona religion, people get married for child bearing as they believe that the family name should continue (Tatira, 2016). If a woman fails to bear children, her parents would be expected to give her husband another woman who would bear them children (*chigadzamapfihwa*) (Tatira, 2016).

Gender and COVID-19 Vaccination

Biologically, it has been proven that men and women respond to many vaccines differently, mainly because of their genes, hormones and probably the dosages (Chirisa, 2021). Researchers such as Chirisa (2021) and Jokwiro (2020) have evidence that more men were dying from COVID-19 but women do experience long-term symptoms and infections. Some social factors are also known to be influencing the burden of COVID-19. Gender barriers are the main effects for the gendered access to COVID-19 vaccines. The immunisation campaigns for COVID-19 vaccinations in Zimbabwe and Buhera South in particular were mostly done by civil servants (teachers) and most of these civil workers (teachers) were women. This was done as a way of supporting the continuity of learning during the pandemic. This idea of providing women with easy and reliable access to COVID-19 vaccines was important in the quest for the communities to achieve herd immunity and have the resilience to recover from the wider social and economic impacts.

The following gender-related barriers to COVID-19 vaccines were found to be vital in COVID-19 vaccine acceptance and/or hesitancy.

Gender Norms

- Women in general and in Buhera South in particular, are central to decision making about family health and caring for the patients so they should be leveraged.
- Women experienced limited decision-making power in health matters.
- Women have limited mobility to reach COVID-19 facilities and healthcare sites, especially in Buhera South.

Information

- Women in Buhera South take care of the family and COVID-19 patients in the home so they should get the right and enough information.
- Because most women in Buhera South have not received high levels of formal Western education they find it difficult to understand COVID-19 vaccine information.

- There seemed to be limited information for people living with disabilities, pregnant women and those living with different diseases like HIV and AIDS.

Accessibility challenges

- Buhera South is a rural setup with transport problems so most people, particularly women, had problems to reach the vaccination sites and other health centres.
- Heath centres in Buhera South have limited health supplies and are over-burdened hence compromised service provision.

Hesitancy

- There are no formal services for information dissemination and other services in Buhera South, meaning that the area is underdeveloped.
- Women have low trust on vaccinations because of the previous controversial immunisation programmes in the country.
- There are very few female healthcare workers in the area that can be used as role models by women.
- There are very few women in power and COVID-19 task force to address gender-related barriers to COVID-19 vaccines.

Lack of information is considered as the most common barrier (Mavhunga, 2020; Jokwiro, 2020) that was preventing women from receiving vaccinations in Buhera South. Most people in the district have misleading information and a lot of myths about the COVID-19 vaccines. Some social norms are discriminatory towards women and children. There are a lot of decisions that block women from being vaccinated. Gender gaps in education and technology also facilitate and widen the gap in literacy. This means that women have little chance of receiving relevant and trustworthy information about COVID-19 vaccinations. From the interviews that were carried out with women in Buhera South, it was noted that women in the district did not get enough information about the COVID-19 vaccinations because of the lockdown measures. Evidence suggested that men have and use cell phones more than women. Women in Buhera South revealed that they do use and rely on their husbands' mobile cell phones for whatever information they need about COVID-19. One unvaccinated woman, **W6**, said: *"Tine foni imwe semhuri asi inogara nababa ndivo muridzi wayo"* (We have one family cell phone but it is always with my husband who is the owner). About 100% of the participants in this study reported that most women were willing to be vaccinated but their husbands were against or were unsure of accepting COVID-19 vaccines. The main reason of such disparities was that some women had limited knowledge about the pandemic and its vaccines. The district has a wider gender gap where most men are more educated than women. This revealed the impact of the restrictive gender norms and barriers that are faced by women and the limited access by these women to

228 *Maradze Viriri, Etwin Machibaya and Cuthbert Pisirai*

COVID-19 information and vaccines (Chirisa, 2021). There is a need for these injustices to be addressed. One participant, female herbalist **(FH1)** who was not vaccinated said: "*Vanhu vari kutipa muchetura usiri chokwadi*" (People are giving us some dangerous and poisonous information which might not be true for sure). Participants also indicated that some government information was considered unreliable. Some said that there were rumours that it was aimed at maintaining government interest.

Physical access to health centres was also cited as a barrier. Buhera South area has a poor transport network. Most women in Buhera South did not have enough time to go to the vaccine sites within the given hours. They were failing to secure a time slot for vaccination mainly because of their domestic roles. The vaccination centre was far for most women and because of the imposed COVID-19 lockdown, transport and permission to travel was a dream to most women. Most people did not get the information correctly. One participant, Village head 1 **(VH1)**, said: "*Ini ndine mibvunzo yakawandisa. Chiinombori chii chaizvo? Mutauro uri kushandiswa wakaoma kuti tinzwisise kupararira kwacho? Tingachipedza sei kuno kwedu?*" (I still have many questions. What exactly is it? The language used is difficult to understand how it is spread? How can we stop it here in our area?) Women as care givers could not stand the social distancing and hygiene policies. Another woman, **W6**, said: "*Pachivanhu chedu ndini ndinoita zvese pamba. Saka kumboenda kunobaiwa ndichisiya muri nenzara hazviite*" (Culturally, I am the care giver here. Leaving my family for vaccination is impossible).

On the overburdening of the health centres in Buhera South, it was noted that there were only four rural district clinics and each had only one qualified nurse and two first aiders because of high brain drain in the country. It was noted that COVID-19 vaccinations require a multifaceted approach that includes community education, training of healthcare professionals and the appropriate vaccine administration infrastructures and venues (Chirisa, 2021). As a result, the government of Zimbabwe had to rehabilitate some of its existing venues/clinics and hospitals to be fit for COVID-19 specifically. As such, in Buhera South, only one clinic was selected to cater for COVID-19 vaccinations. This increased the load and burden of the centre and the selected clinic had no significant human and material resources. Schools were closed and this led to adolescent pregnancies as the girls could not get help from the centre as it was now for COVID-19 only (Mavhunga, 2020). The country had serious shortages of the doses, leading to some people taking longer to get the second dose (Chirisa, 2021). During the first days of COVID-19, the clinics were not able to cope with the demand of the vaccines which were in short supply and rural areas were the ones to suffer most. The country had limited stock of the COVID-19 vaccines (Chirisa, 2021) and corruption also prevented the availability of the vaccines in Buhera South.

Vaccine hesitancy was indicated as another barrier to COVID-19 vaccination in Buhera South. Hannan et al. (2021) observed that misinformation fuelled the COVID-19 pandemic. The study revealed that about one third of the participants demonstrated COVID-19 hesitancy and about one third were willing to get a COVID-19 vaccine, yet one third were undecided or had family refusals. This lack of confidence was noted throughout the country, including Buhera South. The public mistrust of vaccines was mainly because the local people in Buhera South have a strong mistrust of the medical industry trails. One participant, **VH3**, stated that: "*Ndinototya zvangu zvirwere zvinotevera kubaiwa. Zvinonzi munhu anooma mutezo mushure memakore matatu abaiwa*" (I am afraid of the so-called side effects of the COVID-19 vaccines. We heard that one will be paralysed for life after three years). Kramer (2021) says that there were rumours that encouraged participants that as Blacks they had strong immune systems and that they would not succumb to the pandemic. Woman herbalist 2 (**WH2**) said: "*Chirwere ichi hachiuraye isu vanhu vatema. Takasimba*" (This virus cannot affect Black people. We are strong.)

Results from this research also revealed that the vaccination programme was received differently across the gender divide. Interviews carried out with some women participants show that women were willing to participate in the vaccination programme but there are factors which hinder them from executing their wish to get vaccinated. This seems to concur with Swai (2010) who argues that women in any society occupy a special place in the improvement and promotion of healthcare services, mainly because they participate in and manage many healthcare activities that affect the health of their families. One female participant, **W4**, had this to say: "*Isu kubayiwa jekiseni rekudzivirirwa kubva kuchirwere ichi tinoda chose asi kuti bedzi mukana wekuti tiriwane unonetsa nekuti riri kunzi rionopiwa avo vari kumabasa vanoshanda neruzhinji rwevanhu.*" (We want to get vaccinated but for us to get the opportunity to do so is a challenge since priority is being given to front line workers). Another woman, **W6**, said: "*Ndakarambidzwa kubaiwa hanzi hariite kunesu tinoyamwisa.*" (They could not apply it on me. They said it is not good for us who are breast feeding). These sentiments are a true reflection of what is obtaining in Buhera South where there are more males who are employed in government departments compared to women.

Despite the fact that Buhera South is a patriarchal society, this research found out that women were very cooperative in this vaccination programme. Thus, women of Buhera South are moving away from the traditional norm of resisting anything Western by incorporating the vaccination programme. These results seem to contradict the usual norm associated with people who reside in Buhera South who in the past used to resist Western medicine in preference to their traditional herbs. Kaneka et al. (2011: 246) believe that "women especially rural women are negatively affected by prejudices because most men in such areas claim to be the staunch custodians of culture". Athough rural women are often presented as silent, absent and under-appreciated, they represent the world's most strategic untapped natural resource, and they are more than ever before a key to world stability and understanding. Results show that women are not given the opportunity to participate in the vaccination programme as per their wish.

These sentiments are a true reflection of what is obtaining in Buhera South where there are many males who are employed in government departments compared to women. The government made sure that civil servants would get vaccinated first yet the bulk of these civil servants in Buhera South are males. This move by the government meant women were going to lag behind in the COVID-19 vaccination programme. UN (2020) concurs with what this research established when it says that the most common barriers that prevent women from receiving vaccinations are lack of information, social norms that are discriminatory toward women and decisions that fail to prioritise women's health. Gunda (2007) noted that gender gaps in literacy, education and technology mean women are less likely to receive relevant and trustworthy information about COVID-19 vaccination. These results must be interpreted in the context of assertions by Swai (2010), who argues that women in any society occupy a special place in the improvement and promotion of healthcare services, mainly because they participate in and manage many healthcare activities that affect the health of their families.

Results show an overwhelming response by women to the vaccination programme. Out of 10 female participants, 4 were vaccinated and 6 indicated that they wanted to be vaccinated yet they could not since they were not civil servants. On the other hand, of the 10 male participants, 6 had been vaccinated and the remaining 2 said they were not willing to take the jab and the other 2 were not decided.

Another factor that seems to have affected women in the vaccination programme was the lockdown effected by the government which meant limited movement. It emerged that the face-to-face informal network women used to rely on before COVID-19 has been limited by lockdown measures. From the research, it was established that fewer women than men received vaccination jabs for COVID-19. The participant went on to add that they had their own ways of treating diseases in their culture and one of the methods which he singled out was *kunatira* (steaming) and the use of *Zumbani* (Lippia javanica). The participants had different views on the vaccines; some said that the consumption of lemon and other traditional herbs could prevent infection.

Conclusion

This chapter provided an overview of the Shona religion, gender dynamics and their response to COVID-19 vaccination programme. It discussed the significance of the Shona religion's response to COVID-19 vaccination and the gender dynamics associated with the programme at length. It looked at the role of traditional healers, as well as the methods and techniques they used in responding to COVID-19. However, despite the existence of Western methods of healing being available in trying to combat the COVID-19, many traditional Shona Zimbabweans still use traditional healing practices and reported benefiting from them immensely. The traditional Shona healing techniques and approaches are anchored in the wider religious–cultural belief system, thus, they serve the needs of the Shona people. The study found out that some traditional beliefs acted as barriers to achieving herd immunity. The other stumbling block was the physical access to the health centres. Most elderly people involved in the study cited the language used in the campaign against COVID-19 as a barrier. Most of the respondents felt that the medical language used on pamphlets and on social media were too difficult to comprehend given the level of education of the research participants. The research also found out that health care centres in the district under study were understaffed and people had to spend most of their time in queues which had a strong bearing on their farming activities in particular and other domestic chores in general. It is also of paramount importance to note that most of the respondents feared the after-effects of the vaccine. Most of the respondents feared that the vaccine was meant to wipe out the African race as opposed to prevention. The respondents thought that they had a better immune system compared to other races therefore they felt that that it was not necessary for them to get the jab. The study also established that most of the research participants believed in their traditional ways of treating the disease such as the use of steaming and other herbs found in the local environment. Based on the above findings, the study recommends awareness campaigns on the need to be vaccinated. The Ministry of Health and Child Care needs to increase health facilities in the area under study so that there is easy accessibility for all.

References

Bourdillon, M.F.C. 1975. Themes in the understanding of traditional African religion. *Journal of Theology for Southern Africa*, 10, 71–87.

Campbell, H.A. and Zachary, S. 2021. Religious responses to social distancing revealed through memes during COVID-19 pandemic. *Religious*, 12, 787. https://doi.org/10.3390/

Chirisa, I. 2021. The impact of implication of COVID-19: Reflections on the Zimbabwean society. *The journal of Social Sciences & Humanities Open*, 4(1), 100183.

Cohen, L., Manion, L., & Morrison, K. 2011. *Research Methods in Education* (7th Eds). London: Routledge.

Dei, G.J.S. 2006. Introduction: Mapping the retrain – Towards a new politics of resistance. In G.J.S. Dei, and A. Kempf, (Eds), *Anti-colonialism and Education*. Rotterdam, Netherlands: Sense Publishers.

Dei, G.J.S. 2012. Reclaiming our Africanness in the despotized context: The challenge of asserting a critical African personality. *The Journal of Pan African Studies*, 4(10), 42–57.

Gavi, S. 2020. Why a gender lens is needed for the COVID-19 response? www.gaviorg/vaccinework/why-gender-lens-needed-covid19-response

Gunda, R.M. 2007. Christianity, traditional religion and healing in Zimbabwe. *Swedish Missiology Themes*, 95(3), 232. www.scirp.org/(S(351jmbntvnsjt1aadkposzje))/reference/ReferencesPapers.aspx?ReferenceID=2513229

Hannan, A., Syarif, Z., and Yusuf, K.A. 2021. The review of social theology and the science on the benefits of vaccine in the Covid-19 preventive measures, 26(2), 221–240. DOI: 10.32332/akademika.v26i2.3605

Idowu, E.B. 1968. The study of religion with special reference to African Traditional Religion, *Hibbert Journal*, 66(62/63), 89. https://philpapers.org/rec/IDOTSO

Jokwiro, A. 2020. *COVID-19: Which way for Zimbabwe*. www.herald.co.zw/covid-19-which-way-for-zimbabwe

Kanjeke, S., Taba, H., and Teffo, C. 2011. African traditional beliefs. *International Journal of Research in Social Sciences*, 1(4), 254–314.

Kramer, J. 2021. Potent neutralization of SARS Cov-2 variants of concern by an antibody with an uncommon genetic signature and structural mode of spike recognition. In COVID Vaccine Data, LGBTQ People fear Invisibility; *Science Direct:bioRexiv*, 37(1), 109784https://doi.org.1101/2021.05.16.444004

Machinga, M. 2012. Religion, health, and healing in the traditional Shona culture of Zimbabwe. *Emory University*, 4, 1–8.

Magesa, L. 1997. *African Religion*. New York: Orbis Books.

Mavhunga, D. 2020. Lockdown laws draconian, excessive. The Independent online www.theindependent.co.zw/2020/04/03/lockdown-laws-dracion-exessive

Mbiti, J.S. 1975. *New Testament Scatology in an African Background: A Study of the Encounter between Testament Theology and African Traditional Concepts*. XII, Oxford University Press

McMillan, J.H. and Schumacher, S. 2010. *Research in Education: Evidence-based inquiry* (7th Eds). Boston, MA: Pearson Education.

Nabudere, D.W. 2011. *Afrikology, Philosophy and Wholeness*. Pretoria: African Institute of South Africa.

Ndamba, G.T. 2017. Towards a paradigm shift in educational research: A case of post-colonial theory. *Zimbabwe Journal of Educational Research* (ZJER), 29(3), 464–488.

Subedi, B. and Daza, S.L. 2008. The possibilities of postcolonial praxis in education. *Race Ethnicity and Education*, 11(1), 1–10.

Swai, E. (2010). *Beyond Women's Empowerment in Africa: Exploring Dislocation and Agency*. New York: Palgrave MacMillan.

Tatira, L. 2016. The Shona concept of marriage with special reference to procreation and fertility. *South African Journal of African Languages*, 26(1). https://doi.org/10.1080/02572117.2016.1186904

United Nations. 2020. Secretary-General Calls Vaccine Equity Biggest Moral Test for Global Community, as Security Council Considers Equitable Availability of Doses. https://press.un.org/en/2022/sgsm21137.doc.htm

16 From Religion and COVID-19 Vaccination to Religion and Development? A Review

Ezra Chitando, Tenson Muyambo and Fortune Sibanda

Introduction

Literature on religion and development continues to grow, with the United Nations (UN) Sustainable Development Goals (SDGs) providing an added impetus (see e.g. Freston, 2019; Tomalin et al., 2019; Schliesser, 2023). This interest on the potential role of religion spurring development is also expressed in African scholarship (see e.g. Mhaka-Mutepfa and Maundeni, 2019; Chilongozi, 2020; Chitando et al., 2020; Gobo, 2020; Golo and Novieto, 2022). At stake is the issue of whether or how a specific religion on its own, through faith-based organisations (FBOs) (see e.g. Nelson, 2021) or through collective action expressed within interfaith networks (see e.g. Chitando and Gusha, 2022) can contribute to development.

Although appreciable ground has been covered in efforts to uncover the interface between religion and development, there is a need to broaden the horizon by considering how less obvious spheres can help clarify the link. Thus, for example, the COVID-19 pandemic has implications for reflections on religion and development (Boro et al., 2022; Chitando, 2022b). In this chapter, we explore how the responses to COVID-19 vaccinations described in this volume provide valuable insights into the complex relationship between religion and development. This is critical, as it contributes towards more effective initiatives and interventions, given the key role of religion in public life, especially in the Global South. Thus, while there is a growing appreciation of the importance of religion in strategic global institutions such as the World Health Organization (WHO) (see e.g. Winiger and Peng-Keller, 2021), there is a need for more detailed analysis of how religion influences diverse processes. An analysis of religious responses to COVID-19 vaccinations, such as has been undertaken in this volume, is helpful to the extent that it provides leads into the behaviours of religious actors in the face of new developmental initiatives, pandemics or emergencies.

Whereas the extant scholarship on religion and development tends to seek more or less straightforward positions ("religion is a positive force" or "religion is an impediment", or "religion A promotes development while religion Z resists development"), the chapters in this volume demonstrate that the picture

DOI: 10.4324/9781003388630-16

tends to be rather messy. In the wake of the shifting responses to COVID-19 vaccination in Zimbabwe, we argue that religious actors do not generate and retain a permanent position on an emerging (or existing) issue. The chapters in this volume confirm that religious actors are constantly reassessing and adjusting their positions in the light of contemporary experiences and the policies that influence the context in which they operate. This calls for more nuancing of declarations about the relationship between religion and development.

The first section of this chapter summarises the discussion on how COVID-19 vaccination could be regarded as "development". It draws attention to the possibilities and contestations around such an interpretation of the concept of development. It also highlights how such peculiar readings of development affect the responses of particular forms of religious expression, with special reference to Zimbabwe. This is followed by the second section which provides insights into the positive religious responses to the COVID-19 vaccines. The section that follows, the third, summarises religious responses that were associated with COVID-19 vaccine hesitancy. It summarises how religion contributed to COVID-19 vaccine hesitancy in the country. The fourth section is an overview of mixed religious responses to COVID-19 vaccinations in Zimbabwe. We readily concede, however, that the "messy" situation of COVID-19 implies that our allocation of chapters to the different categories must be understood in the context of embracing flexibility in approach. This implies that a good number of chapters could have been assigned to a different category of responses, thereby confirming the complexity of themes under discussion. Overall, the chapter argues that the complex and dynamic religious responses to COVID-19 vaccinations in Zimbabwe constitute valuable data for interpreting the broader interface between religion and development.

COVID-19 Vaccinations in Zimbabwe: Insights for Interpreting the Interface between Religion and Development

We do not assume that our central thesis, namely, that religious responses to COVID-19 vaccinations in Zimbabwe (and elsewhere) constitute a strategic entry point into the discourse on religion and development, is self-evident. Consequently, we do realise that we have to make a case for the standpoint that we have assumed, as well as the assertion that we are making. While space considerations preclude the possibility of a more detailed engagement, we shall draw attention to some of the relevant considerations.

First, in a manner similar to the introduction of COVID-19 vaccinations in Zimbabwe, most communities in the Global South experience "development" (we retain the quotation marks in this specific section due to the contested nature of the concept) as the quest to address a pressing, existential issue (see e.g. Chitando, 2022a for theories of development in Africa). In this regard, we might consider the COVID-19 vaccines themselves either as "development" or as akin to "development". If we consider the COVID-19 vaccinations as "development", we can regard them as having been commissioned to protect and enhance life in the face of a major threat. They were promoted as a critical intervention whose sole purpose was to arrest the high death rates (particularly in the Global North, but also in South Africa) and to protect human lives. However, it is also possible to concentrate on the similarities between the nature of COVID-19 vaccinations and "development". We have chosen the latter option and have sought to explore how the responses of religious actors to COVID-19 vaccinations in Zimbabwe yield helpful data for appreciating their responses to "development".

Second, although this dimension is widely critiqued, both COVID-19 vaccinations and "development" are mostly experienced as exogenous processes. There is a very strong sentiment that the dominant paradigm in both scenarios implies external actors bringing in "development" through processes that overlook local or endogenous values (see e.g. Malunga, 2014). As some of the chapters on religion and vaccine hesitancy in this volume (and summarised below) indicate, suspicions regarding the "invasive" nature of the COVID-19 vaccines and the externally driven concept of "development" are related. Both stem from feeling that those who drive these processes are ensconced in their offices in far-flung places in the Global North and are not really interested in the well-being of everyday people in the Global South. Many religious actors in the Global South tend to approach initiatives that are introduced from outside with a hermeneutics of suspicion.

Third, both COVID-19 vaccines and "development" are mostly mediated by national governments and local political actors. This generates its own dynamic, as citizens are left to confront/engage with their national/local actors, who would be representing or fronting global agendas (that, nonetheless, could still be beneficial to the majority at the national/local level). For example, "development" is often defined and circumscribed by global actors such as the United Nations Development Programme (UNDP), while the WHO championed the uptake of COVID-19 vaccines. However, it is the national and local leadership that has the responsibility of articulating these processes in indigenous terms. Sceptical religious actors at national/local levels ask difficult questions relating to the legitimacy and sustainability of such initiatives that represent the collusion between global and national/local elites.

Fourth, and finally in this section, both COVID-19 vaccines and "development" instigate large-scale community responses. In practice, whether individuals and communities are for or against COVID-19 vaccines and "development" initiatives, they register a response. However, what is less clear (and confirmed by some of the chapters in this volume) is how to characterise these responses. Thus, individuals and communities might initially resist these initiatives, warm up to them gradually as some external factors change, embrace them immediately, appreciate some aspects and resist others, and so on. It is, therefore, problematic to assume that there can be one standard and fairly consistent standpoint that will always define how people respond to various initiatives. In the specific case of COVID-19 vaccines in Zimbabwe, diverse religious actors had varied reactions at different moments, facilitated by unfolding political, legal, administrative and other factors. As we highlight below using selected chapters, this ensured that the paintings of the responses are a kaleidoscope of colours. We argue that this is indicative of the relationship between religion and development.

We must concede, however, that our effort to marry responses to COVID-19 vaccinations and "development" should not be read in a fundamentalist or rigid way. Thus, we are not suggesting that there are only similarities between the two initiatives. Clearly, there are some differences, although this chapter does not focus on these. For example, whereas COVID-19 vaccinations can be approached strictly from a health perspective, "development" is more inclusive and broader. However, we have sought to concentrate on the similarities in order to be better placed to identify the potential implications of religious responses to COVID-19 vaccinations for the interface between religion and development more generally. In the next section, we summarise essays that describe positive responses to COVID-19 vaccines in Zimbabwe from within the faith sector.

Religion and Support for COVID-19 Vaccinations in Zimbabwe: An Overview

The issue of COVID-19 emerged as a challenging one to faith communities in Zimbabwe. To begin with, the ban on religious gatherings meant that faith communities could not fulfil most of their roles, particularly those that promote and sustain a sense of belonging. As Bourdillon (1990) has underscored (following an established tradition within sociology), religion plays the strategic role of establishing and maintaining social bonds. The strict lockdowns also meant that rituals associated with burial could not be observed in full. Given the importance of burial to African Christians (see e.g. Chitando, 1999 and Mwandayi, 2011), this became a major source of frustration and anxiety. When the COVID-19 vaccines were introduced, with the government strongly encouraging (tactfully coercing) citizens to get vaccinated, faith communities found themselves having to make a decision as to whether they would identify with the government and actively support the vaccination drive.

Most leaders of the mainline churches (Catholic and Protestant) and some Pentecostal churches readily accepted the call for citizens/their members to be vaccinated. Adopting a hermeneutic of trust, they embraced the COVID-19 vaccines, set the example by being vaccinated openly and encouraged their members, as well as others, to also do the same. Given the close connection between the missionaries who established the mainline churches, which continued after Independence in 1980 (see e.g. Mhike and Makombe, 2018), it was not surprising that the leaders of mainline churches were very forthcoming in terms of accepting COVID-19 vaccinations in Zimbabwe.

The chapter by Chitando and Chitando in this volume highlights the positive interaction between many religious leaders and public health officials.

While acknowledging that there were some ultra-conservative religious leaders who resisted the COVID-19 vaccines and regarded them as the ultimate test of faith, they show that the dominant narrative had to be that of coordination and harmony between religious leaders and public health officials. According to Chitando and Chitando, the positive response cut across the religious divide and saw leaders from the African Traditional Religions, Christianity, Islam and other religions promoting the uptake of vaccines. They also became reliable sources of information. One significant dimension from their chapter relates to the fact that even when focusing on the positive contribution of faith leaders to the COVID-19 vaccination drive, it remains strategic to acknowledge the existence of resistance and resistors.

The chapter by Hlatywayo and Chirongoma in this volume shows how Ndau Indigenous Knowledge Systems (IKS) facilitated positive responses to COVID-19 vaccines in a rural setting. Whereas the dominant discourse tends to project IKS as conservative and backward, there is a growing scholarly movement championed by African scholars to promote IKS (see e.g. Gumede et al., 2021). Hlatywayo and Chirongoma highlight how IKS facilitated the positive Ndau responses to changes that were necessitated by COVID-19. This is also brought out in the chapter by Taringa and Chirongoma. They trace how the vaDuma had to tweak their burial and post-burial rituals, alongside embracing the COVID-19 vaccines. Their chapter demonstrates that indigenous cultures are not fixed, but are open to modification in the face of emerging challenges. At any rate, every religion represents an open and changing system. It is this adaptability that enables religions to survive and thrive as they embrace new ideas and practices and discard old ones that are no longer fit for purpose. This is also confirmed by the chapter by Mareva and Sibanda where a faith-based organisation, the Apostolic Women's Empowerment Trust (AWET) succeeded in mobilising many Apostolic groups to embrace COVID-19 vaccination.

In the chapter by Tenson Muyambo, Josiah Taru and Fortune Sibanda, the mainline Christian churches' responses to COVID-19 vaccination in Masvingo and Bikita Districts are explored. By using the cases of the Roman Catholic Church and the Reformed Church in Zimbabwe responses to COVID-19 vaccination, they argue that the intervention of the religious leaders played a pivotal role in influencing the majority of the church members and others to embrace the vaccination programme in Bikita and Masvingo Districts. The three scholars proceed to demonstrate that the two mainline Christian churches used the gospel flexibly to speak to the everyday concerns of members whom they encouraged to get vaccinated with available COVID-19 vaccines in order to minimise the risk of the virus. The chapter also notes with great interest that in the context of a health emergency, the mainline faith leaders – in their personal capacities – encouraged members of their churches to test for COVID-19, practice all preventive measures put in place by the government including vaccination, continue with supplicatory prayers and use indigenous remedies to treat colds as a preventive strategy. Therefore, the two churches were pragmatic in that they accepted vaccination within a framework of an integrated health system in Masvingo and Bikita Districts of Zimbabwe.

The chapter by Tobias Marevesa and Fortune Sibanda examines the relevance of the Apostolic Women's Empowerment Trust (AWET) in the context of COVID-19 vaccination in Zimbabwe. The chapter juxtaposes the ultra-conservative view of the Apostolic churches that viewed vaccines as dangerous and a cause of disease and death to AWET's intervention that made some Apostolic members change their mindset, which is something good coming out of Nazareth (the Apostolic adherents). Of interest to note is that women Apostolic members were empowered with information, education communication to promote a healthcare-seeking behaviour to the extent that they confidently expressed their agency and embraced COVID-19 vaccination without fear of reprimand from the church as the best standpoint to promote health and well-being. In their chapter, Marevesa and Sibanda demonstrate that the margins which women Apostles occupy are "spaces of resistance" such that in spite of being the most vulnerable group, they (women Apostles) possessed the ability to respond to processes of marginalisation. Therefore, pertaining to the question: 'Can any good thing or person come from the Apostolic churches in the context of COVID-19 vaccination?', the chapter concludes that vaccination acceptance among some Apostolic members is a good indicator of "changing beliefs and an enduring faith" (see, for example, Cox, 1993), a hermeneutic of trust and openness to modification towards human flourishing under a health emergency in Zimbabwe.

The chapters that analyse positive religious responses to COVID-19 vaccines confirm that the stereotype of religion as an impediment to scientific progress, science and technical issues misrepresents religion. While we do concede that there are instances where religion comes across as highly conservative (see below), it is a misrepresentation to regard this as the one and only side of religion. The chapters that confirm the positive responses to COVID-19 vaccines in this chapter show that the different strands of Christianity and African Traditional Religions were able to embrace the vaccines from the onset. Indeed, Zimbabwe has had a very successful COVID-19 vaccine programme. The role of the faith community in development needs to be appreciated. However, it remains important to pay attention to the vaccine hesitancy and resistance. We discuss this theme in the following section.

Religion and COVID-19 Vaccine Hesitancy in Zimbabwe: A Summary

The foregoing section has described the extent to which various religious actors promoted the uptake of COVID-19 vaccines in Zimbabwe. However, it must be unequivocally stated that while there are some religious groups and individuals which positively responded to initiatives that encouraged people to be vaccinated, it is also important to acknowledge, as some chapters in this volume do, that others were negative. Scholars have argued that positive responses (acceptance) of the vaccines could have been because of coercion (Muyambo and Tendere, 2023), as well as social desirability bias (Anjorin et al., 2021). Due to space considerations and the concluding role of this last chapter, this section summarises the negative responses. The negative responses to COVID-19 vaccination or rather vaccine hesitancy range from myths, misconceptions, mistrust, beliefs and misinformation about the disease (Anjorin et al., 2021).

When COVID-19 was declared a world pandemic by the WHO on 11 March 2020 (Anjorin et al., 2021), there was a casual approach by many people, including those who belong to different religions. For some Christians, it was another example of the work of the devil. They would have reckoned that this was just like the previous pandemics and epidemics that exclusively affect and inflict the evil on the 'sinners'. The 'saints' were immune to such pandemics. They were protected by the word of God and prayers and so for this category of believers, it was business as usual (see Mgovo's chapter). While some believers equated the advent of the pandemic as the end times-biblical apocalypse (Isiko, 2020), others viewed it as punishment from the angry spiritual realm. According to some Christians, the COVID-19 pandemic was punishment from God (Tolmie and Venter, 2021), punishing sinful people for the unsanctioned licentiousness that is rife in the world. For many African traditional practitioners, especially those in the rural areas, the pandemic was an urban pandemic and was not much of a concern to them. However, other traditionalists thought it was the ancestors' vengeance on people's total disregard of them.

Such perceptions about the pandemic did not change either when vaccines were introduced. The issue of vaccines was totally denied in some circles. Many believers and followers of different religions were sceptical about the vaccines. The reason, especially for 'notoriously religious' (Mbiti, 1969: 1) Africans could be that in their worldview, the vaccines catered largely for the body and not the soul (spirit). Kowalczyk et al. (2020) argue that spirituality is very important in the context of healthcare. They further argue that excluding spirituality in the healthcare of people is narrowing human desires to the physical sphere. A man of body dominated over a man of spirit. This could explain vaccine hesitancy witnessed in most of the religious groupings in Zimbabwe. Some of them doubted the origins of the vaccines since the vaccines were predominantly from the West. For instance, in Africa and particularly in Zimbabwe, some people thought this was the continued warfare between the former colonisers and the previously colonised. The formerly colonised thought vaccination was a ploy to exterminate Africans in the long run so as to re-colonise Africa. Such thinking points to the notion that the COVID-19 pandemic was not an African problem (Desmon, 2021). Negative narratives which form part of the conspiracy theories did the rounds. Misinformation, such as becoming infertile once vaccinated or *kuitwa kafira mberi* (prolonged poisoning), were the major fears. Indications were that once vaccinated one would not last for two years. Biswas et al. (2021) are instructive when they argue that vaccine safety and efficacy were found to be major concerns among people of all occupations. These are fears of side effects (Hlongwa et al., 2022).

As such there were utter denials of the vaccines. It is against this backdrop that chapters by Edmore Dube, Wisdom Sibanda, Tarsisio Nyatsanza, Henerietta Mgovo, and Nomatter Sande and Silas Nyadzo in this volume take specific churches' generally negative responses to the COVID-19 vaccination. We summarise their perspectives below.

In Henerietta Mgovo's chapter, African indigenous churches, particularly the Johanne Marange Church, were reluctant to take the vaccines due to their religious beliefs. Mgovo argues that when the government almost made vaccination compulsory by withdrawing certain privileges, the decree posed serious challenges to members of the Johanne Marange Apostolic Church because they do not believe in seeking medication from secular institutions. Her research revealed that there was a clash of conflicting interests between the Johanne Marange Apostolic Church beliefs and the pronouncement made by the Zimbabwe government as well as the WHO. The Church's doctrine does not allow its members to receive help from medical institutions. Still on Johanne Marange Apostolic Church's response to vaccination, Wisdom Sibanda's chapter is framed from the migrant communities' perspective, particularly Johanne Marange Apostolic Church's women refugees at Tongogara Refugee Camp in Chipinge district. The women refugees deny vaccination on religious grounds. Sibanda argues that using religion to evade vaccination is a time bomb and a deadly 'comedy of errors', which makes the women refugees potential super spreaders of the disease. He concludes that despite the effort by the host government to allow refugees to benefit from national vaccination programmes, religion and general apathy to inoculation among the migrant communities has been the major obstacle to the success of the programme among refugee communities.

Edmore Dube's exploration of the Muslim community in Zimbabwe regarding COVID-19 vaccination, what he calls immunisation, reveals an overall negative perception of the uptake of the vaccines. This is evidently seen in the low response to vaccination (less than a third of the population in twelve months). Dube argues that it is not surprising that Muslims have not been forthcoming despite theological encouragement. The prohibitive conspiracy theories are worsened by some of the outlets of the vaccines, including China and India, where Muslim populations are maltreated and live with fear of decimation. Arguing from a power contestation perspective, Tarsisio Nyatsanza, in his chapter, avers that there has been a 'Big Brother' syndrome on the collection, collation and predictions of the 'data' captured through the super-information highways and technologies pertaining to COVID-19. For him vaccination became controversial because of the conspiracies and the doubt of its efficacy in harnessing the pandemic. Previous experiences of racism and marginalisation informed vaccine hesitancy in Zimbabwe and Africa, demonstrating the need to appreciate historical and ideological factors when discussing religion and vaccination in Zimbabwe and Africa. He further argues that while COVID-19 has been and continues to be a global pandemic, there are complex reasons and permutations of reactions and the hesitancy to vaccination based on conspiracy theories and religious beliefs in particular. In their chapter, Nomatter Sande and Silas Nyadzo tackled the experiences of the diasporic Zimbabweans in the United Kingdom as a case of 'disconcerting vaccination voices'. They show that COVID-19 vaccination uptake triggered the underlying issues of racism, inequality and discrimination in the developed society, and further unveil the lessons that developing nations like Zimbabwe can learn when dealing with epidemics and vaccination hesitancy. They emphasise how African Pentecostals in the UK prioritised prayer in times of crises as the means to an end. The same slant of negativity is explored by Chireshe and Macheka's chapter, 'Vaccination Uptake and Power Dynamics: Insights from African Initiated Churches and Traditional Healers in Masvingo Province, Zimbabwe'. The next section looks at the mixed reactions to COVID-19 vaccination.

Mixed Reactions to COVID-19 Vaccinations by Religious Actors in Zimbabwe

Whereas the preceding sections have summarised chapters that discuss positive and negative responses to COVID-19 vaccinations in Zimbabwe, in this section we focus on mixed reactions from within the faith community. This emerges from our observation that for the most part, the same religious entity (individual/group/community/denomination) can have different positions on the same phenomenon depending on a number of factors. The available scientific evidence, the intensity of and access to opposing ideologies (e.g. the conspiracy theories, mostly circulating through social media), the impact of the pandemic or challenge (e.g. high death rate), level of political pressure (e.g. government insistence on vaccination), logistical issues (e.g. availability of the COVID-19 vaccines) and others had a bearing on when and whether some individuals, groups, communities or denominations accepted the COVID-19 vaccines.

The chapter by Bowa in this volume confirms the extent to which the Bible was deployed to both support and resist COVID-19 vaccines. Bowa demonstrates how each camp appealed to the sacred text to justify their preferred stance. This ambivalence of the sacred texts (and the religions that hold them in high esteem) is a consistent feature in studies on religion and development globally. The chapters by Humbe on African Independent Churches (AICs), as well as by Viriri et al. (African traditional religion and gender) confirm this pattern. Thus, the different religious actors were in some instances opposed to COVID-19 vaccines, then in others they were supportive of the same.

The chapters that discuss the mixed responses by the diverse religious actors suggest that it is critical for researchers and development practitioners to adopt a more nuanced approach. While a certain degree of generalisation is unavoidable, it is strategic to adopt a more refined and particular approach when seeking to describe responses by religious actors in greater detail. Thus, blanket statements such as, "religion does this ...", or "AICs are like this ...", or "African religions are like ..." can be less helpful when seeking to understand responses to emerging issues such as COVID-19 vaccines. This is due to the fact that, as outlined at the beginning of this section that is analysing mixed religious responses to COVID-19 vaccines, the responses of religious actors to emerging issues is not determined solely by religious factors. Since religion does not occur in a vacuum, it is affected by historical, political, economic, geographical and various other relevant factors (including position in the movement, educational attainment, gender, age, etc.). Hence it is possible for a religious individual or community in one context to embrace what a fellow religionist in the same religion abhors and resists.

Insights for the Discourse on Religion and Development

Having outlined the diverse religious reactions to COVID-19 vaccinations in Zimbabwe in the preceding sections, in this section we seek to highlight some key points for the discourse on religion and development. First, it is critical for scholarship to challenge the idea that African Traditional Religions/African spirituality/IKS are somehow intrinsically and permanently opposed to modernity or new initiatives. The notion that conservative religio-cultural beliefs in Africa frustrated the COVID-19 drive (see e.g. Mugari and Obioha, 2021) needs to be relativised in the wake of the more complicated pattern that has been described in this volume. Although there were aspects of resistance to the COVID-19 vaccines by African Traditional Religions/African spirituality/ IKS, for the most part they demonstrated remarkable flexibility in terms of adjusting rituals to reflect the reality and demands of COVID-19. In addition, they were mostly accepting COVID-19 vaccines. Further, researches into African Traditional Religions/African spirituality/IKS and development (see e.g. Awuah-Nyakye, 2012) will be highly strategic.

Second, the religious response to COVID-19 vaccines in Zimbabwe underscores the need to invest in appreciating the possible impact of non-religious factors when engaging in scholarly reflections on religion and development. While the dominance of the religionist ideology in the study of religion and development, particularly in Africa is understandable (see e.g. Cox, 1993), it remains helpful to invest in understanding the contribution of factors beyond religion in influencing the interface between religion and development. Religion is not disembodied, but occurs in concrete historical, socio-economic, political, ideological, gendered, etc. contexts. The chapters in this volume have demonstrated that the religious responses to the COVID-19 vaccines in Zimbabwe were coloured by various factors, including the government's strict approach towards the vaccines. Similarly, how, whether and the extent to which religion will interface with development will be influenced by various external factors.

Third, as we noted in our analysis of mixed approaches to religion and the COVID-19 vaccines in Zimbabwe, researchers must be constantly open to the openness and diversity of religious actors. Although scholars have been forced to embrace the rarefied concept of "religion", it remains critical to recognise the diversity that it masks. For example, chapters in this volume highlighted how different AICs in Zimbabwe responded to the COVID-19 vaccines. While some embraced the vaccines, others were militantly opposed to them. Consequently, it is not possible to generate a general statement regarding the responses of AICs to the COVID-19 vaccines. This is a valuable reminder to scholars focusing on AICs and development, namely, that there is great diversity within the movement. Consequently, researchers need to be acutely aware of, and acknowledge, this diversity in their research and publications.

Fourth, and finally, the dominant trend has been to regard "religion" as the variable that is laden with spiritual notions, while "development" is seen as fairly neutral. However, as the ideological resistance to COVID-19 vaccines confirms, in Africa and most parts of the Global South, there is deep suspicion (deriving from the historical and contemporary interactions) that initiatives that emanate from the Global North are crafted to further the interests of the latter. In this regard, vaccine hesitancy can be equated to "development hesitancy". Both processes are informed by a hermeneutics of suspicion on the part of various actors in the Global South and a call to critique and resist domination by the Global North. Reflections on religion and development in Africa, therefore, must contend with this reality.

Conclusion

The introduction of COVID-19 vaccines was regarded by most public health experts as a significant development in the overall response to the pandemic. Promoting the uptake of the vaccines became an urgent undertaking. Political leaders and public health experts joined hands to encourage religious and cultural leaders to mobilise their constituencies to embrace the COVID-19 vaccines. In this chapter, we have summarised how the specific responses to the COVID-19 vaccines by religious leaders provide useful insights in the context of the discourse on religion and development. We highlighted how the positive, negative and mixed religious responses to the COVID-19 vaccines in Zimbabwe present a useful model for approaching religion and development. Further, we identified other dimensions that emerge from the religious responses to the COVID-19 vaccines that can assist in clarifying the religion-development interface. Given the strategic importance of the theme of religion and development to the Global South, we recommend ongoing and in-depth analysis of this theme, including searching for insights in unexpected areas.

References

Anjorin, A.A. et al. 2021. Will Africans take COVID-19 vaccination? *PLoS ONE*, 16(12), 1–15. https://doi.org/10.1371/ journal.pone.0260575
Awuah-Nyamekye, S. 2012. Religion and development: African Traditional Religion's perspective. *Religious Studies and Theology*, 31(1), 75–90.

Biswas, M.R. et al. 2021. Scoping review to find out worldwide COVID-19 vaccine hesitancy and its underlying determinants. *Vaccines*, 9(1243), 1–20. https://doi.org/10.3390/

Boro, E. et al. 2022. The role and impact of faith-based organisations in the management of and response to COVID-19 in low-resource settings. *Religion and Development*, 1(1), 132–146.

Bourdillon, M.F.C. 1990. *Religion and Society: A Text for Africa*. Gweru: Mambo Press.

Chilongozi, M.N. 2020. The role of religion in sustainable development: Theological reflections on sustainable development goals and Mother Earth, in N.P. Matholeni, G.K. Boateng, and M. Manyonganise (Eds), *Mother Earth, Mother Africa & African Indigenous Religions*. Stellenbosch: SUN Press, DOI:10.18820/9781928480730/10

Chitando, E. 1999. Deathly concern: African Christians and cremation in Zimbabwe. *Missionalia*, 27(1), 10–19.

Chitando, E. 2022a. Africa and the quest for sustainable development: A critical review. In E. Chitando and E. Kamaara (Eds), *Values, Identity, and Sustainable Development in Africa*. Cham: Palgrave Macmillan, 69–84.

Chitando, E. 2022b. Religion and COVID-19 in Southern Africa: Implications for the discourse on religion and development. In F. Sibanda, T. Muyambo, and E. Chitando (Eds), *Religion and the COVID-19 Pandemic in Southern Africa*. London: Routledge, 244–256.

Chitando, E., Gunda, M.R., and Togarasei, L. (Eds). 2020. *Religion and Development in Africa*. Bamberg: University of Bamberg Press.

Chitando, E. and Gusha, I.S. (Eds). 2022. *Interfaith Networks and Development: Case Studies from Africa*. Cham: Palgrave Macmillan.

Cox, J.L. 1993. *Changing Beliefs and an Enduring Faith: A Reformulation of Christian Beliefs in Response to Five Major Obstacles for Faith*. Gweru: Mambo Press.

Desmon, S. *Stigma Related to COVID-19 May Thwart Prevention Efforts*. Available online:https://ccp.jhu.edu/2021/02/08/covid-stigma-prevention-ivory-coast/(Accessed25 March 2023).

Freston, P. 2019. Religion and the Sustainable Development Goals. In S. Dalby et al., (Eds), *Achieving the Sustainable Development Goals: Global Governance Challenges*. London: Routledge, pp. 152–169.

Gobo, P. 2020. Rethinking religion and sustainable development in Africa. *East African Journal of Traditions, Culture and Religion*, 2(1), 60–71.

Golo, B-W.K. and Novieto, E. 2022. Religion and Sustainable Development in Africa: Neo-Pentecostal economies in perspectives. *Religion and Development*, 1(1), 73–93.

Gumede, V., Muchie, M., and Shafi, A. (Eds). 2021. *Indigenous Systems and Africa's Development*. Pretoria: Africa Institute of South Africa.

Hlongwa, M., Afolabi, A.A., and Dzinamarira, T. 2022. Hesitancy towards a COVID-19 vaccine in selected countries in Africa: Causes, effects and strategies for improving COVID-19 vaccine uptake. *Global Biosecurity*, 3(1), 1–5.

Isiko, A.P. 2020. Religious construction of disease: An exploratory appraisal of religious responses to the COVID-19 pandemic in Uganda. *Journal of African Studies and Development*, 12(3), 77–96.

Kowalczyk, O., Roszkowski, K., Montane, X., Pawliszak, W., Tylkowski, B., and Bajek, A. 2020. Religion and faith perception in a pandemic of COVID-19. *Journal of Religion and Health*, 59, 2671–2677. https://doi.org/10.1007/s10943-020-01088-3

Malunga, C. 2014. Identifying and understanding African norms and values that support endogenous development in Africa. *Development in Practice*, 24(5/6), 623–636.

Mbiti, J.S. 1969. *African Religions and Philosophy.* Nairobi: Heinemann.

Mhaka-Mutepfa, M. and Maundeni, T. 2019. The role of faith (spirituality/religion) in resilience in Sub-Saharan African children. *The International Journal of Community and Social Development*, 1(3), 211–233. https://doi.org/10.1177/2516602619859961

Mhike, I. and Makombe, E.K. 2018. Mission and state health institutions: "Invisible" public-private partnerships in Zimbabwe, 1980–1999. *Studia Historiae Ecclesiasticae*, 44(1), 12. Available at www.scielo.org.za/pdf/she/v44n1/03.pdf

Mugari, I. and Obioha, E.E. 2021. African beliefs and citizens' disposition towards COVID-19 vaccines: The belief guided choice. *African Journal of Governance and Development*, 10(1.1), 277–293.

Muyambo, T. and Tendere, J. 2023. Beyond the COVID-19 pandemic: Is rethinking the interface religion and science possible in the Zimbabwean context. In Molly Manyonganise (Ed.), *Religion and Health in a COVID-19 Context: Experiences from Zimbabwe.* Bamberg: University of Bamberg Press, 285–304.

Mwandayi, C. 2011. *Death and After-life Rituals in the Eyes of the Shona: Dialogue with Shona Customs in the Quest for Authentic Inculturation.* Bamberg: University of Bamberg Press.

Nelson, P.J. 2021. *Religious Voices in the Politics of International Development Faith-Based NGOs as Non-state Political and Moral Actors.* Cham: Palgrave Macmillan.

Schliesser, C. 2023. *On the Significance of Religion for the SDGs: An Introduction.* London: Routledge.

Tolmie, F. and Venter, R. 2021. Making sense of the COVID-19 pandemic from the Bible-Some perspectives. *HTS Teologiese Studies/Theological Studies*, 77(4), a6493. https://doi.org/10.4102/hts.v77i4.6493

Tomalin, E., Haustein, J., and Kidy, S. 2019. Religion and the Sustainable Development Goals. *Review of Faith & International Affairs*, 17(2), 102–118.

Winiger, F. and Peng-Keller, S. 2021. Religion and the World Health Organization: an evolving relationship. *BMJ Global Health*, 6:e004073. DOI:10.1136/bmjgh-2020-004073

Index

2019-nCov *see* COVID-19 pandemic

Abrus precatorius (water lily) 38
African Apostolic Church 211
African communalism (*Hunhu/Ubuntu*)
  142
African Independent Churches (AICs)
  77, 88–90, 94, 204, 208, 241; awareness
  campaign programs 93; AWET
  advocacy for COVID-19 vaccination
  in 90–2; bad death 213; childhood
  and adult vaccination programs
  92; communities 87; confusion
  213; COVID-19 vaccination 204–6,
  209; definition of 208; embrace
  vaccination 212; forests/mountains
  213; healing 216; Johanne Marange
  Apostolic churches 149, 182; middle-
  aged female AIC faith healer 210;
  Nazareth 13; notion of strictness
  206; social networks 217; stance on
  COVID vaccines 88; strictness 205;
  vaccination of women in 85; ZANU-
  PF government 207, 208; in Zimbabwe
  243; *see also* African Initiated
  Churches (AICs); African Instituted
  Churches (AICs)
African Indigenous Religions (AIRs) 99,
  101
African Initiated Churches (AICs) 13,
  21, 143, 168, 169, 179, 181, 182, 208;
  church leaders as pro-vaccination
  agents 209–12; in the context of
  COVID-19 pandemic 141–3; effects of
  lockdowns on 143–4; health matters
  confronted by COVID-19 208–9;
  ideology of 207–8, 212; infrastructural
  developments 150; integration of 142;
  Johanne Masowe Apostolic Church

144; leaders leading by example 212–
  13; no to vaccination 214–15; painful
  death, issue of 213–14; Paul Mwazha
  Church 144; prophecy on COVID-19
  215; regretting for being vaccinated
  215–16; social distancing 142; 'strict'
  churches ideological framework 206–7;
  on use of scientific medicines 143;
  vaccination rollout, in Zimbabwe 140;
  Zion Apostolic Church 214
African Instituted Churches (AICs) 21
African Pentecostal church 25, 155, 193
African religion, religious practices 6,
  27–8, 221, 242
African spirituality 131, 134, 183, 242
African traditional medicine (ATM) 75,
  132; COVID-19 and 36–9; resurgence
  in the use of 37
African Traditional Religions/African
  spirituality/IKS 24, 131, 156, 160, 237,
  242
AIDS *see* HIV/AIDS
American Anthropological Association 73
Anjorin, A. A. 6
Annual Paschal Festivals 110
Anthropology Southern Africa Ethical
  Guidelines 73
anti-COVID-19 vaccines 9
antiretrovirals (ARVs) 8
anti-vaccination: campaign 120;
  conspiracy theories 170; information
  99; myths 121; supporters 205
anti-vax 12
anti-vaxxers 13
antiviral drugs, lack of 34, 37
anxiety 92, 114, 134, 151, 158, 236
Apostolic Church *see* African
  Independent Churches (AICs)
Apostolic faith community 90